PHARMACY ESSENTIALS

A Compact Guide for Students and Practitioners

Dr. Amit Kumar
Dr. Ravi Prakash Degala
Mr. Prakash Nathaniel Kumar Sarella
Mrs. Vinny Therissa Mangam
Dr. Ajmal Tariq Hussain

ISBN: 9788198765727

Scan to view online

Editors

Dr. Amit Kumar

Dr. Ravi Prakash Degala

Mr. Prakash Nathaniel Kumar Sarella

Mrs. Vinny Therissa Mangam

Dr. Ajmal Tariq Hussain

First Edition: 2025

ISBN: 9788198765727

Maximum Retail Price: Rs. 1000/- (Inclusive of all taxes)

Published by ThinkPlus Pharma Publications,
9-15/1, Indrapalem, Kakinada, AP-533006, India.
Website: www.books.jopir.in

Cover Page Illustration: Kiran Priyam Kumar Sarella

Printed at Tarangini Printing Works, Subhadra Arcade, Bhanugudi, Kakinada, AP-533003, India.

DEDICATION

This textbook is dedicated to

The pharmacy students of today and tomorrow, whose passion for learning and commitment to patient care will shape the future of our profession. The educators who inspire and mentor the next generation of pharmacists, imparting not only knowledge but also the values and critical thinking skills essential to pharmaceutical care.

The practicing pharmacists who daily demonstrate the vital role of pharmacy in healthcare through their clinical expertise, compassionate patient interactions, and tireless advocacy for optimal medication therapy.

The patients whose needs remain at the center of our professional purpose, reminding us that behind every prescription is a person deserving of our best care.

And to all who strive to advance the science and practice of pharmacy in service of human health and wellbeing.

"May this book serve as a trusted companion in your professional journey"

CONTENTS

ACKNOWLEDGMENTS

The creation of this textbook has been a collaborative journey that would not have been possible without the contributions, expertise, and support of the authors. The editors wish to express their sincere gratitude to all the authors who have played a role in bringing this textbook to fruition.

We are grateful to the students who participated in focus groups and pilot testing of educational materials contained within these pages. Their perspective has been crucial in creating a student-centered resource that addresses learning needs at various stages of pharmacy education.

Special recognition is due to the pharmacy organizations and institutions that provided access to resources, clinical practice guidelines, and case studies that enrich this work. Their commitment to advancing pharmacy education aligns with our vision for this textbook.

We acknowledge the editorial and production staff whose attention to detail, design expertise, and tireless efforts have transformed manuscript pages into a polished, accessible educational tool.

Finally, we express our gratitude to our families, colleagues, and mentors who supported us throughout this project with their patience, encouragement, and understanding. Their unwavering support made this collaborative endeavor possible.

While we have strived hard for accuracy and comprehensiveness, we welcome feedback from readers as we continuously seek to improve future editions of this work.

CHAPTER 1

FUNDAMENTALS OF PHARMACY PRACTICE

Author

Dr. Amit Kumar, Associate Professor, Department of Pharmacy Practice, Amity Institute of Pharmacy, Amity University, Lucknow, India

Abstract

Pharmacy practice operates at the intersection of healthcare delivery, legal compliance, and ethical decision-making. Professional ethics in pharmacy establishes core values including beneficence, non-maleficence, autonomy, and justice, guiding pharmacists through moral dilemmas in patient care and business operations. Pharmacy laws create a regulatory framework spanning controlled substances management, dispensing requirements, and practice standards, with federal statutes like the Controlled Substances Act working alongside state-specific regulations that define scope of practice. Contemporary healthcare systems position pharmacists as medication experts within interdisciplinary teams, with roles expanding beyond traditional dispensing to include medication therapy management, immunizations, and direct patient care services in various practice settings. Effective communication serves as the foundation for patient-centered care, with pharmacists employing active listening, cultural sensitivity, and health literacy assessment to convey complex medication information, conduct motivational interviewing, and navigate challenging interactions with both patients and healthcare colleagues. These elements create the system within which pharmacy professionals deliver patient care, maintain legal compliance, and uphold the profession's commitment to public health.

Keywords: *Professional Responsibility; Medication Safety; Scope of Practice; Patient-Centered Care; Healthcare Collaboration*

Learning Objectives

After completion of the chapter, the learners should be able to:

- Apply principles of autonomy, beneficence, non-maleficence, and justice to resolve ethical dilemmas in pharmacy practice scenarios.
- Differentiate between federal and state pharmacy regulations, including requirements for controlled substance dispensing under the Controlled Substances Act.
- Analyze the expanding scope of pharmacy practice across various healthcare settings, including clinical services beyond traditional dispensing roles.
- Demonstrate effective patient counseling techniques that address health literacy barriers and promote medication adherence.
- Implement strategies for interprofessional communication that optimize patient care coordination within healthcare teams.
- Evaluate situations requiring mandatory reporting and methods to maintain patient confidentiality while complying with HIPAA regulations.

PROFESSIONAL ETHICS

Professional ethics forms the cornerstone of pharmacy practice, providing the moral framework through which pharmacists navigate their responsibilities to patients, colleagues, and society. The ethical foundation of pharmacy practice is codified in various professional codes, most notably the Code of Ethics established by professional pharmacy organizations worldwide. These codes articulate the fundamental values that guide pharmaceutical care: beneficence, non-maleficence, justice, and respect for autonomy.

The principle of beneficence obligates pharmacists to act in the best interest of patients, optimizing therapeutic outcomes while minimizing risks. This principle manifests in daily practice through medication reviews, therapeutic recommendations, and patient education. Non-maleficence—the obligation to avoid causing harm—requires pharmacists to exercise vigilance in detecting potential medication errors, drug interactions, and inappropriate prescribing. Together, these principles underscore the pharmacist's primary commitment to patient welfare.

Justice in pharmacy practice encompasses fair allocation of healthcare resources and equitable treatment of all patients regardless of socioeconomic status, cultural background, or other personal characteristics. This principle becomes particularly salient when addressing healthcare disparities and access to essential medications. Respect for patient autonomy honors the individual's right to make informed decisions about their health. Pharmacists uphold this principle by providing comprehensive medication counseling that enables patients to understand their treatment options and participate meaningfully in their care.

Table 1.1: Principles of Pharmacy Ethics

Ethical Principle	Description
Autonomy	Respecting patients' right to make their own healthcare decisions
Beneficence	Acting in the best interest of patients
Nonmaleficence	Avoiding harm to patients ("first, do no harm")
Justice	Distributing healthcare resources fairly
Veracity	Telling the truth and not deceiving patients
Fidelity	Keeping promises and maintaining confidentiality
Respect for persons	Treating all individuals with dignity and respect
Confidentiality	Protecting patient information from unauthorized disclosure
Accountability	Taking responsibility for professional decisions and actions
Integrity	Adhering to moral and ethical principles in all situations

Ethical Decision-Making in Pharmacy

The complexity of modern healthcare frequently presents pharmacists with ethical dilemmas that require systematic resolution approaches. These dilemmas may involve conflicts between ethical principles, such as balancing respect for patient autonomy with concerns about medication safety, or navigating tensions between business interests and professional obligations.

Ethical decision-making frameworks provide structured approaches to resolving such dilemmas. These frameworks typically involve identifying the ethical problem, gathering relevant information, analyzing available options against ethical principles, consulting colleagues or ethics committees when appropriate, implementing the chosen course of action, and reflecting on outcomes to inform future decisions.

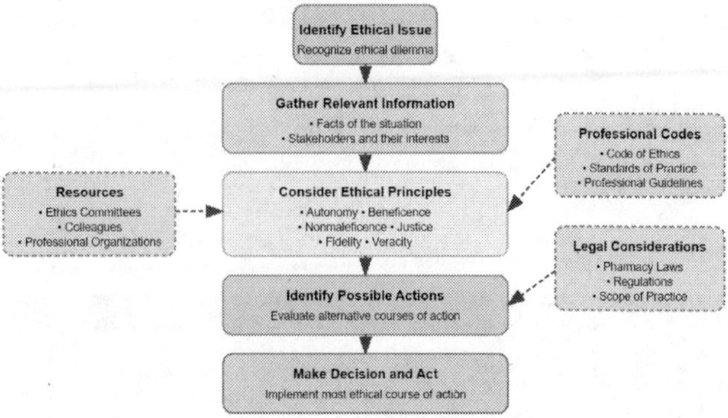

Figure 1.1 Ethical Decision-Making Framework in Pharmacy Practice

Confidentiality and Privacy

Pharmacists are entrusted with sensitive patient information, making confidentiality a fundamental ethical obligation. This extends beyond legal requirements to respect the dignity and privacy of those seeking pharmaceutical care. The pharmacist-patient relationship is predicated on trust, which is strengthened when patients are confident their personal health information will be protected.

The advent of electronic health records and integrated pharmacy systems has introduced new dimensions to privacy considerations. Pharmacists must remain vigilant about data security while balancing the benefits of information sharing for coordinated care. Ethical practice requires ongoing attention to evolving standards for information management, with particular sensitivity to vulnerable populations whose privacy concerns may be heightened.

PHARMACY LAWS

The legal framework governing pharmacy practice serves to protect public health and ensure professional standards. Pharmacy law encompasses federal, state, and local regulations that address prescription requirements, controlled substances, licensing standards, and other aspects of pharmaceutical care. Understanding this legal landscape is essential for compliant practice and professional longevity.

2.1 Regulatory Bodies and Their Functions

Multiple regulatory agencies oversee different aspects of pharmacy practice. At the federal level, the Food and Drug Administration (FDA) regulates drug approval, manufacturing standards, and labeling requirements. The Drug Enforcement Administration (DEA) establishes and enforces controls on substances with abuse potential.

Table 1.2: Federal Pharmacy Legislations

Legislation	Year	Primary Purpose
Pure Food and Drug Act	1906	Prohibited misbranded and adulterated foods and drugs
Food, Drug, and Cosmetic Act	1938	Required drug safety before marketing
Durham-Humphrey Amendment	1951	Defined prescription vs. OTC medications
Kefauver-Harris Amendment	1962	Required proof of drug efficacy and safety
Comprehensive Drug Abuse Prevention & Control Act	1970	Established controlled substance schedules
Orphan Drug Act	1983	Encouraged development of drugs for rare diseases
Drug Price Competition & Patent Term Restoration Act	1984	Established ANDA process for generic drugs
Prescription Drug Marketing Act	1987	Restricted drug sample distribution
Omnibus Budget Reconciliation Act	1990	Required patient counseling for Medicaid patients
Health Insurance Portability and Accountability Act	1996	Protected patient health information
Medicare Modernization Act	2003	Created Medicare Part D prescription benefit
Affordable Care Act	2010	Expanded healthcare coverage and services
Drug Quality and Security Act	2013	Enhanced drug supply chain security
SUPPORT for Patients and Communities Act	2018	Addressed opioid crisis with multiple provisions

State boards of pharmacy hold primary authority for licensing pharmacists, pharmacy technicians, and pharmacy facilities, while also establishing practice standards specific to their jurisdictions. The interplay between these regulatory bodies creates a complex compliance environment that requires pharmacists to maintain current knowledge of evolving requirements. Regulatory agencies increasingly emphasize a risk-based approach to oversight, focusing resources on areas with the greatest potential impact on public health.

Prescription Requirements and Record-Keeping

Legal requirements for valid prescriptions vary somewhat by jurisdiction but typically include prescriber information, patient identification, drug name, strength, dosage form, quantity, directions for use, and appropriate authorization for refills. Electronic prescribing has introduced additional authentication requirements to ensure security and prevent fraud.

Record-keeping obligations are particularly stringent for controlled substances, requiring specific documentation of inventory, dispensing, and disposal. These records must be maintained for specified periods and made available for inspection by regulatory authorities. Beyond controlled substances, pharmacists must maintain records of all prescription medications dispensed, patient counseling provided, and interventions made to address therapeutic concerns.

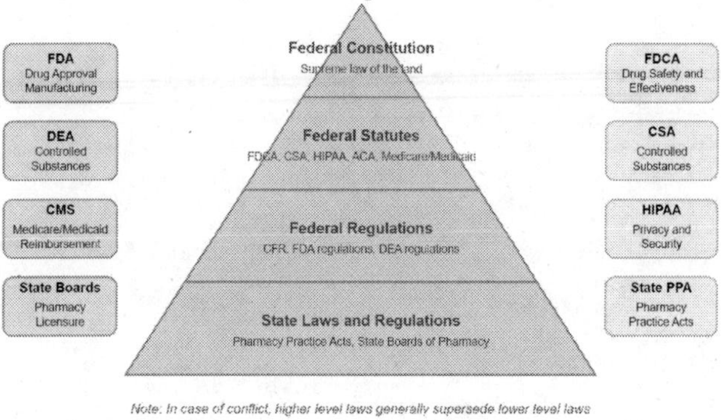

Figure 1.2 Hierarchy of Pharmacy Regulatory Laws

Liability and Risk Management

Professional liability represents a significant concern for practicing pharmacists. The expanding scope of pharmacy practice, with its focus on patient care services beyond dispensing, has introduced new liability considerations. Pharmacists may be held liable for negligence in medication dispensing, inadequate patient counseling, failure to detect dangerous drug interactions, or inappropriate recommendations for therapy management.

Risk management strategies include maintaining comprehensive documentation of patient care activities, adhering to established practice standards, pursuing continuing education to remain current with therapeutic developments, and obtaining appropriate professional liability insurance. Many pharmacies implement quality assurance programs that systematically identify and address potential sources of error.

HEALTHCARE SYSTEMS AND PHARMACIST ROLE

The configuration of healthcare delivery systems significantly influences how pharmacy services are provided and reimbursed. These systems vary considerably across countries and even within regions, reflecting different approaches to financing healthcare, prioritizing services, and organizing providers. Understanding these systems is essential for pharmacists to function effectively within them and advocate for optimal patient care.

Evolution of Pharmacy Practice Models

Pharmacy practice has undergone remarkable evolution from its historical focus on medication compounding and dispensing to its current emphasis on patient-centered care. This transformation reflects growing recognition of medication therapy as a complex intervention requiring specialized expertise to optimize outcomes and minimize risks.

Contemporary pharmacy practice models emphasize the pharmacist's role as a medication therapy expert working collaboratively with other healthcare providers. These models vary across practice settings but share common elements: systematic assessment of medication-related needs, development of care plans addressing those needs, and ongoing evaluation of therapeutic outcomes. The pharmaceutical care model provides a conceptual framework for this approach, defining the pharmacist's responsibility for achieving defined therapeutic goals.

Interprofessional Collaboration

Effective patient care increasingly depends on collaboration among healthcare providers with complementary expertise. Pharmacists contribute specialized knowledge of medication therapy to interprofessional teams, working alongside physicians, nurses, and other professionals to optimize treatment regimens. This collaboration may occur through formal team structures in institutional settings or through communication networks in community practice.

Successful interprofessional collaboration requires mutual understanding of each profession's capabilities and limitations, shared commitment to patient-centered goals, effective communication systems, and organizational support for team-based approaches. Pharmacists must develop both clinical expertise and collaborative skills to function effectively in these environments.

Table 1.3: Pharmacist Roles in Various Healthcare Settings

Practice Setting	Primary Responsibilities
Community Pharmacy	Dispensing medications, patient counseling, OTC recommendations, vaccination
Hospital Pharmacy	Medication distribution, IV preparation, clinical monitoring, formulary management
Ambulatory Care	Medication therapy management, chronic disease management, health screening
Long-term Care	Medication regimen review, consulting services, regulatory compliance
Home Health	Infusion therapy, patient education, care coordination
Managed Care	Formulary development, drug utilization review, cost containment strategies
Nuclear Pharmacy	Preparation of radioactive medications, quality control
Academia	Teaching, research, service, mentoring
Industry	Drug development, clinical trials, regulatory affairs, manufacturing
Government	Public health programs, regulatory oversight, research, policy development
Consulting	Specialized expertise in specific disease states or pharmacy practices
Specialty Pharmacy	Complex medication management for rare or chronic conditions
Informatics	Electronic health record optimization, clinical decision support
Veterinary Pharmacy	Compounding and dispensing medications for animals

Health Insurance and Pharmacy Benefits

Pharmacy benefits constitute a significant component of health insurance coverage, with various mechanisms employed to manage medication access and costs. These include formularies that categorize medications into tiers with different patient cost-sharing requirements, prior authorization processes for certain medications, quantity limits, and step therapy requirements.

Table 1.4: Healthcare Payment Systems and Their Impact on Pharmacy

Payment System	Description	Impact on Pharmacy Practice
Fee-for-Service	Payment for each service provided	Emphasis on prescription volume
Capitation	Fixed payment per patient regardless of services	Focus on cost-effective therapy
Value-Based Payment	Reimbursement tied to quality measures	Increased emphasis on outcomes
Medicare Part D	Prescription drug coverage for Medicare beneficiaries	Complex billing, coverage gaps
Medicaid	State-federal program for low-income individuals	Varied formularies, low reimbursement rates
Private Insurance	Employer or individual health plans	Multiple formularies, prior authorizations
Cash Payment	Direct patient payment without insurance	Price sensitivity, discount programs
Pharmacy Benefit Managers	Third-party administrators of prescription programs	Negotiated reimbursement rates, formularies
Manufacturer Assistance	Programs to help patients afford medications	Complex eligibility requirements
340B Program	Discounted medications for eligible entities	Inventory management challenges
Medication Therapy Management	Reimbursement for clinical pharmacy services	New revenue opportunities
Accountable Care Organizations	Shared savings models for coordinated care	Team-based care opportunities
Pay-for-Performance	Bonuses for meeting quality metrics	Focus on adherence and outcomes

Pharmacists must understand these systems to advocate for appropriate patient access while recognizing legitimate needs for resource stewardship. This requires understanding insurance terminology, reimbursement methodologies, and appeal processes. In many settings, pharmacists also play key roles in designing and implementing pharmacy benefit structures that balance clinical appropriateness with economic considerations.

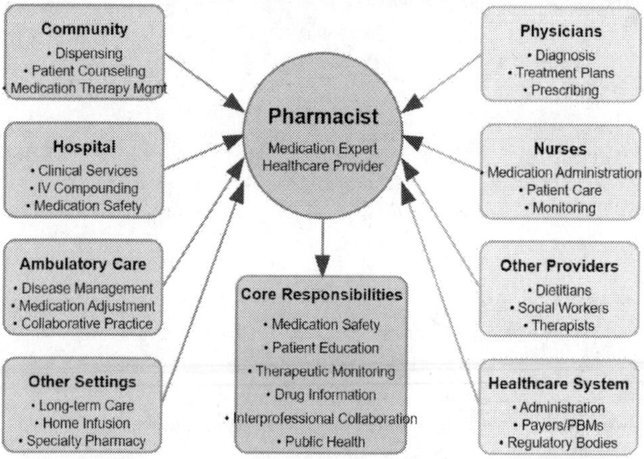

Figure 1.3: Healthcare Systems and Pharmacy Practice Roles

COMMUNICATION SKILLS IN PHARMACY PRACTICE

Effective communication underpins all aspects of pharmacy practice, from patient interactions to collaboration with healthcare colleagues. Communication skills directly influence therapeutic outcomes by affecting medication adherence, patient satisfaction, and interdisciplinary collaboration. These skills can be systematically developed through education, practice, and reflective learning.

Patient-Centered Communication

Patient-centered communication adapts information delivery and interaction styles to meet individual needs and preferences. This approach recognizes patients as active participants in their care rather than passive recipients of services. Key elements include establishing rapport, eliciting patient perspectives on medication experiences and concerns, providing information at appropriate literacy levels, checking comprehension, and engaging patients in shared decision-making.

Table 1.4: Effective Communication Techniques for Pharmacists

Technique	Description	Application
Active Listening	Fully concentrating on speaker, providing feedback	Patient interviews, medication counseling
Open-ended Questions	Questions requiring more than yes/no answers	Gathering comprehensive information
Closed-ended Questions	Questions with specific, limited responses	Confirming understanding, focusing discussion
Empathetic Responses	Acknowledging patient's feelings and concerns	Building rapport with anxious or distressed patients
Nonverbal Communication	Body language, eye contact, facial expressions	Conveying attentiveness and respect
Teach-back Method	Asking patients to explain information in their own words	Confirming understanding of medication instructions
Plain Language	Using simple, clear terms instead of jargon	Explaining complex medication information
Cultural Sensitivity	Respecting cultural differences in communication	Serving diverse patient populations
Motivational Interviewing	Collaborative approach to behavior change	Improving medication adherence
Written Communication	Clear, concise written information	Supplementing verbal counseling
Visual Aids	Pictures, diagrams, charts	Understanding medication use
Electronic Communication	Email, patient portals, telehealth	Providing convenient access to pharmacy
Conflict Resolution	Techniques to address disagreements constructively	Managing difficult patient interactions

Cultural competence represents an essential dimension of patient-centered communication. Pharmacists must recognize how cultural backgrounds influence health beliefs, medication practices, and communication styles. This awareness enables adaptation of counseling approaches to respect cultural perspectives while promoting optimal medication use.

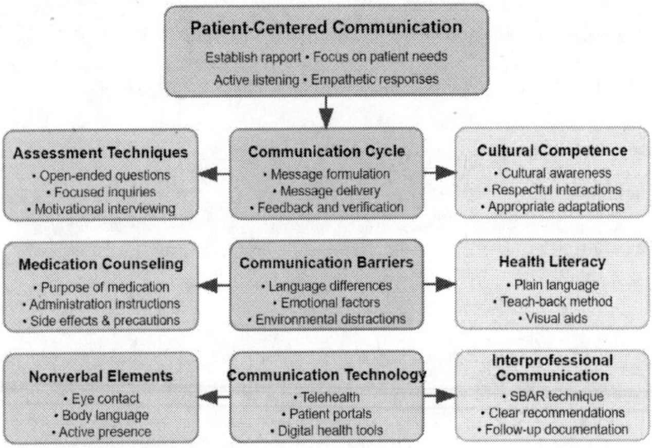

Figure 1.4: Effective Communication Model for Pharmacy Practice

Medication Counseling Techniques

Effective medication counseling transcends mere information transfer to enable patients to use medications safely and appropriately. Structured counseling approaches, such as the Indian Health Service method or the USP medication counseling model, provide frameworks for comprehensive education that addresses key aspects of medication use.

Visual aids, demonstration techniques, and teach-back methods enhance counseling effectiveness, particularly for complex medication regimens or patients with limited health literacy. Written information supplements verbal counseling, providing reference material for later review. Increasingly, digital tools complement traditional counseling approaches, offering resources tailored to diverse learning preferences.

Documentation and Professional Communication

Documentation serves multiple purposes in pharmacy practice: creating legal records of services provided, facilitating continuity of care, demonstrating quality improvement, and supporting reimbursement claims. Effective documentation is concise yet comprehensive, focusing on clinically relevant information and pharmacist interventions that influence patient outcomes.

Communication with healthcare colleagues requires adaptation to different professional cultures and communication preferences. SBAR (Situation-Background-Assessment-Recommendation) and other structured communication frameworks enhance clarity when discussing patient care issues. Electronic communication systems facilitate information exchange but introduce challenges related to message security, information overload, and potential misinterpretation.

Managing Challenging Communications

Pharmacy practice inevitably involves difficult conversations: delivering unwelcome news about medication coverage limitations, addressing medication misuse concerns, responding to dissatisfied patients, or communicating with healthcare providers about prescribing concerns. These situations require advanced communication skills that balance empathy with appropriate boundaries.

Conflict resolution approaches emphasize focusing on the problem rather than the person, seeking to understand underlying concerns, generating multiple potential solutions, and working toward mutually acceptable outcomes. De-escalation techniques help manage emotionally charged interactions by maintaining a calm demeanor, acknowledging emotions without judgment, and redirecting conversation toward constructive problem-solving

Summary

Pharmacy practice combines ethical principles, legal guidelines, healthcare system roles, and communication strategies essential for effective patient care. Core bioethical values—autonomy, beneficence, non-maleficence, and justice—guide decision-making when confronting confidentiality concerns, conflicts of interest, and resource allocation challenges. These principles operate within a comprehensive regulatory structure established by federal legislation including the Controlled Substances Act, Food, Drug, and Cosmetic Act, and HIPAA, alongside state-specific practice acts governing licensure requirements and scope of practice boundaries. The pharmacist's role has evolved substantially beyond medication dispensing to encompass clinical services such as medication therapy management, collaborative practice protocols, immunization delivery, and care transitions across diverse settings from community pharmacies to hospitals and specialty practices. Effective patient communication represents a critical competency, requiring adaptation to varying health literacy levels, cultural backgrounds, and emotional states. Techniques including motivational interviewing facilitate behavioral change, while structured counseling approaches ensure comprehension of complex medication regimens. Equally important is interprofessional communication, which enables coordinated care through clear documentation, SBAR (Situation-Background-Assessment-Recommendation) methodology, and conflict resolution strategies. Together, these fundamental elements create the professional foundation upon which pharmaceutical care is delivered, empowering pharmacists to serve as medication experts within healthcare teams while maintaining ethical standards and regulatory compliance in service of improved patient outcomes.

Multiple Choice Questions

1. Which of the following best describes the principle of beneficence in pharmacy ethics?
   a) Respecting a patient's right to make their own healthcare decisions
   b) Acting in a way that benefits patients and promotes their welfare
   c) Treating all patients equally regardless of background
   d) Maintaining patient confidentiality at all times
2. Under federal law, which schedule of controlled substances has the highest potential for abuse with no currently accepted medical use?
   a) Schedule I
   b) Schedule II
   c) Schedule III
   d) Schedule IV
3. A pharmacist receives a prescription for hydrocodone/acetaminophen that is missing the prescriber's DEA number. What is the appropriate action?
   a) Fill the prescription and document the missing DEA number
   b) Fill the prescription but reduce the quantity by half
   c) Contact the prescriber to obtain the DEA number before dispensing
   d) Refuse to fill the prescription and refer the patient elsewhere

4. Which regulatory body is primarily responsible for approving new drugs for marketing in the United States?
a) Drug Enforcement Administration (DEA)
b) Food and Drug Administration (FDA)
c) State Board of Pharmacy
d) Centers for Medicare and Medicaid Services (CMS)
5. In the context of patient autonomy, which of the following actions by a pharmacist would be considered most appropriate?
a) Dispensing a medication despite known patient allergies because the doctor prescribed it
b) Refusing to dispense emergency contraception due to personal beliefs without referring the patient
c) Providing complete information about medication risks and benefits to allow informed decision-making
d) Making medication decisions for elderly patients without consultation
6. Which of the following services falls under the category of Medication Therapy Management (MTM)?
a) Automated refill reminder calls
b) Comprehensive medication review
c) Routine dispensing of medications
d) Immunization administration
7. A pharmacist is discussing a new antihypertensive medication with a patient who has limited health literacy. Which communication technique would be most effective?
a) Providing detailed written materials explaining the medication's pharmacology
b) Using medical terminology to emphasize the importance of adherence
c) Using the teach-back method to confirm understanding of key instructions
d) Speaking loudly to ensure the patient hears all information
8. Under HIPAA regulations, which of the following would be considered a permissible disclosure of protected health information without specific patient authorization?
a) Sharing medication history with the patient's family members without permission
b) Discussing a celebrity patient's prescription with

pharmacy staff not involved in their care
c) Providing information to another healthcare provider for treatment purposes
d) Posting de-identified patient cases on social media for educational purposes

9. Which payment model reimburses healthcare providers based on patient health outcomes rather than the volume of services provided?
a) Fee-for-service
b) Value-based care
c) Capitation
d) Direct patient billing

10. In interprofessional healthcare teams, the pharmacist's primary role typically includes:
a) Diagnosing medical conditions
b) Performing physical assessments
c) Providing medication expertise and optimizing drug therapy
d) Directing the overall treatment plan

Self-Assessment Questions

1. Describe a scenario where patient autonomy conflicts with beneficence in pharmacy practice, and explain how you would resolve this ethical dilemma while balancing professional obligations and patient welfare.
2. Analyze the concept of "duty to care" as it applies to pharmacists during public health emergencies, discussing the ethical considerations that guide a pharmacist's responsibility to provide services despite personal risk.
3. Explain how the Controlled Substances Act's scheduling system categorizes medications, and describe the specific record-keeping, inventory, and dispensing requirements that apply to Schedule II medications.
4. Compare and contrast the regulatory roles of the State Board of Pharmacy, the FDA, and the DEA in overseeing pharmacy practice, highlighting how their jurisdictions overlap and differ.
5. Describe the evolution of the pharmacist's role from traditional dispensing functions to current clinical responsibilities, identifying specific services that exemplify this transition and the legal frameworks enabling expanded practice.
6. Analyze the structure of the U.S. healthcare system, explaining how different payment models (fee-for-service, value-based care, capitation) impact pharmacy operations and patient access to medications.
7. Describe how a medication therapy management service differs from traditional dispensing activities, detailing the specific components, documentation requirements, and potential outcomes of a comprehensive medication review.
8. Explain techniques for effectively communicating with patients who have limited health literacy, providing specific strategies to ensure comprehension of complex medication instructions.
9. Describe how you would apply motivational interviewing techniques to address medication non-adherence, providing examples of specific questions and responses that demonstrate the core principles of this communication approach.
10. Analyze the barriers and solutions to effective interprofessional communication in healthcare settings, explaining how structured communication tools (such as SBAR) improve patient care coordination across disciplines.

Bibliography

1. Gallagher CT, Greenland VAM, Hickman AC. Ethical dilemmas in pharmacy practice: A survey of difficulty and incidence. Int J Pharm Pract. 2019;27(5):459-466.
2. Qato DM, Zenk S, Wilder J, Harrington R, Gaskin D, Alexander GC. The availability of pharmacies in the United States: 2007-2015. PLoS One. 2017;12(8):e0183172.
3. Bader LR, McGrath S, Rouse MJ, Anderson C. A conceptual framework toward identifying and analyzing challenges to the advancement of pharmacy. Res Social Adm Pharm. 2017;13(2):321-331.
4. Guirguis LM, Chewning BA. Role theory: Literature review and implications for patient-pharmacist interactions. Res Social Adm Pharm. 2005;1(4):483-507.
5. Blumenthal KJ, Chang Y, Ferris TG, Spetz J, Vogeli C, Wagle N, et al. Using a self-reported global health measure to identify patients at high risk for future healthcare utilization. J Gen Intern Med. 2017;32(8):877-882.
6. Wheeler JS, Chisholm-Burns M. The benefit of continuing professional development for continuing pharmacy education. Am J Pharm Educ. 2018;82(3):6461.
7. McDonough RP, Bennett MS. Improving communication skills of pharmacy students through effective precepting. Am J Pharm Educ. 2006;70(3):58.
8. Gabay M. The Federal Controlled Substances Act: Schedules and pharmacy registration. Hosp Pharm. 2013;48(6):473-474.
9. Hepler CD, Strand LM. Opportunities and responsibilities in pharmaceutical care. Am J Hosp Pharm. 1990;47(3):533-543.
10. Nunes-da-Cunha I, Arguello B, Martinez FM, Fernandez-Llimos F. A comparison of patient-centered care in pharmacy curricula in the United States and Europe. Am J Pharm Educ. 2016;80(5):83.

CHAPTER 2

PHARMACEUTICAL CALCULATIONS

Author

Miss Farsiya Fatima, Associate Professor, Department of Pharmaceutics, Sultan ul Uloom College of Pharmacy, Banjara Hills, Hyderabad, Telangana, India

Abstract

Pharmaceutical calculations form the mathematical foundation of medication preparation, dispensing, and administration. Basic mathematical principles essential to pharmacy practice include measurement systems (metric, apothecary, household), unit conversions, ratio expressions, proportions, and alligation calculations that ensure accurate medication processing. Dosage calculations translate prescribed amounts into practical administration instructions, incorporating body weight and surface area considerations for pediatric and specialized populations, while accounting for creatinine clearance in renally eliminated medications. Compounding calculations support formulation development through percentage strength determinations, dilution ratios, molecular weight conversions, and accurate measurement of active and inactive ingredients to create customized medications. Concentration and dilution calculations enable pharmacists to prepare solutions of specified strengths, adjust existing concentrations, and perform isotonicity calculations ensuring physiological compatibility of parenteral preparations. These mathematical skills directly impact patient safety by preventing medication errors, enabling accurate dosing across diverse patient populations, and supporting the precise preparation of both routine and specialized pharmaceutical products.

Keywords: *Dosage Determination; Mathematical Accuracy; Measurement Conversion; Formulation; Preparation; Solution Concentration*

Learning Objectives

After completion of the chapter, the learners should be able to:

- Convert measurements accurately between metric, apothecary, and household systems using appropriate conversion factors.
- Calculate pediatric medication doses using body weight, body surface area, and age-based methods.
- Determine quantities of ingredients needed for compounded preparations based on prescription requirements and formulation records.
- Solve concentration problems involving percentage strength, ratio strength, and parts per million expressions.
- Calculate isotonicity values and adjustments required for parenteral preparations to ensure physiological compatibility.
- Perform alligation and dilution calculations to prepare solutions of specified strengths from available stock concentrations.

BASIC MATHEMATICAL PRINCIPLES

Pharmaceutical calculations rely on a solid foundation of mathematical principles that underpin every aspect of medication preparation, dispensing, and administration. These principles ensure accuracy and precision in pharmaceutical practice, where even minor calculation errors can lead to significant therapeutic consequences. Mastery of these fundamentals is therefore essential for safe and effective pharmacy practice.

The metric system serves as the primary measurement system in pharmaceutical practice worldwide due to its decimal-based structure and internal consistency. This system employs standard units for mass (gram), volume (liter), and length (meter), along with their decimal multiples and submultiples. Conversion within the metric system involves simple multiplication or division by powers of ten, facilitating accurate measurement across scales from nanograms to kilograms. Despite the predominance of the metric system, pharmacists must also maintain familiarity with other measurement systems, particularly the apothecary and avoirdupois systems, which may still appear in certain clinical contexts or historical literature.

Pharmaceutical calculations frequently require conversion between measurement systems. These conversions rely on established equivalence factors, such as 1 grain being equivalent to 64.8 milligrams or 1 fluid ounce corresponding to approximately 29.57 milliliters. When performing such conversions, it is imperative to use exact conversion factors rather than rounded approximations to maintain calculation accuracy, particularly when dealing with medications that have narrow therapeutic indices.

Table 2.1: Essential Mathematical Concepts for Pharmacy

Concept	Definition	Pharmacy Application
Fractions	Parts of a whole expressed as ratios	Tablet splitting, partial doses
Decimals	Numbers expressed in base 10	Medication dosing, measurements
Percentages	Parts per hundred	Concentration expressions, solutions
Ratios	Relationship between two quantities	Drug dilutions, compounding
Proportions	Equality between two ratios	Dosage calculations, aliquots
Significant Figures	Digits that contribute to precision	Analytical measurements, quality control
Scientific Notation	Expressing numbers as powers of 10	Very large or small quantities
Dimensional Analysis	Method using conversion factors	Converting between units
Rounding	Reducing digits to specified precision	Practical dosing, measurements
Estimation	Approximate calculations	Verifying calculated results
Alligation	Method to determine mixture properties	Calculating mixture concentrations
Logarithms	Exponents expressing order of magnitude	pH calculations, drug stability
Exponents	Powers to which numbers are raised	Drug concentration decay
Basic Statistics	Mean, median, mode, standard deviation	Quality control, clinical trials

Significant Figures and Scientific Notation

The concept of significant figures addresses the inherent limitations in measurement precision and calculation accuracy. In pharmaceutical calculations, the number of significant figures in a measurement indicates its precision, while the number of significant figures in a calculated result should reflect the precision of the least precise input value. This principle prevents the communication of false precision that might lead to dosing errors.

Scientific notation provides an elegant solution for expressing very large or very small values that are common in pharmaceutical contexts. By representing numbers in the form of a coefficient multiplied by a power of ten (e.g., 1.5×10^{-3} rather than 0.0015), scientific notation simplifies calculations and reduces transcription errors. This notation is particularly valuable when working with molecular weights, microdose medications, or pharmacokinetic parameters that often involve multiple orders of magnitude.

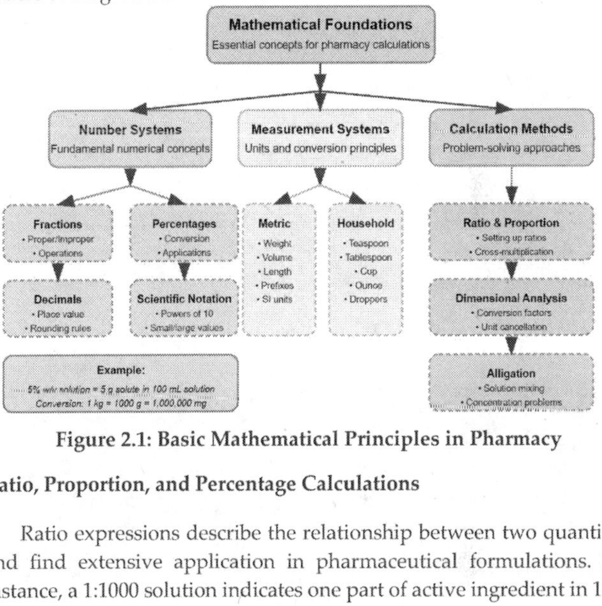

Figure 2.1: Basic Mathematical Principles in Pharmacy

Ratio, Proportion, and Percentage Calculations

Ratio expressions describe the relationship between two quantities and find extensive application in pharmaceutical formulations. For instance, a 1:1000 solution indicates one part of active ingredient in 1000 parts of solution. Understanding how to interpret and manipulate these ratios is crucial for accurate preparation of medications and solutions.

Proportional relationships form the basis for many pharmaceutical calculations, allowing pharmacists to determine unknown values when other related values are known. The principle that the ratio of corresponding values remains constant across equivalent relationships enables the use of cross-multiplication techniques to solve for unknown quantities in medication adjustments, alligation calculations, and dose conversions.

Percentage calculations appear throughout pharmacy practice in contexts ranging from drug concentration expressions to dose adjustments. These calculations can represent weight-in-weight (w/w), weight-in-volume (w/v), or volume-in-volume (v/v) relationships, with each type requiring specific interpretation. For example, a 5% w/v solution contains 5 grams of solute per 100 milliliters of solution, while a 5% v/v solution contains 5 milliliters of solute per 100 milliliters of solution.

Logarithmic and Exponential Functions

Logarithmic and exponential functions are indispensable in pharmaceutical calculations related to pharmacokinetics, chemical stability, and pH determinations. The logarithmic function, as the inverse of the exponential function, allows the conversion of multiplicative relationships to additive ones, simplifying complex calculations.

The pH scale exemplifies the practical application of logarithmic functions in pharmacy, where pH is defined as the negative logarithm of hydrogen ion concentration. This transformation converts a wide range of concentration values (spanning multiple orders of magnitude) into a more manageable scale typically ranging from 0 to 14. Understanding the logarithmic nature of the pH scale is essential for pharmaceutical buffer preparation, stability assessment, and formulation development.

DOSAGE CALCULATIONS

Dosage calculations represent perhaps the most critical application of pharmaceutical mathematics, directly impacting patient safety and therapeutic outcomes. These calculations ensure that patients receive the appropriate amount of medication based on various factors including body weight, age, organ function, and the specific characteristics of the drug itself.

Weight-Based Dosing

Weight-based dosing involves calculating medication doses based on a patient's body weight, typically expressed in milligrams per kilogram (mg/kg) or micrograms per kilogram (μg/kg). This approach is particularly important for pediatric patients, where developmental differences in drug metabolism and body composition necessitate individualized dosing.

The calculation typically follows the formula: Dose = (Weight in kg × Dose in mg/kg). For example, if a child weighing 20 kg requires amoxicillin at 40 mg/kg/day divided into three doses, the calculation would be: (20 kg × 40 mg/kg/day) ÷ 3 = 266.67 mg per dose. Depending on available formulation strengths, this might be rounded to 250 mg or 275 mg, with consideration for the drug's therapeutic index and available dosage forms.

Weight-based dosing extends beyond pediatrics to include certain adult medications such as chemotherapeutic agents, anticoagulants, and critical care medications. In these contexts, precise weight measurement and careful calculation are essential to avoid potentially severe adverse effects while ensuring therapeutic efficacy.

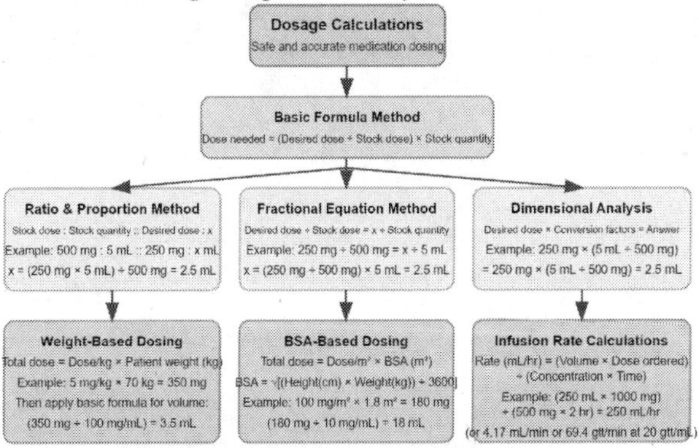

Figure 2.2: Dosage Calculation Methods

Body Surface Area Calculations

Body surface area (BSA) provides an alternative basis for dose individualization that accounts for both weight and height. BSA-based dosing is particularly valuable for medications with significant toxicity potential, such as antineoplastic agents, where the relationship between BSA and drug clearance often proves more reliable than weight alone.

Several formulas exist for calculating BSA, with the Mosteller formula (BSA (m^2) = $\sqrt{[(\text{Height (cm)} \times \text{Weight (kg)})/3600]}$) representing a commonly used approach due to its relative simplicity and accuracy across patient populations. Once the BSA is determined, the dose calculation follows the formula: Dose = BSA (m^2) × Dose per m^2.

For example, calculating the dose of doxorubicin (50 mg/m^2) for a patient with a BSA of 1.8 m^2 would yield: 1.8 m^2 × 50 mg/m^2 = 90 mg. The precision required in these calculations reflects the narrow therapeutic window characteristic of many medications dosed according to BSA.

Creatinine Clearance and Renal Dosing

Renal function significantly influences the elimination of many medications, necessitating dose adjustments for patients with impaired kidney function. Creatinine clearance (CrCl) serves as a clinical estimate of glomerular filtration rate, providing the basis for such adjustments.

The Cockcroft-Gault equation represents the most widely used method for estimating creatinine clearance in adults:

CrCl (ml/min) = [(140 - Age) × Weight (kg) × (0.85 if female)] ÷ [72 ×

Serum Creatinine (mg/dL)]

Table 2.2: Dosage Calculation Formulas and Examples

Calculation Type	Formula	Example
Weight-Based Dosing	Dose = (mg/kg) × Patient Weight	5 mg/kg × 70 kg = 350 mg
Body Surface Area Dosing	Dose = BSA (m^2) × Dose/m^2	1.8 m^2 × 100 mg/m^2 = 180 mg
Creatinine Clearance	CrCl = [(140-age) × weight] ÷ (72 × SCr)	[(140-65) × 70] ÷ (72 × 1.2) = 47.7 mL/min
Pediatric Dose (Clark's rule)	Child's dose = (Child's weight ÷ 70) × Adult dose	(25 kg ÷ 70) × 500 mg = 178.6 mg
Infusion Rate	Rate (mL/hr) = (Dose × Volume) ÷ (Concentration × Time)	(1000 mg × 250 mL) ÷ (5 mg/mL × 60 min) = 833.3 mL/hr
Drip Rate	Drops/min = (Volume × Drop factor) ÷ Time (min)	(1000 mL × 15 gtt/mL) ÷ 480 min = 31.3 gtt/min
Dosage Frequency	Frequency = 24 hr ÷ Dosing interval	24 hr ÷ 8 hr = 3 doses per day
Insulin Units	Units = Blood glucose - 100 ÷ Correction factor	(250 - 100) ÷ 30 = 5 units
Loading Dose	LD = Target Cp × Vd	10 mg/L × 35 L = 350 mg
Maintenance Dose	MD = Cl × Target Cp × τ	0.1 L/hr × 10 mg/L × 12 hr = 12 mg
Ideal Body Weight (IBW)	Male: IBW = 50 kg + 2.3 kg(height in inches - 60)	50 kg + 2.3 kg(70 - 60) = 73 kg
Adjusted Body Weight	ABW = IBW + 0.4(TBW - IBW)	70 kg + 0.4(100 kg - 70 kg) = 82 kg
Bioavailability Adjustment	Dose = (Desired dose ÷ Bioavailability)	100 mg ÷ 0.5 = 200 mg

Dose adjustments based on creatinine clearance may involve reduced doses, extended dosing intervals, or both, depending on the drug's pharmacokinetic properties and therapeutic index. For example, a medication normally dosed at 500 mg every 8 hours might be adjusted to 250 mg every 8 hours or 500 mg every 12 hours for a patient with moderate renal impairment, depending on its elimination characteristics.

Pediatric Dosing

Pediatric dosing requires special consideration beyond simple weight-based calculations. Developmental changes in absorption, distribution, metabolism, and excretion necessitate age-specific approaches to dose determination.

Various rules and formulas have been developed to estimate pediatric doses from adult doses, including Young's rule (Child's dose = [Age in years ÷ (Age + 12)] × Adult dose) and Clark's rule (Child's dose = [Weight in pounds ÷ 150] × Adult dose). However, these rules provide only rough approximations and have largely been supplanted by evidence-based, pediatric-specific dosing guidelines for most medications.

Medication administration in pediatric settings often requires additional calculations to determine appropriate volumes for liquid formulations. These calculations must account for the concentration of the medication and the precision of available measuring devices to ensure accurate dosing.

COMPOUNDING CALCULATIONS

Pharmaceutical compounding involves the preparation of customized medications to meet specific patient needs not addressed by commercially available products. The calculations associated with compounding ensure that these preparations contain the correct quantities of active and inactive ingredients, exhibiting appropriate physicochemical properties for their intended use.

Weighing and Measuring

Accurate weighing and measuring form the foundation of pharmaceutical compounding. These processes require selection of appropriate equipment based on the quantity being measured and the precision required. Analytical balances capable of measuring to 0.1 mg may be necessary for potent medications, while prescription balances with sensitivity to 5 mg might suffice for less critical components.

The principle of minimizing weighing errors by working with larger quantities when possible guides many compounding procedures. This approach might involve preparing a larger batch than immediately needed (with appropriate stability considerations) or using geometric dilution techniques when incorporating small quantities of active ingredients into larger masses.

Volume measurements in compounding utilize graduated cylinders, conical graduates, pipettes, and syringes, each selected based on the volume to be measured and the accuracy required. The meniscus reading technique, where the bottom of the concave liquid surface is aligned with the calibration mark at eye level, ensures accurate volume determination for transparent liquids.

Table 2.3: Compounding Calculation Methods

Method	Description	Example Calculation
Master Formula	Recipe for preparing compound	Prepare 100 g of 5% salicylic acid ointment
Percentage Strength	Parts per hundred	For 5% w/w: 5 g salicylic acid + 95 g base = 100 g
Parts per Million (ppm)	Parts per 1,000,000	1 ppm = 1 mg/L or 1 μg/mL
Parts per Billion (ppb)	Parts per 1,000,000,000	1 ppb = 1 μg/L or 1 ng/mL
Ratio Strength	Component:Total	1:1000 = 1 g per 1000 g (0.1%)
Milliequivalents	Measure of chemical activity	mEq = mg ÷ (molecular weight ÷ valence)
Molarity	Moles per liter	1 M NaCl = 58.44 g/L
Molality	Moles per kg solvent	1 m NaCl = 58.44 g/1000 g water
Normality	Gram-equivalents per liter	1 N H_2SO_4 = 49.04 g/L
Dilution	Reducing concentration	$C_1V_1 = C_2V_2$
Aliquot Method	Using portion of stock	10 mL of 1:100 solution to make 100 mL of 1:1000
Geometric Dilution	Progressive incorporation	Mix 1 g drug with 1 g base, then 2 g more base, etc.
Alligation	Determining mixture ratios	Mixing 10% and 2% solutions to create 5% solution
Density Adjustments	Converting volume to weight	100 mL × 0.9 g/mL = 90 g

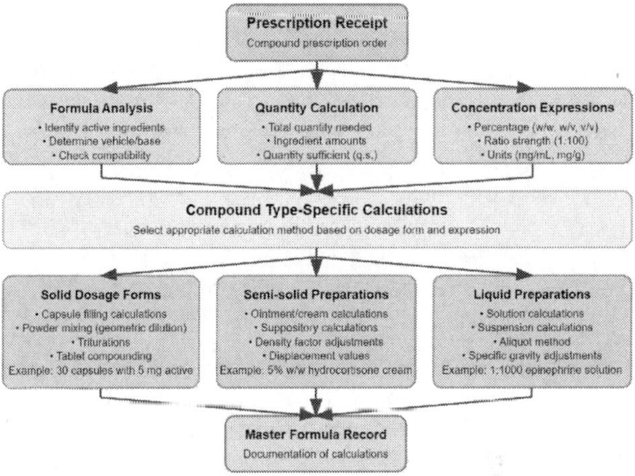

Figure 2.3: Compounding Calculations

Aliquot Method and Geometric Dilution

The aliquot method provides an approach for accurately measuring very small quantities by working with a larger, more manageable amount. This technique involves preparing a solution or mixture of known concentration, then using a precisely measured portion (aliquot) of this preparation to obtain the desired amount of ingredient.

For example, to incorporate 1 mg of a potent drug into a formulation, a pharmacist might prepare a 1 mg/mL solution, then measure 1 mL of this solution rather than attempting to directly weigh 1 mg of the pure drug. This approach significantly reduces measurement error, particularly when working with quantities below the reliable limit of available balances.

Geometric dilution addresses the challenge of uniformly incorporating a small quantity of active ingredient into a larger mass of base material. This technique involves sequential dilution, where the active ingredient is first mixed with an approximately equal quantity of base, then this mixture is combined with another equal portion of base, continuing until the entire quantity of base has been incorporated. This progressive dilution ensures homogeneous distribution of the active ingredient throughout the preparation.

Capsule and Suppository Calculations

Capsule preparation requires calculation of the total formula weight and the weight per capsule. The formula weight encompasses all active and inactive ingredients in the formulation, while the weight per capsule must account for capsule capacity constraints.

For instance, if preparing 30 capsules containing 25 mg of active ingredient per capsule, with a diluent density that allows 300 mg total weight per capsule, the calculation would indicate 750 mg total active ingredient (30 × 25 mg) and 8.25 g total diluent [(300 mg - 25 mg) × 30], yielding a total formula weight of 9 grams.

Suppository calculations similarly require determination of total formula weight, but must also account for density displacement values when incorporating active ingredients into the suppository base. The displacement value represents the weight of base displaced by a given weight of active ingredient, allowing for adjustment of the base quantity to maintain consistent suppository size.

CONCENTRATION AND DILUTION CALCULATIONS

Concentration and dilution calculations permeate pharmaceutical practice, from the preparation of intravenous admixtures to the formulation of topical preparations. These calculations ensure that medications are delivered at appropriate concentrations for their intended routes of administration and therapeutic purposes.

Table 2.4: Concentration and Dilution Calculations

Concentration Type	Definition	Calculation Method
Weight/Weight (w/w)	Grams of solute per 100 g of product	% w/w = (g solute ÷ g total) × 100
Weight/Volume (w/v)	Grams of solute per 100 mL of solution	% w/v = (g solute ÷ mL solution) × 100
Volume/Volume (v/v)	mL of solute per 100 mL of solution	% v/v = (mL solute ÷ mL solution) × 100
Molarity (M)	Moles of solute per liter of solution	M = moles ÷ liters
Normality (N)	Gram-equivalents per liter	N = (grams × valence) ÷ (molecular weight × liters)
Molality (m)	Moles of solute per kg of solvent	m = moles ÷ kg solvent
Millimoles (mmol)	One-thousandth of a mole	mmol = mg ÷ (molecular weight ÷ 1000)

Concentration Type	Definition	Calculation Method
Milliequivalents (mEq)	Millimoles × valence	mEq = (mg × valence) ÷ molecular weight
Parts per Million (ppm)	mg solute per kg or L solution	ppm = (mg solute ÷ kg solution) × 10^6
Parts per Billion (ppb)	μg solute per kg or L solution	ppb = (μg solute ÷ kg solution) × 10^9
Ratio Strength	Component: Total	1:1000 = 1 g per 1000 g = 0.1%
Serial Dilution	Stepwise concentration reduction	Each 1:10 dilution reduces concentration 10-fold
Stock Solution	Concentrated solution for dilution	Stock × Volume = Final concentration × Final volume
Simple Dilution	Direct dilution of stock	$C_1V_1 = C_2V_2$
Multiple Dilutions	Series of simple dilutions	Overall dilution = Product of individual dilutions

Concentration Expressions

Pharmaceutical concentrations can be expressed in multiple formats, each with specific applications. Percentage concentrations include weight-in-weight (w/w), weight-in-volume (w/v), and volume-in-volume (v/v) expressions. For example, a 2% w/v lidocaine solution contains 2 grams of lidocaine in 100 mL of solution, while a 2% v/v alcohol solution contains 2 mL of alcohol in 100 mL of solution.

Ratio strengths express concentration as a ratio of one part to a certain number of parts. A 1:1000 epinephrine solution indicates 1 gram of epinephrine in 1000 mL of solution (equivalent to 0.1% w/v). This expression format is particularly common for certain emergency medications and antiseptic solutions.

Molarity, expressing concentration as moles of solute per liter of solution, finds application in situations where chemical equivalence is important, such as buffer preparation or osmolarity calculations. Related expressions include normality (equivalents per liter) and molality (moles per kilogram of solvent).

Parts per million (ppm) and parts per billion (ppb) provide concentration expressions for very dilute solutions, particularly in contexts such as water purification standards or trace element analysis.

These units represent mg/L and μg/L, respectively, in aqueous solutions.

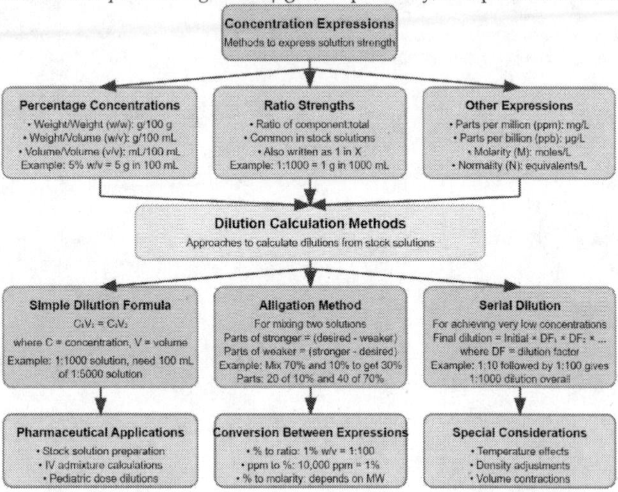

Figure 2.4: Concentration and Dilution Calculation Methods

Dilution Methods

Dilution calculations determine the volumes of stock solution and diluent needed to prepare a solution of desired concentration. The fundamental relationship governing these calculations is $C_1V_1 = C_2V_2$, where C represents concentration and V represents volume, with subscripts 1 and 2 indicating initial and final values, respectively.

For example, to prepare 500 mL of a 0.45% sodium chloride solution from a 0.9% stock solution, the calculation would be: $(0.9\% \times V_1) = (0.45\% \times 500 \text{ mL})$, yielding $V_1 = 250$ mL. This indicates that 250 mL of the 0.9% solution should be diluted with sufficient water to make 500 mL of final solution.

Serial dilution involves stepwise dilution to achieve very low concentrations or to prepare a series of solutions with systematically varying concentrations. Each step typically involves a consistent dilution factor, such as 1:10, allowing for the preparation of solutions spanning several orders of magnitude in concentration.

Alligation Calculations

Alligation provides a method for determining the proportions in which solutions of different concentrations should be mixed to achieve a desired intermediate concentration. This method is particularly valuable when preparing solutions from available stock solutions of higher and lower concentrations than the target.

The alligation medial formula calculates the final concentration when mixing solutions of known concentrations in specified proportions: Final concentration = [(Volume$_1$ × Concentration$_1$) + (Volume$_2$ × Concentration$_2$)] ÷ (Volume$_1$ + Volume$_2$).

Table 2.5: Common Pharmacy Measurement Conversions

Measurement Type	Conversion Factors	Examples
Weight	1 kg = 1000 g	2.2 kg = 2200 g
	1 g = 1000 mg	0.5 g = 500 mg
	1 mg = 1000 µg	2 mg = 2000 µg
	1 kg = 2.2 lb	70 kg = 154 lb
	1 lb = 454 g	10 lb = 4540 g
	1 oz = 28.35 g	4 oz = 113.4 g
	1 grain = 64.8 mg	5 grain = 324 mg
Volume	1 L = 1000 mL	2.5 L = 2500 mL
	1 mL = 1 cc	5 mL = 5 cc
	1 fl oz = 29.57 mL	8 fl oz = 236.6 mL
	1 tablespoon = 15 mL	3 tbsp = 45 mL
	1 teaspoon = 5 mL	2 tsp = 10 mL
	1 pint = 473 mL	2 pints = 946 mL
	1 gallon = 3.785 L	0.5 gallon = 1.89 L
Temperature	°F = (°C × 9/5) + 32	25°C = 77°F
	°C = (°F - 32) × 5/9	98.6°F = 37°C
Length	1 m = 100 cm	1.8 m = 180 cm
	1 cm = 10 mm	5 cm = 50 mm
	1 inch = 2.54 cm	6 inches = 15.24 cm
	1 foot = 30.48 cm	5 feet = 152.4 cm

Conversely, the alligation alternate method determines the proportions needed to achieve a specific target concentration. This approach involves calculating the difference between the target concentration and each of the stock concentrations, then setting these differences in inverse proportion to the required volumes.

Isotonicity Calculations

Isotonic solutions have the same osmotic pressure as body fluids, making them appropriate for parenteral administration, ophthalmic preparations, and other applications where tissue irritation must be minimized. Calculations to achieve isotonicity ensure that preparations exert appropriate osmotic effects.

The sodium chloride equivalent method represents one approach to isotonicity calculations, based on the principle that a 0.9% w/v sodium chloride solution is isotonic with blood. Using published sodium chloride equivalent values for various compounds, pharmacists can calculate the amount of additional tonicity-adjusting agent needed to achieve isotonicity.

For example, if preparing an isotonic ophthalmic solution containing 1% w/v of a drug with a sodium chloride equivalent of 0.2, the calculation would indicate that the drug contributes the equivalent of 0.2% sodium chloride to tonicity. To achieve isotonicity, additional sodium chloride or other tonicity agent would be needed to provide the equivalent of 0.7% sodium chloride (0.9% - 0.2% = 0.7%).

Freezing point depression calculations offer an alternative approach to isotonicity determination, based on the relationship between osmotic pressure and colligative properties of solutions. This method employs the principle that an isotonic solution depresses the freezing point of water by 0.52°C, allowing calculation of required tonicity adjustments based on molecular properties of the solutes.

Summary

Mathematical principles form the backbone of safe medication preparation, dispensing, and administration across all pharmacy settings. Fundamental concepts including arithmetic operations, significant figures, scientific notation, ratio relationships, and dimensional analysis create the framework for accurate pharmaceutical calculations. Measurement system conversions between metric, apothecary, and household units are essential skills, particularly when interpreting prescriptions or providing patient instructions. These basics support complex patient-specific dosing determinations including weight-based pediatric calculations, body surface area formulas for chemotherapy, creatinine clearance estimations guiding renal adjustments, and parenteral therapy rate calculations involving concentration parameters and flow rates. Compounding mathematics presents unique challenges requiring precision in ingredient quantities, including aliquot preparation methods for potent substances, displacement value considerations for suppositories, capsule density adjustments, and geometric dilution techniques ensuring uniform distribution. Concentration expressions appear in multiple formats including percentage strength (weight-in-weight, weight-in-volume, volume-in-volume), ratio strength, parts per million, and molarity—each requiring specific calculation approaches. Additional specialized calculations include isotonicity adjustments for ophthalmic and parenteral preparations, alligation methods for preparing desired concentrations from available stock solutions, and reconstitution determinations for antibiotic suspensions. Mastery of these mathematical principles safeguards against medication errors while enabling accurate preparation of both manufactured and custom-compounded medications.

Multiple Choice Questions

1. A prescription calls for amoxicillin 40 mg/kg/day divided into three doses for a child weighing 22 kg. How many milligrams of amoxicillin should be administered per dose?
   a) 293 mg
   b) 880 mg
   c) 40 mg
   d) 66 mg
2. A pharmacist needs to prepare 120 mL of a 1:4000 solution. How many grams of active ingredient are needed?
   a) 0.03 g
   b) 0.3 g
   c) 3 g
   d) 30 g
3. A patient is to receive vancomycin 15 mg/kg IV every 12 hours. If the patient weighs 70 kg, how many grams of vancomycin will the patient receive in 24 hours?
   a) 1.05 g
   b) 2.1 g
   c) 10.5 g
   d) 21 g
4. A stock solution contains 10% w/v dextrose. How many milliliters of this solution should be used to prepare 500 mL of a 5% w/v dextrose solution?
   a) 50 mL
   b) 100 mL
   c) 250 mL
   d) 500 mL
5. A patient's creatinine clearance is calculated using the Cockcroft-Gault equation. If the patient is a 72-year-old female weighing 65 kg with a serum creatinine of 1.8 mg/dL, what is her estimated creatinine clearance? (Use 0.85 as the correction factor for females)
   a) 24 mL/min
   b) 28 mL/min
   c) 33 mL/min
   d) 39 mL/min

6. A pharmacy receives a prescription for 30 capsules, each containing 0.5 mg of a drug. The pharmacy has 50 mg of the pure drug powder. How much inert diluent should be added to prepare the capsules?
   a) 15 mg
   b) 35 mg
   c) 450 mg
   d) 4950 mg
7. How many milliliters of a 1:100 stock solution are needed to prepare 250 mL of a 1:2000 solution?
   a) 1.25 mL
   b) 12.5 mL
   c) 20 mL
   d) 125 mL
8. A medication order calls for gentamicin 5 mg/kg/day divided into doses given every 8 hours. For a patient weighing 80 kg, how many milligrams should be administered per dose?
   a) 133 mg
   b) 400 mg
   c) 133.3 mg
   d) 240 mg
9. A pharmacist needs to prepare a solution that is isotonic with blood (equivalent to 0.9% sodium chloride). If the E value of a drug is 0.18, what percentage concentration of the drug would make an isotonic solution?
   a) 0.9%
   b) 5%
   c) 9%
   d) 0.18%
10. Using the alligation method, in what proportion should 70% alcohol and 30% alcohol be mixed to prepare 50% alcohol?
   a) 1 part 70% and 1 part 30%
   b) 2 parts 70% and 1 part 30%
   c) 1 part 70% and 2 parts 30%
   d) 3 parts 70% and 2 parts 30%

Self-Assessment Questions

1. Explain the concept of significant figures as it applies to pharmaceutical calculations, and describe how rounding errors could potentially impact patient safety when preparing medications with narrow therapeutic indices.
2. Describe the process of dimensional analysis for solving pharmaceutical calculations, and demonstrate how this method could be used to convert a medication order from micrograms per kilogram per minute to milligrams per hour for a patient weighing 70 kg.
3. Analyze the differences between ratio strength, percentage strength, and parts per million expressions of concentration, providing examples of when each would be most appropriately used in pharmacy practice.
4. Explain how to calculate the correct volume needed when preparing an intravenous infusion that must deliver 10 mg/kg/day of a medication for a 65 kg patient, using a premixed solution containing 5 mg/mL.
5. Describe the mathematical adjustments needed when calculating pediatric dosages using different methods (mg/kg, body surface area, Clark's rule), and analyze the clinical situations where each method would be most appropriate.
6. Explain the calculations involved in determining the creatinine clearance for a 72-year-old female patient weighing 65 kg with a serum creatinine of 1.8 mg/dL, and describe how this value would influence medication dosing decisions.
7. Describe the aliquot method of pharmaceutical compounding, explaining when it would be necessary and detailing the calculations required to prepare 30 capsules containing 0.5 mg of a drug using a 50 mg/mL stock solution.
8. Analyze the calculations needed to account for drug displacement values when preparing suppositories, explaining why this adjustment is necessary and how failing to consider it would affect the final product.
9. Describe the calculations involved in preparing an isotonic ophthalmic solution using sodium chloride as a tonicity agent, explaining the concept of freezing point depression and E values in determining appropriate concentrations.
10. Explain the alligation method and demonstrate how it would be used to determine the quantities needed to prepare 500 mL of a 35% alcohol solution using available stock solutions of 70% and 20% alcohol.

Bibliography

1. Ansel HC, Stoklosa MJ. Pharmaceutical calculations. 15th ed. Philadelphia: Wolters Kluwer; 2017.
2. Brown MC, Conway J, Fike DS. Impact of a problem-based learning approach to teaching pharmaceutical calculations. Curr Pharm Teach Learn. 2020;12(10):1213-1221.
3. Shepler BM. 3-Step approach to calculations for critical care nursing. Crit Care Nurse. 2018;38(4):e1-e6.
4. Johnson PJ, Barrett DA, Rowe RC. The measurement of tablet friability: A comparison of different test conditions. Drug Dev Ind Pharm. 1997;23(10):1065-1073.
5. Nahata MC, Pai VB, Hipple TF. Pediatric drug formulations. 5th ed. Cincinnati: Harvey Whitney Books; 2004.
6. Lesar TS. Medication calculation errors associated with direct infusion rates. Hosp Pharm. 1996;31(9):1089-1094.
7. Wang XM, Tang KL, Shang XL, Li C, Tang YL, Lin JH. Evaluation of intravenous preparations based on mathematical calculation of osmotic pressure. Drug Deliv. 2018;25(1):1951-1957.
8. Phillips LD, Gorski LA. Manual of IV therapeutics: Evidence-based practice for infusion therapy. 6th ed. Philadelphia: F.A. Davis Company; 2014.
9. Zaveri M, Patel V, Vidyasagar G, Solanki S. Development of simple spectrophotometric methods for estimation of famotidine in bulk and tablet formulation. Pharm Methods. 2010;1(1):43-46.
10. Myers AL, Kawedia JD, Champlin RE, Kramer MA, Nieto Y, Ghose R, et al. Clarifying busulfan dosing and pharmacokinetics in high-dose chemotherapy to improve clinical outcomes: A new model for dose individualization. Biol Blood Marrow Transplant. 2017;23(3):445-454.

CHAPTER 3

PHARMACEUTICAL CHEMISTRY

Author

Miss Pratiksha P. Yawalkar, Lecturer, Department of Quality Assurance, Dr. Rajendra Gode Institute of Pharmacy, Amravati, Maharashtra, India

Abstract

Pharmaceutical chemistry links chemical principles with drug development, formulation, and clinical application. Drug structure fundamentally determines pharmacological activity through functional groups that influence receptor binding, with structural modifications strategically employed to enhance potency, selectivity, and pharmacokinetic properties. Chemical kinetics principles govern drug stability and degradation pathways, including hydrolysis, oxidation, and photolysis reactions, informing appropriate storage conditions, beyond-use dating, and formulation strategies to maximize shelf life. Quality control methodologies employ analytical techniques including chromatography, spectroscopy, and dissolution testing to verify identity, purity, and potency of pharmaceutical products, ensuring batch consistency and conformance with established specifications. Pharmaceutical salt forms represent deliberate modifications of parent compounds through acid-base chemistry, enhancing solubility, stability, and bioavailability of otherwise problematic drugs, with selection among hydrochlorides, sulfates, and other salt variations significantly impacting formulation characteristics and therapeutic outcomes. These chemical principles directly influence clinical medication use by determining drug behavior in biological systems, manufacturing techniques, storage requirements, and ultimately therapeutic effectiveness across various patient populations.

Keywords: *Molecular Structure; Degradation Pathways; Analytical Methods; Chemical Stability; Bioavailability Modification*

Learning Objectives

After completion of the chapter, the learners should be able to:

- Correlate chemical structures with pharmacological activity by identifying functional groups that influence receptor binding.
- Predict stability challenges for medications based on their chemical properties and potential degradation pathways.
- Select appropriate analytical methods to verify identity, purity, and potency of pharmaceutical compounds.
- Compare the physicochemical properties of different salt forms and their impact on solubility, dissolution rate, and bioavailability.
- Evaluate how structural modifications alter drug pharmacokinetic properties including absorption, distribution, and elimination.
- Apply principles of stereochemistry to explain differences in pharmacological activity between enantiomers and diastereomers.

DRUG STRUCTURE AND PROPERTIES

The molecular structure of pharmaceutical compounds determines their physical, chemical, and biological properties, ultimately influencing their pharmacological activity, stability, and formulation characteristics. Understanding these structure-property relationships enables rational drug design, optimization of formulations, and prediction of drug behavior in biological systems.

Organic chemistry principles govern the architecture of most pharmaceutical molecules, which typically consist of carbon frameworks decorated with various functional groups. These functional groups—including amines, carboxylic acids, alcohols, esters, amides, and heterocyclic rings—serve as recognition elements for receptor binding, influence water solubility and lipophilicity, and provide sites for chemical modification during drug metabolism. The three-dimensional arrangement of these structural components creates the molecular topography that determines receptor complementarity and biological activity.

Stereochemistry in Drug Action

Stereochemistry exerts profound influence on drug-receptor interactions, as biological receptors exhibit inherent chirality that results in stereoselective recognition. Enantiomers, which are mirror-image molecules with identical physical properties but different spatial arrangements, often display dramatically different pharmacological profiles. For instance, S-ibuprofen exhibits significantly greater anti-inflammatory activity than its R-enantiomer, while S-fluoxetine has a markedly different metabolic profile than R-fluoxetine.

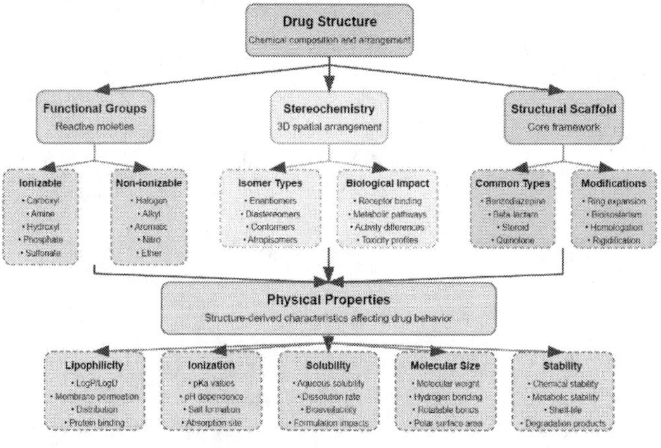

Figure 3.1: Drug Structure-Activity Relationship

The thalidomide tragedy stands as a sobering historical reminder of stereochemistry's importance, where one enantiomer provided therapeutic antiemetic effects while the other caused devastating teratogenic outcomes. This case catalyzed regulatory changes requiring stereochemical characterization of chiral drugs and evaluation of individual enantiomers. Modern pharmaceutical development frequently pursues single-enantiomer formulations (enantiopure drugs) to optimize efficacy and safety profiles, although racemic mixtures remain common when stereoselectivity offers limited therapeutic advantage or when interconversion occurs *in vivo*.

Diastereomers—stereoisomers that are not mirror images—exhibit different physical properties and biological activities from one another. This property finds application in prodrug design, where inactive diastereomers convert to active forms through enzymatic transformations, enabling targeted drug delivery or sustained release profiles. The conformational flexibility of molecular structures adds another dimension to stereochemical considerations, as many drugs can adopt multiple conformations with varying receptor affinities.

Physicochemical Properties and Bioavailability

The bioavailability of pharmaceutical compounds depends substantially on their physicochemical properties, particularly solubility and lipophilicity. These properties influence absorption, distribution, metabolism, and excretion (ADME) processes that determine drug concentration at target sites.

Solubility in aqueous media generally enhances absorption from the gastrointestinal tract but may limit membrane permeability. Conversely, lipophilicity facilitates membrane penetration but can reduce aqueous solubility and increase protein binding, potentially limiting the free drug concentration available for receptor interaction. This paradoxical relationship underpins Lipinski's Rule of Five, which identifies molecular characteristics associated with favorable oral bioavailability: molecular weight less than 500 Da, no more than 5 hydrogen bond donors, no more than 10 hydrogen bond acceptors, and calculated log P (octanol-water partition coefficient) less than 5.

Ionization state significantly affects drug absorption and distribution by altering solubility and membrane permeability characteristics. The Henderson-Hasselbalch equation describes the relationship between pH and ionization for acidic and basic drugs:

- For acids: $pH = pKa + \log([A^-]/[HA])$
- For bases: $pH = pKa + \log([B]/[BH^+])$

Weakly acidic drugs remain predominantly un-ionized in the acidic environment of the stomach, facilitating absorption, while weakly basic drugs show enhanced absorption in the more alkaline environment of the small intestine. Understanding these relationships enables strategic formulation decisions to optimize bioavailability for different drug classes.

Structure-Activity Relationships

Structure-activity relationships (SAR) establish correlations between molecular structure and biological activity, providing a framework for rational drug design and optimization. These relationships guide molecular modifications to enhance potency, selectivity, bioavailability, or metabolic stability while minimizing undesired effects.

Table 3.1: Functional Groups in Drug Structures

Functional Group	Structure	Example Drugs	Pharmaceutical Significance
Hydroxyl	-OH	Ethanol, Propranolol	Hydrogen bonding, solubility enhancement
Carboxyl	-COOH	Aspirin, NSAIDs	Acidity, salt formation, solubility
Amine	$-NH_2$, -	Amphetamine,	Basicity, salt

Functional Group	Structure	Example Drugs	Pharmaceutical Significance
	NHR, -NR$_2$	Fluoxetine	formation, solubility
Amide	-CONH$_2$	Acetaminophen, Lidocaine	Stability, hydrogen bonding
Ester	-COOR	Aspirin, Local anesthetics	Lipophilicity, hydrolysis susceptibility
Ether	-O-	Diphenhydramine, Morphine	Stability, lipophilicity
Carbonyl	-C=O	Ketoprofen, Cyclophosphamide	Reactivity, hydrogen bonding
Halogen	-F, -Cl, -Br, -I	Haloperidol, Fluoroquinolones	Lipophilicity, metabolic stability
Sulfhydryl	-SH	Captopril, Penicillamine	Oxidation susceptibility, binding
Phosphate	-PO$_4$	Fosinopril, Nucleotides	Solubility, charged state
Sulfonate	-SO$_3$	Mesalamine, Docusate	Strong acidity, solubility
Nitro	-NO$_2$	Chloramphenicol, Metronidazole	Electron withdrawing, reduction potential
Nitrile	-C≡N	Anastrozole, Citalopram	Metabolic stability, lipophilicity
Azide	-N$_3$	Zidovudine	Reactivity, stability
Phenyl	-C$_6$H$_5$	Most benzodiazepines	Lipophilicity, metabolism pathways

Quantitative structure-activity relationships (QSAR) extend this approach by developing mathematical models that predict biological activity based on structural descriptors. These descriptors may include physicochemical parameters (partition coefficients, electronic properties, steric parameters) or computational characteristics (molecular orbital energies, electrostatic potential maps). Modern QSAR approaches employ sophisticated computational methods, including machine learning algorithms that identify complex, non-linear relationships between structural features and biological responses.

Bioisosteric replacement represents a strategic application of SAR principles, where functional groups with similar physicochemical properties substitute for one another to maintain biological activity while modifying other properties such as metabolic stability or toxicity. Classical bioisosteres include exchangeable groups such as -COOH/-CONHR/-COOR/-COSR or $-NH_2$/-OH/-SH, while non-classical bioisosteres involve more substantial structural modifications that preserve essential binding interactions.

CHEMICAL KINETICS AND STABILITY

Chemical stability determines the shelf life of pharmaceutical products and influences dosage form design, packaging requirements, and storage conditions. Understanding the kinetics of degradation reactions enables prediction of stability profiles and development of strategies to minimize degradation during manufacturing, storage, and use.

Reaction Kinetics in Pharmaceutical Systems

Degradation reactions in pharmaceutical systems generally follow first-order, second-order, or pseudo-first-order kinetics. First-order reactions, where the rate depends linearly on the concentration of a single reactant, characterize many hydrolytic degradation pathways. The integrated first-order rate equation, $\ln[A]_{(t)} = \ln[A]_{(0)} - kt$, enables calculation of the concentration remaining after a specified time or determination of the time required for a certain percentage of degradation to occur.

Half-life ($t_1/_2$), representing the time required for 50% of the drug to degrade, provides a practical parameter for comparing stability profiles. For first-order reactions, $t_1/_2 = 0.693/k$, where k represents the rate constant. This relationship remains constant regardless of initial concentration, while for second-order reactions, half-life varies inversely with initial concentration.

Arrhenius relationship describes the temperature dependence of degradation rates:

$k = Ae^{(-Ea/RT)}$

Where k is the rate constant, A is the frequency factor, Ea is the activation energy, R is the gas constant, and T is absolute temperature.

This relationship allows extrapolation of stability data to different storage conditions and serves as the foundation for accelerated stability testing. Generally, a 10°C increase in temperature increases reaction rates 2-5 fold, though this rule of thumb requires verification for specific degradation pathways.

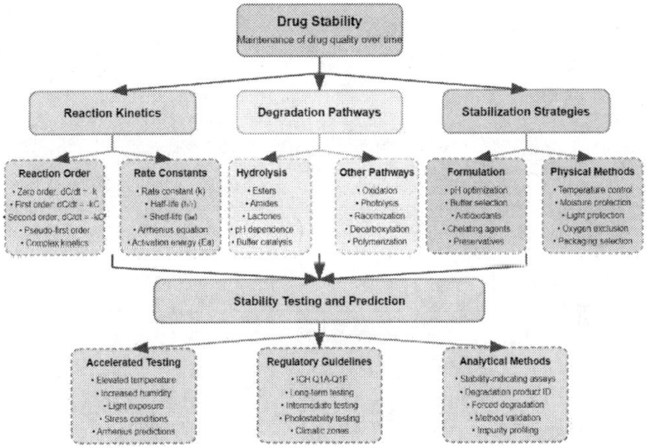

Figure 3.2: Chemical Kinetics and Drug Stability Factors

Hydrolytic Degradation

Hydrolysis represents the most common degradation pathway for pharmaceuticals, particularly affecting functional groups such as esters, amides, lactones, lactams, imides, and carbamates. Water acts as both solvent and reactant in these processes, cleaving susceptible bonds to form degradation products with altered activity and potential toxicity.

The rate of hydrolytic degradation depends on several factors, including pH, buffer composition, ionic strength, and solvent system. Many drugs exhibit pH-rate profiles with distinct regions of maximum stability, reflecting the different reactivities of ionized and un-ionized species. For instance, aspirin undergoes hydrolysis catalyzed by both hydrogen ions (specific acid catalysis) and hydroxide ions (specific base catalysis), resulting in a U-shaped pH-rate profile with maximum stability around pH 2.5-3.0. Buffer catalysis occurs when buffer components directly participate in the degradation reaction, beyond their effect on pH maintenance. This phenomenon necessitates careful selection of buffer systems for liquid formulations, particularly for drugs susceptible to general acid or general base catalysis.

Table 3.2: Chemical Kinetics and Stability Parameters

Parameter	Definition	Significance in Pharmacy
Rate Constant (k)	Proportionality constant in rate equation	Quantifies reaction speed
Half-life ($t_{1/2}$)	Time for 50% of drug to degrade	Expiration dating, storage requirements
Shelf-life (t_{90})	Time for 10% of drug to degrade	Product expiration determination
Arrhenius Equation	$k = A \times e^{(-Ea/RT)}$	Predicts temperature effects on degradation
Activation Energy (Ea)	Energy barrier for reaction	Higher Ea means greater stability
Zero-order Kinetics	Rate independent of concentration	Linear degradation over time
First-order Kinetics	Rate proportional to concentration	Exponential degradation over time
Second-order Kinetics	Rate proportional to square of concentration	Less common in drug degradation
pH-rate Profile	Degradation rate vs. pH	Determines optimal pH for stability
Hydrolysis	Degradation by reaction with water	Common in esters, amides
Oxidation	Degradation by reaction with oxygen	Common in unsaturated compounds
Photolysis	Degradation by light exposure	Requires light-protective packaging
Q_{10} Rule	Rate change with 10°C temperature change	Approximate stability predictions
Accelerated Stability	Testing at elevated temperature/humidity	Predicts long-term stability

The total rate of hydrolysis can be expressed as:

$$\text{Rate} = k_0[\text{Drug}] + kH[H^+][\text{Drug}] + kOH[OH^-][\text{Drug}] + kB[\text{Buffer}][\text{Drug}]$$

Where the individual k terms represent rate constants for uncatalyzed, acid-catalyzed, base-catalyzed, and buffer-catalyzed degradation, respectively.

Oxidative and Photolytic Degradation

Oxidative degradation affects drugs containing susceptible functional groups such as phenols, catechols, thiols, polyunsaturated compounds, and certain heterocyclic rings. These reactions typically involve free radical mechanisms initiated by oxygen, peroxides, or metal ion catalysts, and may proceed through complex pathways involving multiple intermediates.

Antioxidants inhibit oxidative degradation by scavenging free radicals (primary antioxidants such as butylated hydroxytoluene) or preventing radical formation (secondary antioxidants such as EDTA, which chelates metal ions). Selection of appropriate antioxidants requires consideration of solubility, pH compatibility, and potential interactions with active ingredients and packaging materials.

Photolytic degradation occurs when drugs absorb light energy, promoting electrons to higher energy states that facilitate chemical reactions not possible in ground states. Compounds containing aromatic rings, conjugated double bonds, carbonyl groups, and nitro groups typically exhibit photosensitivity. Photodegradation often follows complex kinetics influenced by light intensity, wavelength distribution, and the presence of photosensitizers or quenchers.

Protection strategies include amber or opaque containers to block light transmission, coating tablets with light-resistant films, incorporating UV absorbers in formulations, and providing patient instructions regarding proper storage. Packaging design must balance protection against environmental factors with considerations of cost, convenience, and environmental impact.

Stabilization

Solid-state stability generally exceeds that of solutions due to reduced molecular mobility and limited water availability. Consequently, conversion to solid dosage forms represents a primary stabilization strategy for labile compounds. When liquid formulations are necessary, stability optimization may involve pH adjustment to minimize degradation rate, selection of appropriate buffer systems, addition of stabilizing excipients, or use of co-solvent systems to reduce water activity.

Chemical modification of the drug molecule itself sometimes offers a solution to stability challenges. Prodrugs, which convert to active forms *in vivo*, may incorporate protective groups that shield labile functionalities during storage and administration. Similarly, salt or ester formation can enhance stability by modifying susceptibility to hydrolysis or oxidation.

The concept of microenvironmental pH recognizes that the pH experienced by a drug molecule may differ from the bulk pH of a formulation due to interactions with excipients or localized environments within dosage forms. This concept explains why certain excipients exert stabilizing or destabilizing effects beyond their influence on bulk properties, and guides rational selection of formulation components for optimal stability.

DRUG ANALYSIS AND QUALITY CONTROL

Analytical methods in pharmaceutical chemistry ensure the identity, purity, potency, and performance of drug substances and products throughout their lifecycle. These methods range from classical wet chemistry techniques to sophisticated instrumental approaches capable of detecting and quantifying analytes at extremely low concentrations.

Spectroscopic Methods

Ultraviolet-visible (UV-Vis) spectroscopy represents one of the most widely used analytical techniques in pharmaceutical analysis due to its simplicity, speed, and cost-effectiveness. This method exploits the absorption of light by chromophores within drug molecules, with the Beer-Lambert law establishing the linear relationship between absorbance and concentration:

$$A = \varepsilon bc$$

Where A is absorbance, ε is the molar absorptivity, b is the path length, and c is the concentration. While simple in principle, practical applications must address potential interferences from excipients, degradation products, or other components in complex matrices.

Table 3.3: Common Drug Analysis Methods

Analytical Method	Applications	Advantages	Limitations
UV-Visible Spectroscopy	Quantitative analysis, dissolution testing	Simple, inexpensive, rapid	Limited specificity, interferences
HPLC	Assay, impurity testing, stability studies	High resolution, sensitivity, versatility	Expensive equipment, method development

Analytical Method	Applications	Advantages	Limitations
UPLC	Same as HPLC with faster analysis	Faster, higher resolution than HPLC	Very high pressure requirements
Mass Spectrometry	Structure elucidation, impurity identification	Highly specific, sensitive	Expensive, complex interpretation
IR Spectroscopy	Identity testing, polymorphism	Structural information, fingerprinting	Limited quantitative applications
NMR Spectroscopy	Structure elucidation, purity	Detailed structural information	Expensive, limited sensitivity
TLC	Identity, purity, stability	Simple, inexpensive, visual	Limited resolution, semi-quantitative
GC	Residual solvents, volatile impurities	High efficiency, sensitivity	Limited to volatile compounds
Karl Fischer Titration	Moisture content analysis	Specific for water, accurate	Interferences possible
Polarimetry	Chiral purity, concentration	Simple, specific for chirality	Limited application range
DSC/Thermal Analysis	Polymorphism, purity, compatibility	Physical state information	Indirect measurement
X-ray Diffraction	Polymorphism, crystal properties	Definitive for crystal structure	Requires crystalline material
Dissolution Testing	Bioavailability prediction	*In vitro-in vivo* correlation	Variable correlation to bioavailability
Potentiometry	pH, ion-selective analysis	Simple, continuous monitoring	Limited to ionic species

Infrared (IR) spectroscopy provides structural information based on the absorption of infrared radiation by covalent bonds, causing vibrational excitation. The resulting IR spectrum serves as a molecular fingerprint useful for identity confirmation, polymorphism detection, and compatibility assessment. Fourier transform infrared spectroscopy (FTIR) offers advantages in resolution and signal-to-noise ratio compared to traditional dispersive instruments, while attenuated total reflectance (ATR) accessories facilitate analysis of diverse sample types without extensive preparation.

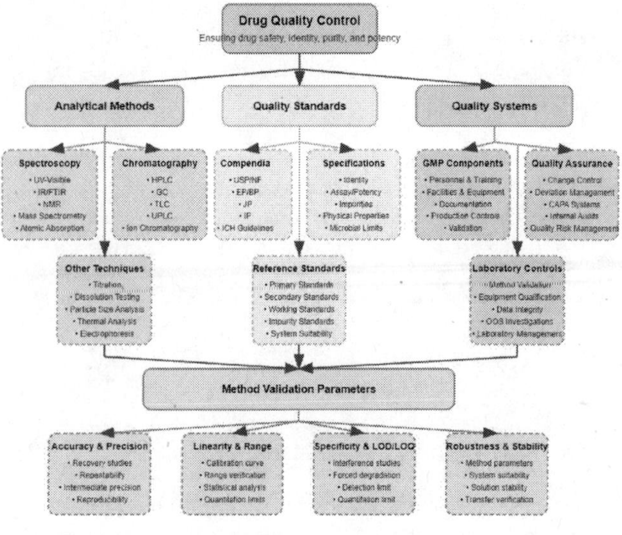

Figure 3.3: Drug Analysis and Quality Control Framework

Nuclear magnetic resonance (NMR) spectroscopy exploits the magnetic properties of certain atomic nuclei (particularly ^1H and ^{13}C) to provide detailed structural information about organic molecules. This technique reveals the electronic environment surrounding specific nuclei, enabling determination of molecular structure, confirmation of synthetic pathways, identification of impurities, and analysis of complex mixtures. Quantitative NMR (qNMR) offers advantages for purity determination, as signal intensity directly relates to the number of nuclei contributing to the signal, obviating the need for reference standards of identical chemical composition.

Mass spectrometry (MS) provides information about molecular weight and structural fragments, facilitating identification of unknown compounds and detection of trace impurities. Modern MS techniques coupled with chromatographic separation methods (LC-MS, GC-MS) enable sensitive and specific analysis of complex pharmaceutical mixtures. High-resolution MS distinguishes compounds with very similar molecular weights, while tandem MS (MS/MS) provides structural information through controlled fragmentation of selected ions.

Chromatographic Techniques

High-performance liquid chromatography (HPLC) stands as the cornerstone of pharmaceutical analysis, offering versatility for diverse compounds and matrices. This technique separates mixture components based on their differential distribution between a stationary phase (typically bonded silica) and a mobile phase (liquid). Detection methods include UV-Vis absorption, fluorescence, electrochemical detection, and mass spectrometry, each offering different sensitivity and selectivity profiles.

Reversed-phase HPLC, employing non-polar stationary phases and polar mobile phases, predominates in pharmaceutical analysis due to its broad applicability and robustness. Method development involves optimization of mobile phase composition, pH, temperature, and flow rate to achieve adequate resolution of all components of interest. Validation parameters include specificity, linearity, range, accuracy, precision, detection limit, quantitation limit, and robustness, ensuring method reliability for intended applications.

Gas chromatography (GC) provides exceptional separation efficiency for volatile compounds, making it particularly valuable for analysis of residual solvents, volatile impurities, and certain drug substances. This technique separates components based on their vapor pressure and interaction with the stationary phase, typically requiring derivatization for compounds with poor volatility or thermal stability. Detector options include flame ionization detection (FID), electron capture detection (ECD), and mass spectrometry, each offering different sensitivity and selectivity characteristics.

Thin-layer chromatography (TLC) continues to serve important roles in pharmaceutical analysis despite technological advances in other techniques. Its advantages include simplicity, low cost, minimal sample preparation, and ability to analyze multiple samples simultaneously. Modern high-performance TLC (HPTLC) with densitometric scanning provides quantitative capabilities approaching those of HPLC for many applications, while requiring less sample and generating less waste.

Table 3.4: Quality Control Parameters and Specifications

Test Parameter	Purpose	Typical Specification	Method
Assay	Active ingredient content	90.0-110.0% of label claim	HPLC, UV spectroscopy
Dissolution	Drug release rate	Q = 75-80% in specified time	USP apparatus, HPLC
Disintegration	Tablet/capsule breakdown	Complete in specified time	USP disintegration tester
Impurities	Related substances	Individual: ≤0.2%, Total: ≤1.0%	HPLC, TLC
Residual Solvents	Organic volatile impurities	Class-dependent limits	GC, headspace GC
Water Content	Moisture determination	Product-specific limits	Karl Fischer titration
Microbial Limits	Bioburden assessment	Total count limits, absence of pathogens	USP microbial tests
Sterility	Absence of microorganisms	No growth observed	USP sterility test
Bacterial Endotoxins	Pyrogen testing	≤5 EU/kg body weight	LAL test
Particulate Matter	Visible/subvisible particles	Size and count limits	Light obscuration, microscopy
pH	Hydrogen ion concentration	Product-specific range	pH meter
Weight Variation	Dosage unit consistency	±5-10% from average weight	Analytical balance
Hardness	Tablet crushing strength	Product-specific target	Hardness tester
Friability	Tablet resistance to abrasion	≤1.0% weight loss	Friability tester

Pharmacopoeial Standards and Specifications

Pharmacopoeias establish legally enforceable standards for pharmaceutical substances and products, including specifications for identity, purity, strength, and performance. These compendiums describe standardized analytical methods and acceptance criteria that ensure consistent quality across manufacturers and jurisdictions. Major pharmacopoeias include the United States Pharmacopeia-National Formulary (USP-NF), European Pharmacopoeia (Ph. Eur.), British Pharmacopoeia (BP), and Japanese Pharmacopoeia (JP), with ongoing harmonization efforts reducing discrepancies among these standards.

The International Council for Harmonisation of Technical Requirements for Pharmaceuticals for Human Use (ICH) develops guidelines that complement pharmacopoeial standards, addressing aspects of pharmaceutical quality such as impurity control, stability testing, and analytical method validation. These guidelines establish a scientific basis for regulatory expectations and promote consistency in pharmaceutical development and quality control across regions.

Specifications for drug substances typically include tests for appearance, identification, assay, impurities, water content, residual solvents, and physical properties such as particle size or polymorphic form. Drug product specifications extend these requirements to include content uniformity, dissolution or disintegration, microbial limits, and dosage form-specific tests. Acceptance criteria balance feasibility of manufacturing with clinical requirements for safety and efficacy.

Stability-Indicating Methods

Stability-indicating methods specifically detect and quantify degradation products that may form during storage or use, providing a reliable measure of drug substance or product stability. Development of these methods typically involves forced degradation studies that deliberately stress samples under conditions of heat, humidity, oxidation, photolysis, and extreme pH to generate degradation products that might form during normal shelf life.

Method specificity represents the most critical attribute of stability-indicating assays, requiring demonstration that degradation products, excipients, and impurities do not interfere with quantification of the active ingredient. This typically necessitates high-resolution chromatographic techniques with optimized separation conditions to resolve all potential interfering species. The method must also demonstrate linearity, accuracy, precision, and robustness across the expected range of degradation.

Mass balance considerations require that the sum of the active ingredient and all degradation products should approximate the initial drug concentration, accounting for analytical variability. Significant deviations from mass balance may indicate formation of undetected degradation products, necessitating further method development or additional detection techniques such as MS to capture all degradation pathways.

PHARMACEUTICAL SALT FORMS

Salt formation represents one of the most common and effective strategies for modifying the physicochemical properties of ionizable drug molecules. Approximately half of all drugs used clinically are administered as salts, reflecting the significant advantages this approach offers for improving solubility, dissolution rate, stability, and manufacturability.

Principles of Salt Formation

Salt formation involves the interaction of acidic or basic drugs with suitable counterions to form ionic compounds. Acidic drugs (containing carboxylic acid, phenolic, or other acidic functional groups) typically form salts with basic counterions such as sodium, potassium, calcium, or organic bases like ethanolamines. Basic drugs (containing amine or other basic functionalities) form salts with acidic counterions such as hydrochloride, sulfate, maleate, or fumarate.

The feasibility of salt formation depends on the relative strength of the acid and base involved, typically requiring a difference of at least 2-3 units between the pKa of the drug and the pKa of the counterion. This principle, known as the "rule of three," predicts that stable salt formation occurs when:

- For acidic drugs: pKa (drug) < pKa (counterion) - 3
- For basic drugs: pKa (drug) > pKa (counterion) + 3

Salt formation significantly alters the physicochemical properties of the parent compound, particularly its solubility profile across different pH environments. The pH-solubility behavior of drug salts can be predicted using the Henderson-Hasselbalch relationship, with consideration of the salt's solubility product. The pH of maximum solubility typically occurs at values where the drug exists primarily in its ionized form.

Selection of Appropriate Salt Forms

Salt selection involves consideration of multiple factors including solubility enhancement, stability, hygroscopicity, melting point, crystallinity, and compatibility with intended formulation components. No single counterion proves optimal for all drugs or all purposes, necessitating systematic evaluation of multiple salt forms during pharmaceutical development.

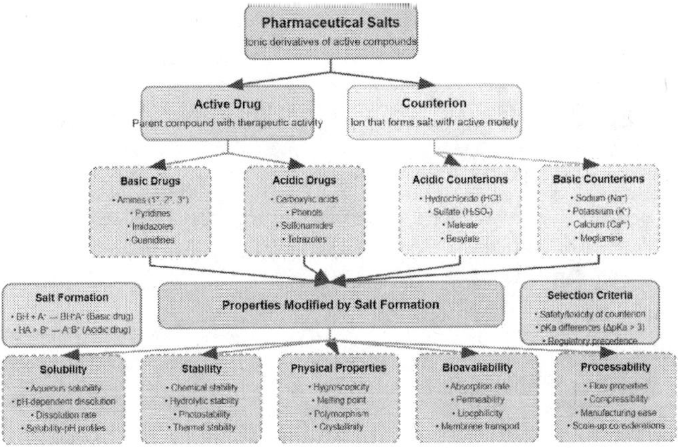

Figure 3.4: Pharmaceutical Salt Forms and their Properties

Solubility and dissolution rate often represent primary considerations in salt selection, particularly for poorly water-soluble drugs with dissolution-limited bioavailability. Different counterions can produce dramatically different solubility profiles; for example, hydrochloride salts typically exhibit higher aqueous solubility than free bases but may show reduced solubility in gastric fluid due to the common ion effect.

Solid-state properties significantly influence manufacturing processes and product performance. High melting point salts generally exhibit better chemical stability but may present challenges for thermal processing methods. Crystallinity affects physical stability, with highly crystalline salts typically showing reduced hygroscopicity and better stability under stress conditions compared to amorphous forms.

Regulatory considerations influence salt selection decisions, with preference often given to counterions with established safety profiles and regulatory precedent. The FDA's GRAS (Generally Recognized As Safe) list includes commonly used counterions with acceptable safety profiles, simplifying the regulatory pathway for salts incorporating these species.

Physicochemical Characterization of Salt Forms

Comprehensive characterization of pharmaceutical salts requires multiple analytical approaches addressing different aspects of their physical and chemical properties. X-ray diffraction techniques provide definitive evidence of salt formation and crystalline structure, distinguishing true salts from co-crystals, polymorphs, or amorphous dispersions with similar macroscopic properties.

Table 3.5: Pharmaceutical Salt Forms and Their Properties

Salt Form	Parent Drug Example	Solubility
Hydrochloride	Diphenhydramine HCl	High in water, low in alcohols
Sodium	Naproxen sodium	Very high water solubility
Potassium	Penicillin K	High water solubility
Calcium	Alendronate calcium	Moderate water solubility
Sulfate	Morphine sulfate	Good water solubility
Mesylate	Deferoxamine mesylate	Very high water solubility
Besylate	Amlodipine besylate	High water solubility
Tosylate	Tamsulosin tosylate	Moderate water solubility
Maleate	Brompheniramine maleate	Good water solubility
Tartrate	Metoprolol tartrate	High water solubility
Citrate	Sildenafil citrate	Moderate water solubility
Acetate	Fludrocortisone acetate	Moderate water solubility
Phosphate	Dexamethasone phosphate	Very high water solubility
Fumarate	Quetiapine fumarate	Moderate water solubility

Thermal analysis methods, including differential scanning calorimetry (DSC) and thermogravimetric analysis (TGA), characterize melting behavior, phase transitions, desolvation processes, and thermal stability. These techniques help identify hydrates, solvates, and metastable forms that might influence product performance or stability during processing or storage.

Hygroscopicity—the tendency to absorb atmospheric moisture—significantly affects the physical stability and processing characteristics of pharmaceutical salts. Dynamic vapor sorption (DVS) quantifies moisture uptake across different relative humidity conditions, enabling prediction of behavior during manufacturing and storage. Highly hygroscopic salts may require specialized processing techniques, protective packaging, or conversion to alternate salt forms.

Dissolution testing under biorelevant conditions provides insight into the likely *in vivo* performance of different salt forms. These tests employ media simulating gastric and intestinal fluids, incorporating physiologically relevant pH values, buffer capacities, and surfactant concentrations to predict dissolution behavior in the gastrointestinal tract.

Pharmaceutical Applications of Different Salt Forms

Hydrochloride salts represent the most commonly employed salt form for basic drugs, offering advantages including high aqueous solubility, good stability, and established safety profile. However, these salts sometimes exhibit disadvantages including hygroscopicity, reduced solubility in gastric fluid due to the common ion effect, and potential for corrosion of processing equipment.

Sulfate salts typically exhibit good chemical stability and lower hygroscopicity compared to hydrochlorides, making them valuable alternatives when moisture sensitivity presents concerns. Their higher molecular weight results in lower drug content per unit weight, potentially necessitating larger dosage forms for high-dose medications.

Organic acid salts, including citrates, tartrates, fumarates, and maleates, offer diverse physicochemical properties addressing specific formulation challenges. These counterions generally demonstrate good compatibility with common excipients and may provide advantages for taste masking or controlled release applications. However, some organic acid salts exhibit limited aqueous solubility or chemical stability issues requiring careful evaluation during development.

Sodium and potassium salts of acidic drugs typically provide excellent aqueous solubility and often serve as bases for injectable formulations. Their rapid dissolution can achieve high plasma concentrations quickly, benefiting situations requiring fast onset of action. However, these salts often exhibit hygroscopicity and may undergo chemical degradation more readily than the corresponding free acids.

Salt disproportionation—the conversion of a salt to its free acid or base form during processing or storage—represents a significant concern for pharmaceutical development. This phenomenon occurs when environmental conditions (pH, humidity, excipient interactions) favor the non-ionized form, potentially altering dissolution, bioavailability, or stability characteristics. Understanding the factors influencing disproportionation enables formulation strategies to maintain salt integrity throughout the product lifecycle

Summary

Pharmaceutical chemistry connects molecular structure to therapeutic function through fundamental relationships between drug properties and clinical effects. Structural elements including functional groups, stereochemistry, and molecular configuration directly influence receptor binding, absorption characteristics, and metabolic pathways. Understanding atomic arrangement provides insights into structure-activity relationships that drive drug development and modification for enhanced efficacy or reduced toxicity. Chemical kinetics principles govern drug stability considerations, quantifying degradation rates through zero-order, first-order, and second-order reactions while identifying pathways including hydrolysis, oxidation, photolysis, and racemization that compromise medication integrity. These stability factors inform proper storage conditions, packaging requirements, and expiration dating to maintain potency throughout the product lifecycle. Quality control methodologies employ analytical techniques including high-performance liquid chromatography, mass spectrometry, ultraviolet spectroscopy, and infrared analysis to verify identity, purity, potency, and dissolution characteristics according to established pharmacopeial standards. Salt forms represent a critical formulation strategy, where selection of appropriate counter-ions modifies solubility, dissolution rate, stability, and bioavailability of active pharmaceutical ingredients. Common modifications include hydrochloride, sulfate, sodium, and mesylate forms, each offering distinct advantages for specific administration routes and therapeutic applications. These pharmaceutical chemistry principles provide the scientific foundation for understanding medication behavior in biological systems, formulation considerations for optimal delivery, and quality assurance measures ensuring consistent therapeutic performance throughout the medication use process.

Multiple Choice Questions

1. Which of the following functional groups is most likely to increase the water solubility of a drug molecule?
   a) Methyl group
   b) Halogen (F, Cl, Br)
   c) Carboxylic acid
   d) Benzene ring
2. The process by which a racemic mixture is separated into its individual enantiomers is called:
   a) Recrystallization
   b) Resolution
   c) Racemization
   d) Distillation
3. Which of the following statements about stereoisomers is correct?
   a) Enantiomers always have identical pharmacological activity
   b) Diastereomers have identical physical properties
   c) Enantiomers rotate plane-polarized light in equal but opposite directions
   d) Meso compounds contain multiple chiral centers but are optically inactive
4. A drug follows first-order degradation kinetics. If 20% of the drug degrades in 6 months, approximately what percentage will remain after 18 months?
   a) 40%
   b) 60%
   c) 51.2%
   d) 48.8%
5. Which analytical technique separates compounds based on their differential partitioning between a stationary phase and a mobile phase?
   a) Mass spectrometry
   b) Nuclear magnetic resonance
   c) High-performance liquid chromatography
   d) Infrared spectroscopy
6. The pKa of a weak acid drug is 5.5. At which pH would this drug be approximately 50% ionized?
   a) 2.5
   b) 5.5

c) 7.4
d) 8.5

7. Converting a drug into its salt form typically affects which of the following properties?
   a) Pharmacological activity at the receptor level
   b) Metabolic pathway
   c) Solubility and dissolution rate
   d) Molecular weight of the active moiety
8. Which degradation pathway would most likely affect a drug containing an ester functional group?
   a) Oxidation
   b) Hydrolysis
   c) Racemization
   d) Photolysis
9. In drug development, which modification to a lead compound might increase its lipophilicity?
   a) Adding a hydroxyl group
   b) Adding a carboxylic acid group
   c) Replacing a hydrogen with a methyl group
   d) Converting to a quaternary ammonium salt
10. Which technique would be most appropriate for determining the molecular weight of a newly synthesized drug compound?
    a) Thin-layer chromatography
    b) Mass spectrometry
    c) UV-visible spectroscopy
    d) Melting point determination

Self-Assessment Questions

1. Analyze how modifications to functional groups in a benzodiazepine molecule might affect its lipophilicity, receptor binding affinity, and metabolism, providing specific examples of structural changes and their predicted pharmacological consequences.
2. Describe the relationship between stereochemistry and drug action, explaining how enantiomers can exhibit different pharmacological properties and providing examples of medications where stereoisomerism significantly impacts safety or efficacy.
3. Explain the principles of structure-activity relationships in drug development, describing how systematic modifications to a lead compound can optimize therapeutic properties while minimizing undesirable effects.
4. Analyze the chemical factors affecting drug stability, explaining how pH, temperature, light exposure, and oxidation influence degradation rates and describing specific protective measures for sensitive medications.
5. Compare and contrast zero-order, first-order, and second-order reaction kinetics in pharmaceutical degradation, explaining how each affects shelf-life determination and providing examples of drugs following each kinetic pattern.
6. Describe the specific chemical degradation pathways (hydrolysis, oxidation, photolysis, racemization) that commonly affect medications, identifying structural features that increase vulnerability to each pathway and appropriate stabilization strategies.
7. Analyze the principles and applications of high-performance liquid chromatography (HPLC) in pharmaceutical analysis, explaining how this technique separates and quantifies drug substances and impurities based on their chemical properties.
8. Explain how spectroscopic techniques are used to identify pharmaceutical compounds, describing the specific molecular information provided by each method.
9. Describe the chemical rationale for developing pharmaceutical salt forms, explaining how ionization state affects solubility, dissolution rate, stability, and bioavailability of active pharmaceutical ingredients.
10. Analyze the chemical properties and therapeutic implications of different salt forms (hydrochloride, maleate, sodium, besylate) of the same active drug, explaining how salt selection might be optimized for specific administration routes or patient populations

Bibliography

1. Patrick GL. An introduction to medicinal chemistry. 6th ed. Oxford: Oxford University Press; 2017.
2. Baertschi SW, Alsante KM, Reed RA. Pharmaceutical stress testing: Predicting drug degradation. 2nd ed. London: Informa Healthcare; 2011.
3. Yoshioka S, Stella VJ. Stability of drugs and dosage forms. New York: Kluwer Academic/Plenum Publishers; 2000.
4. Berge SM, Bighley LD, Monkhouse DC. Pharmaceutical salts. J Pharm Sci. 1977;66(1):1-19.
5. Wermuth CG, Aldous D, Raboisson P, Rognan D. The practice of medicinal chemistry. 4th ed. Amsterdam: Elsevier/Academic Press; 2015.
6. Ahuja S, Scypinski S. Handbook of modern pharmaceutical analysis. 2nd ed. Amsterdam: Elsevier Academic Press; 2010.
7. Alsante KM, Ando A, Brown R, Ensing J, Hatajik TD, Kong W, et al. The role of degradant profiling in active pharmaceutical ingredients and drug products. Adv Drug Deliv Rev. 2007;59(1):29-37.
8. Serajuddin AT. Salt formation to improve drug solubility. Adv Drug Deliv Rev. 2007;59(7):603-616.
9. Qiu Y, Chen Y, Zhang GGZ, Liu L, Porter W. Developing solid oral dosage forms: Pharmaceutical theory and practice. 2nd ed. Amsterdam: Academic Press; 2016.
10. Baboota S, Agarwal SP. Formulation of sustained release diltiazem hydrochloride tablets using different viscosity grades of HPMC and its *in vitro* release characteristics. Curr Drug Deliv. 2006;3(4):429-434.

CHAPTER 4

PHARMACEUTICS AND DRUG DELIVERY

Author

Mr. Mushraff Ali Khan M, Associate Professor,
Department of Pharmaceutics, Sultan-ul-Uloom College of Pharmacy, Banjara Hills, Hyderabad, Telangana, India

Abstract

Pharmaceutics converts an active pharmaceutical ingredient into effective dosage forms through scientific principles of drug delivery. Dosage form design balances pharmacological requirements with patient factors, creating solid forms (tablets, capsules), liquid preparations, semisolids, and specialized delivery systems, each requiring specific formulation approaches addressing stability, release kinetics, and manufacturing scalability. Drug absorption mechanisms determine therapeutic effectiveness through complex processes influenced by physicochemical properties, physiological variables, and formulation factors, with bioavailability measures quantifying the fraction of administered drug reaching systemic circulation. Novel drug delivery systems extend beyond conventional formulations to provide targeted delivery, controlled release, and enhanced stability through liposomal encapsulation, nanoparticle carriers, transdermal patches, implantable systems, and 3D-printed medications tailored to individual patient needs. Pharmaceutical excipients serve essential functions beyond merely completing formulations, acting as diluents, binders, disintegrants, lubricants, coating materials, preservatives, and solubilizers, with careful selection required to ensure compatibility, stability, and proper drug release while avoiding potential allergic reactions or interactions.

Keywords: *Formulation; Drug Release; Delivery Systems; Physicochemical Properties; Product Development*

Learning Objectives

After completion of the chapter, the learners should be able to:

- Classify dosage forms based on physical state, route of administration, and release characteristics.
- Analyze factors affecting drug dissolution, absorption, and bioavailability across different physiological barriers.
- Compare controlled-release technologies including matrix systems, reservoir devices, and osmotic pump mechanisms.
- Select appropriate excipients for specific formulations based on their functional properties and compatibility with active ingredients.
- Evaluate novel drug delivery approaches including nanoparticles, liposomes, and targeted delivery systems for specific therapeutic applications.
- Design appropriate beyond-use dating for compounded preparations based on stability considerations and USP guidelines.

DOSAGE FORM DESIGN

Dosage form design involves the systematic development of drug delivery systems that optimize therapeutic outcomes while addressing patient needs, manufacturing considerations, and commercial viability. This multidisciplinary process integrates pharmaceutical science with engineering principles to create formulations that deliver medications effectively, safely, and conveniently.

The rational design of dosage forms begins with preformulation studies that characterize the physicochemical properties of the active pharmaceutical ingredient (API). These properties—including solubility, partition coefficient, pKa, crystal structure, particle size, and stability profile—establish constraints and opportunities that guide formulation decisions. For instance, a drug with poor aqueous solubility might benefit from particle size reduction, amorphization, or incorporation into lipid-based delivery systems, while a moisture-sensitive compound might require protective coating or packaging strategies.

Patient-centered considerations significantly influence dosage form selection and design. The target patient population's characteristics—including age, comorbidities, dexterity limitations, and medication adherence challenges—inform decisions regarding route of administration, dosage form size, taste characteristics, and ease of use. Pediatric formulations, for example, often prioritize taste masking, flexible dosing options, and age-appropriate administration routes, while geriatric formulations might emphasize ease of swallowing, simplified dosing regimens, and packaging that accommodates limited dexterity.

Table 4.1: Common Dosage Forms and Their Characteristics

Dosage Form	Onset of Action	Advantages	Disadvantages
Tablets	30-60 minutes	Convenience, stability, accurate dosing	First-pass effect, GI irritation
Capsules	30-60 minutes	Taste masking, easy to swallow	Manufacturing complexity
Solutions	15-30 minutes	Rapid absorption, easy administration	Stability issues, taste concerns
Suspensions	15-30 minutes	Taste masking, insoluble drugs	Sedimentation, shaking required
Immediate-release	30-60 minutes	Rapid effect, simple formulation	Short duration, frequent dosing
Extended-release	1-2 hours	Reduced dosing frequency, steady levels	Complex formulation, higher cost
Delayed-release	Variable	Targeted release, protect from acid	Manufacturing complexity
Injections	Seconds to minutes	Rapid effect, high bioavailability	Pain, sterility requirements
Inhalers	5-15 minutes	Direct to target, reduced systemic effects	Technique-dependent, local irritation

Dosage Form	Onset of Action	Advantages	Disadvantages
Transdermal	Hours	Extended delivery, avoids first-pass	Skin irritation, limited applicability
Suppositories	15-30 minutes	Avoids first-pass, useful when NPO	Patient acceptance, melting concerns
Creams	Variable	Easy application, moisturizing	Greasy feel, limited penetration
Ointments	Variable	Occlusive, enhanced penetration	Greasy, staining potential
Gels	Variable	Less greasy, transparent	Drying effect, stinging potential
Patches	Hours	Controlled release, convenience	Adhesion issues, skin irritation
Lozenges	15-30 minutes	Local effect, slow dissolution	Limited to certain drugs
Implants	Days to months	Extended release, adherence	Surgical procedure, removal concerns

Solid Oral Dosage Forms

Tablets remain the most widely used pharmaceutical dosage form due to their manufacturing efficiency, dosing precision, stability advantages, and patient acceptance. Tablet design involves selection and optimization of multiple components: active ingredients, diluents, binders, disintegrants, lubricants, glidants, and potentially coating materials. Each component serves specific functions that collectively determine the tablet's physical integrity, disintegration profile, dissolution characteristics, and ultimately its *in vivo* performance.

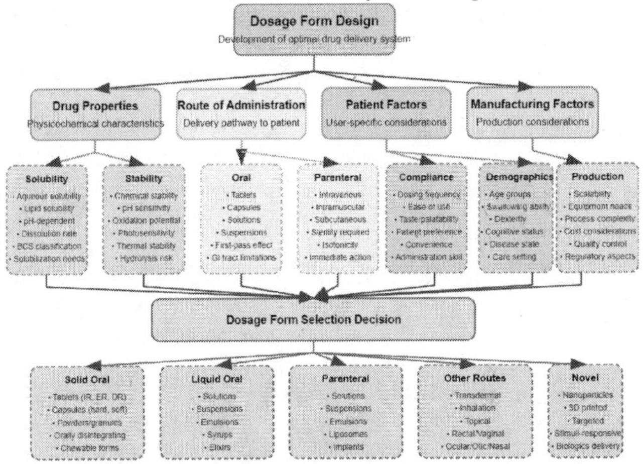

Figure 4.1: Dosage Form Design Decision

Direct compression represents the simplest and most economical tablet manufacturing method, suitable for stable, freely flowing materials with good compressibility. This approach involves simple blending of ingredients followed by compression, avoiding the complexity and potential stability challenges associated with wet processes. However, many APIs lack the flow and compression properties necessary for direct compression, necessitating alternative approaches.

Wet granulation improves the flow and compression characteristics of powder blends by creating larger agglomerates with more uniform composition. This process involves mixing the API with excipients, adding a granulating liquid to form a moist mass, wet-milling or screening to achieve uniform granule size, drying to remove the granulating liquid, and finally dry-milling to optimize granule size distribution. While more complex than direct compression, wet granulation accommodates a wider range of drug properties and often produces tablets with superior content uniformity.

Dry granulation provides an intermediate option for moisture-sensitive materials, using mechanical pressure rather than liquid to create granules. Roller compaction, the most common dry granulation method, compresses powder blends between counter-rotating rollers to form dense sheets (ribbons) that are subsequently milled into granules. This approach improves flow properties and content uniformity without exposure to moisture or heat, though typically producing granules with lower binding capacity than wet granulation methods.

Capsules provide an alternative solid oral dosage form, particularly valuable for drugs with poor compression properties or requirements for rapid dissolution. Hard gelatin capsules accommodate powder blends or granules, while soft gelatin capsules typically contain liquid or semi-solid formulations that enhance solubility and dissolution of poorly water-soluble compounds. Both capsule types offer advantages including taste masking, reduced irritant contact with oral mucosa, and distinctive appearance that aids product identification.

Liquid Dosage Forms

Solutions represent the simplest liquid dosage forms, with the drug completely dissolved in a suitable solvent system. These formulations offer rapid drug availability and dosing flexibility but often present stability challenges and may require inclusion of preservatives, antioxidants, buffers, or other functional excipients. The selection of solvent systems balances considerations of drug solubility, stability, palatability, and toxicity, often necessitating co-solvent mixtures to achieve optimal performance.

Suspensions contain finely divided solid drug particles dispersed in a liquid vehicle, providing options for drugs with limited solubility or stability in solution. The physical stability of suspensions depends on particle size control, viscosity adjustment, and incorporation of surfactants or polymers that modify particle-particle interactions. Structured vehicles containing thixotropic agents help prevent sedimentation during storage while allowing flow during administration, improving dose uniformity and patient acceptability.

Emulsions consist of two immiscible liquids, with one dispersed as droplets within the other, stabilized by emulsifying agents. Oil-in-water (o/w) emulsions typically offer better palatability and can be diluted with aqueous fluids, while water-in-oil (w/o) emulsions provide prolonged contact with absorption surfaces and protection for water-sensitive compounds. Microemulsions and self-emulsifying drug delivery systems (SEDDS) represent advanced approaches that enhance bioavailability of poorly water-soluble drugs through formation of small droplets with high surface area and solubilization capacity.

Parenteral solutions and suspensions require exceptional quality standards due to their administration routes that bypass natural protective barriers. These formulations must meet requirements for sterility, endotoxin limits, particulate matter control, and compatibility with body tissues and fluids. Tonicity adjustment prevents tissue damage from osmotic effects, while pH adjustment optimizes stability and minimizes injection pain. Selection of appropriate preservatives for multi-dose formulations requires careful balance between antimicrobial efficacy and tissue compatibility.

Semi-solid Dosage Forms

Ointments provide occlusive, water-repellent vehicles for topical drug delivery, based on hydrocarbon (oleaginous), absorption, water-removable, or water-soluble bases. These formulations prolong drug contact with application sites and enhance permeation of lipophilic compounds through the stratum corneum. The rheological properties of ointments significantly influence their spreading characteristics, retention at application sites, and patient acceptance.

Creams represent emulsified systems for topical application, with oil-in-water (hydrophilic) or water-in-oil (hydrophobic) structures offering different cosmetic and functional properties. Hydrophilic creams typically provide better acceptability due to their non-greasy feel and washability, while hydrophobic creams offer greater occlusion and water resistance. The selection between these types depends on drug solubility characteristics, required depth of penetration, and application site considerations.

Gels consist of liquid phases within three-dimensional polymeric networks that provide structural integrity. Hydrogels incorporate water within hydrophilic polymer matrices, creating elegant formulations with cooling effects upon application. Organogels utilize non-aqueous solvents within their structures, often providing enhanced permeation for lipophilic drugs. Both gel types offer advantages of transparency, ease of application, and non-occlusive properties that support various therapeutic applications.

Transdermal delivery systems extend the principles of topical formulations to achieve systemic drug effects through controlled skin permeation. These systems typically combine drug reservoirs with rate-controlling membranes or matrix structures that modulate release over extended periods. Adhesive properties ensure consistent skin contact, while permeation enhancers may overcome the barrier function of the stratum corneum for drugs with suboptimal skin penetration characteristics.

Modified Release Dosage Forms

Extended-release formulations maintain therapeutic drug concentrations over prolonged periods, reducing dosing frequency and fluctuations in drug levels. Matrix systems embed drugs within polymeric structures that control release through diffusion, erosion, or combined mechanisms. Hydrophilic matrices (e.g., HPMC, sodium alginate) form gel layers upon hydration, creating diffusion barriers that retard drug release, while hydrophobic matrices (e.g., waxes, insoluble polymers) release drugs primarily through erosion or pore diffusion pathways.

Reservoir systems encapsulate drug cores within rate-controlling membranes that determine release kinetics through permeability characteristics. These systems can achieve near-zero-order release profiles independent of drug concentration and provide robust control over release rates. However, membrane defects present risks of dose dumping, necessitating rigorous quality control during manufacturing.

Delayed-release formulations target drug release to specific regions of the gastrointestinal tract by incorporating pH-dependent polymers that remain intact in gastric acid but dissolve at higher pH environments of the intestine. Enteric coatings protect acid-labile drugs from degradation, reduce gastric irritation from aggressive compounds, or target release to intestinal sites for local action or improved absorption. Common enteric polymers include cellulose acetate phthalate, methacrylic acid copolymers, and hydroxypropyl methylcellulose phthalate, each offering different dissolution profiles across pH ranges.

Pulsatile delivery systems provide programmed release after specific lag times, mimicking circadian rhythms or targeting drug delivery to coincide with symptom manifestation. These sophisticated formulations utilize approaches such as rupturable coatings, erodible plugs, or osmotic mechanisms to achieve precisely timed release independent of physiological variables. Chronotherapeutic applications include management of early morning symptoms in conditions like rheumatoid arthritis or asthma, where anticipatory dosing enhances therapeutic outcomes.

DRUG ABSORPTION AND BIOAVAILABILITY

Drug absorption represents the process by which medications enter the systemic circulation from administration sites, while bioavailability quantifies the rate and extent of active drug reaching the circulation. These parameters fundamentally determine the onset, intensity, and duration of therapeutic effects, linking dosage form performance to clinical outcomes.

Absorption Mechanisms and Barriers

Passive diffusion constitutes the predominant absorption mechanism for most drugs, driven by concentration gradients across biological membranes. This process follows Fick's first law, where flux is proportional to concentration gradient, diffusion coefficient, membrane surface area, and inversely proportional to membrane thickness. Lipophilic compounds typically traverse cell membranes directly through the lipid bilayer, while small hydrophilic molecules may utilize paracellular pathways between adjacent cells, limited by tight junction restrictions.

Carrier-mediated transport involves specialized membrane proteins that facilitate movement of specific substances across biological barriers. Active transport systems require energy expenditure to move substances against concentration gradients, while facilitated diffusion accelerates movement along existing gradients without direct energy input. These transport systems demonstrate substrate specificity, saturation kinetics, and potential for competitive or non-competitive inhibition by structurally related compounds, creating opportunities for drug-drug interactions.

Vesicular transport mechanisms, including endocytosis and transcytosis, enable absorption of macromolecular drugs or particulate delivery systems. Receptor-mediated endocytosis offers particularly promising approaches for targeted delivery by exploiting specific cellular receptors that trigger internalization. These mechanisms circumvent traditional permeability limitations but generally provide lower absorption efficiency than passive diffusion for small molecules.

The gastrointestinal tract presents multiple barriers to oral drug absorption. The mucus layer, though protective against harmful substances, may trap or bind certain drugs, reducing their access to absorption surfaces. Epithelial cell monolayers with tight junctions restrict paracellular passage, while enzymatic activity within the intestinal lumen and enterocytes may degrade susceptible compounds before they reach the circulation. Additionally, efflux transporters such as P-glycoprotein actively pump certain drugs back into the intestinal lumen, reducing their net absorption.

Table 4.2: Factors Affecting Drug Absorption and Bioavailability

Factor	Effect on Absorption/Bioavailability	Example
Solubility	↑ solubility → ↑ dissolution → ↑ absorption	Griseofulvin absorption ↑ with fatty meal
Particle Size	↓ particle size → ↑ surface area → ↑ dissolution	Micronized griseofulvin has better absorption
pKa	Affects ionization, unionized forms better absorbed	Weak acids absorb better in stomach
Lipophilicity	↑ lipophilicity → ↑ membrane permeation	Benzodiazepines cross BBB readily
Salt Form	Different salts have different dissolution rates	Diclofenac sodium dissolves faster than potassium

Crystal Form	Polymorphs have different solubility	Form I of chloramphenicol palmitate isn't absorbed
First-pass Metabolism	Reduces bioavailability of orally administered drugs	Propranolol has only 30% bioavailability
GI Transit Time	↑ transit time → variable absorption	Metoclopramide accelerates transit, reducing absorption
Food Effects	Can increase/decrease/delay absorption	Tetracycline absorption decreased by calcium in food
Disease States	Alter GI physiology affecting absorption	Crohn's disease reduces absorption area
Age	Affects GI physiology and organ function	Elderly have reduced first-pass metabolism
Gastric pH	Affects drug ionization and dissolution	PPIs reduce absorption of weak bases
Gastric Emptying	Delays absorption of drugs absorbed in intestine	Opioids slow gastric emptying
Intestinal Efflux	P-gp pumps drugs back into intestinal lumen	Cyclosporine absorption limited by P-gp
Drug Formulation	Controlled release alters absorption profile	ER formulations provide slower, sustained absorption
Drug Interactions	Competition for absorption or metabolism	Calcium reduces tetracycline absorption
Intestinal Metabolism	CYP3A4 in intestinal wall reduces bioavailability	Significant first-pass for midazolam

Factors Affecting Oral Bioavailability

Physicochemical properties of drugs significantly influence their absorption potential. Solubility in gastrointestinal fluids represents a prerequisite for absorption of most drugs, with dissolution rate often limiting the absorption of poorly soluble compounds. The Biopharmaceutics Classification System (BCS) categorizes drugs based on solubility and permeability characteristics, providing a framework for predicting absorption behavior and guiding formulation strategies.

Lipophilicity, typically quantified by octanol-water partition coefficient (log P), correlates with membrane permeability for many drugs. However, excessive lipophilicity can reduce aqueous solubility and increase binding to plasma proteins, potentially limiting free drug concentration available for pharmacological action. The relationship between lipophilicity and absorption follows a parabolic pattern, with optimal absorption typically occurring at intermediate log P values (approximately 2-3).

Ionization state, determined by drug pKa and environmental pH, substantially affects both solubility and membrane permeability. According to the pH-partition hypothesis, un-ionized forms generally demonstrate superior membrane permeability, while ionized forms typically exhibit better aqueous solubility. This principle explains the preferential absorption of weak acids in the acidic environment of the stomach and weak bases in the more alkaline environment of the intestine.

Formulation factors can significantly modify drug bioavailability through effects on dissolution rate, solubilization capacity, gastrointestinal transit time, or permeation enhancement. Particle size reduction increases surface area available for dissolution, while amorphous solid dispersions disrupt crystal lattice energy barriers to dissolution. Solubilizing excipients such as surfactants or cyclodextrins enhance dissolution of poorly water-soluble drugs, while permeation enhancers temporarily modify epithelial barrier properties to increase absorption.

Physiological variables introduce significant inter- and intra-individual variability in drug absorption. Gastric emptying time affects how quickly drugs reach the small intestine, the primary absorption site for most compounds. This parameter demonstrates considerable variability based on factors including meal composition, fluid volume, emotional state, and disease conditions. Intestinal motility influences residence time at absorption sites, while intestinal pH and buffer capacity affect drug ionization state and dissolution. First-pass metabolism by intestinal and hepatic enzymes may substantially reduce bioavailability of susceptible compounds, necessitating formulation strategies that protect drugs from enzymatic degradation or bypass first-pass effects.

Bioavailability Assessment

Plasma concentration-time profiles provide the fundamental data for bioavailability assessment, reflecting the combined influences of absorption, distribution, metabolism, and excretion processes. These profiles typically display an absorption phase with rising concentrations, a peak representing maximum concentration (Cmax), and an elimination phase with declining concentrations. Mathematical modeling of these data enables determination of pharmacokinetic parameters that characterize the rate and extent of absorption.

Area under the plasma concentration-time curve (AUC) quantifies the extent of drug absorption, reflecting total drug exposure over time. This parameter, calculated by numerical integration methods such as the trapezoidal rule, serves as the primary metric for bioavailability assessment. Absolute bioavailability (F) compares the AUC after extravascular administration to that following intravenous dosing (normalized for dose differences), while relative bioavailability compares AUC between different extravascular formulations.

Maximum plasma concentration (Cmax) and time to maximum concentration (Tmax) provide information about absorption rate, complementing the AUC's indication of absorption extent. These parameters influence the onset and intensity of therapeutic effects, with rapid-acting formulations typically exhibiting higher Cmax values and shorter Tmax intervals than extended-release alternatives.

Bioequivalence studies compare the bioavailability of different formulations to establish therapeutic equivalence without requiring full clinical efficacy trials. Regulatory standards typically consider products bioequivalent when the 90% confidence intervals for the ratios of geometric means (test/reference) for AUC and Cmax fall within 80-125%. These studies employ crossover designs to minimize the influence of inter-subject variability, with washout periods between treatments to eliminate carryover effects.

In vitro dissolution testing provides valuable predictive information about *in vivo* performance, particularly for BCS Class I (high solubility, high permeability) and Class III (high solubility, low permeability) drugs where dissolution rather than permeability limits absorption. *In vitro-in vivo* correlations (IVIVC) establish mathematical relationships between dissolution profiles and bioavailability parameters, enabling quality control decisions based on dissolution testing and supporting biowaivers for certain formulation changes.

Bioavailability Enhancement

Physical modifications that enhance dissolution rate represent first-line approaches for improving bioavailability of poorly water-soluble drugs. Micronization reduces particle size to increase surface area available for dissolution, while more aggressive size reduction to nanoscale dimensions can substantially increase saturation solubility through effects on surface curvature and vapor pressure. Amorphous solid dispersions distribute drugs within hydrophilic polymer matrices in non-crystalline states, eliminating the crystal lattice energy barrier to dissolution and often incorporating polymers that inhibit recrystallization.

Chemical modifications including prodrug formation and salt selection can address specific bioavailability limitations. Prodrugs incorporate metabolically labile groups that enhance solubility or membrane permeability, with subsequent enzymatic conversion releasing the active parent compound. This approach has proven particularly valuable for improving intestinal permeability of drugs containing carboxylic acid or hydroxyl groups that limit passive diffusion. Salt formation enhances dissolution rate and apparent solubility of ionizable drugs, with appropriate counterion selection balancing considerations of solubility enhancement, stability, hygroscopicity, and processing characteristics.

Lipid-based delivery systems exploit natural lipid absorption pathways to enhance bioavailability of lipophilic drugs. Self-emulsifying drug delivery systems (SEDDS) combine oils, surfactants, and co-solvents that spontaneously form fine oil-in-water emulsions upon contact with gastrointestinal fluids, presenting drugs in solubilized form with high surface area for absorption. These systems additionally may promote lymphatic transport, bypass hepatic first-pass metabolism, inhibit efflux transporters, and increase intestinal membrane permeability, providing multiple mechanisms for bioavailability enhancement.

Permeation enhancers temporarily modify epithelial barrier properties to increase drug absorption. These compounds operate through various mechanisms including disruption of intercellular tight junctions, alteration of membrane fluidity, inhibition of efflux transporters, or opening of transient hydrophilic pores. While effective, these approaches require careful balancing of enhancement effects against potential mucosal irritation or systemic toxicity, limiting the concentration and exposure duration to minimize adverse effects.

NOVEL DRUG DELIVERY SYSTEMS

Novel drug delivery systems extend beyond conventional formulations to achieve targeted delivery, controlled release kinetics, enhanced stability, or improved patient compliance. These sophisticated approaches apply advanced materials science and engineering principles to overcome limitations of traditional dosage forms and expand therapeutic possibilities.

Nanoparticulate Drug Delivery Systems

Polymeric nanoparticles consist of drugs entrapped within nanoscale polymer matrices, offering versatile platforms for controlled release and targeted delivery. These systems utilize biodegradable polymers such as poly(lactic-co-glycolic acid) (PLGA), polycaprolactone, or chitosan that release encapsulated drugs through diffusion, polymer degradation, or combined mechanisms. Surface modification with hydrophilic polymers like polyethylene glycol (PEGylation) reduces recognition by the reticuloendothelial system, prolonging circulation time, while conjugation with targeting ligands directs nanoparticles to specific tissues or cellular receptors.

Lipid-based nanocarriers include liposomes, solid lipid nanoparticles, and nanostructured lipid carriers, each offering distinct advantages for drug delivery. Liposomes—phospholipid vesicles with aqueous cores—can accommodate both hydrophilic (in the aqueous core) and lipophilic (in the bilayer) drugs, with composition and surface charge influencing stability, circulation time, and tissue distribution. Solid lipid nanoparticles provide enhanced physical stability compared to liposomes while maintaining good biocompatibility, though often limited in drug loading capacity. Nanostructured lipid carriers incorporate liquid lipids into solid lipid matrices, creating imperfections that accommodate higher drug loads while maintaining structural integrity.

Inorganic nanoparticles including gold, silver, iron oxide, and mesoporous silica offer unique properties for drug delivery applications. Gold nanoparticles provide opportunities for photothermal therapy through surface plasmon resonance, while their easily functionalized surfaces accommodate targeting ligands and therapeutic molecules. Magnetic nanoparticles enable externally directed targeting through applied magnetic fields and provide contrast enhancement for diagnostic imaging. Mesoporous silica nanoparticles offer exceptionally high surface areas and pore volumes for drug loading, with pore size and surface chemistry modifications controlling release kinetics.

Nanotherapeutics face significant translation challenges despite their promising performance in preclinical studies. Scalable

Table 4.3: Novel Drug Delivery Systems and Technologies

Delivery System	Description	Advantages
Liposomes	Phospholipid vesicles	Targeted delivery, reduced toxicity
Nanoparticles	Sub-micron colloidal carriers	Enhanced solubility, targeting
Microemulsions	Thermodynamically stable dispersions	Improved solubilization
Microspheres	Spherical matrix systems	Controlled release, targeting
Transdermal Systems	Drug delivery through skin	Avoids first-pass, sustained delivery
Buccal/Sublingual	Absorption through oral mucosa	Rapid onset, avoids first-pass
Pulmonary Delivery	Inhalation to lungs	Direct to target, rapid absorption
Osmotic Pumps	Osmotic pressure-driven release	Zero-order release, predictable
Ion-Exchange Resins	Drug bound to resin	Taste masking, controlled release
Floating Systems	Gastric retention devices	Extended absorption window
Bioadhesive Systems	Adhere to biological surfaces	Prolonged contact time
Implantable Devices	Surgically placed systems	Long-term delivery, compliance
Microneedles	Minimally invasive skin delivery	Pain-free, enhanced penetration
3D Printing	Additive manufacturing of dosage forms	Personalized medicine, complex structures
Smart Polymers	Respond to environmental stimuli	Targeted, controlled release
Dendrimers	Branched, monodisperse polymers	High drug loading, targeting
Microbial Vectors	Bacteria/viruses for gene delivery	Gene therapy, vaccination

manufacturing with consistent physicochemical properties requires sophisticated process controls beyond those typical for conventional formulations. Regulatory requirements for nanomedicines continue to evolve, with particular attention to characterization of particle size distribution, surface properties, drug loading, release kinetics, and potential for complement activation or immunogenicity.

Stimuli-Responsive Drug Delivery

pH-responsive systems exploit pH variations across anatomical sites or pathological conditions to trigger selective drug release. These systems typically incorporate polymers with ionizable groups that undergo conformational or solubility changes in response to environmental pH shifts. Polyacidic polymers (e.g., polyacrylic acid, polymethacrylic acid) remain collapsed at gastric pH but swell or dissolve at intestinal pH, enabling targeted intestinal delivery. Conversely, polybasic polymers (e.g., chitosan, polyethylenimine) exhibit opposite behavior, swelling at acidic pH and contracting at neutral or alkaline conditions. These properties enable targeted delivery to tumors, infected tissues, or inflammation sites that exhibit lower pH than surrounding healthy tissues.

Temperature-sensitive systems utilize polymers that undergo phase transitions at specific temperatures, typically employing materials with lower critical solution temperature (LCST) or upper critical solution temperature (UCST) behavior. Poly(N-isopropylacrylamide) (PNIPAM) exemplifies LCST polymers, transitioning from hydrophilic to hydrophobic states above its transition temperature (approximately 32°C), causing collapse of hydrogel structures and expulsion of entrapped drugs. These systems enable externally triggered release through localized heating or exploitation of elevated temperatures in pathological sites such as tumors or infections.

Enzyme-responsive delivery systems leverage differential enzyme expression between normal and pathological tissues to achieve targeted release. These approaches incorporate enzyme-cleavable linkages within delivery system structures, allowing specific enzymatic activity to trigger drug release or carrier degradation. For example, matrix metalloproteinase-responsive systems target tumor microenvironments where these enzymes show elevated expression, while phospholipase or glycosidase-sensitive systems target bacterial infection sites based on their distinct enzymatic profiles.

Externally triggered systems respond to non-physiological stimuli including light, ultrasound, or magnetic fields, offering precise spatial and temporal control over drug release. Photosensitive systems incorporate chromophores or photocleavable groups that undergo structural changes upon light exposure at specific wavelengths, triggering drug release or carrier destabilization. Ultrasound-responsive systems utilize acoustic cavitation effects to temporarily disrupt carrier structures or enhance membrane permeability, while magnetically responsive systems employ ferromagnetic materials that generate localized heating under alternating magnetic fields through hysteresis effects.

Targeted Drug Delivery

Passive targeting exploits the enhanced permeability and retention (EPR) effect observed in tumors and inflammatory tissues, where abnormal vasculature with enlarged endothelial gaps permits preferential accumulation of nanoparticles. This phenomenon provides the basis for many nanomedicine approaches in oncology, allowing localization of therapeutic agents at tumor sites without specific molecular recognition elements. Nanocarrier properties including size, shape, and surface characteristics significantly influence the efficiency of passive targeting, with particles approximately 50-200 nm typically showing optimal EPR accumulation.

Active targeting employs specific ligand-receptor interactions to direct drug carriers to particular cell types or tissues. These approaches conjugate targeting moieties—including antibodies, antibody fragments, peptides, aptamers, or small molecules—to carrier surfaces, enabling recognition of cell-specific surface markers. For example, folate receptor targeting directs carriers to various cancer cells overexpressing this receptor, while transferrin receptor targeting facilitates blood-brain barrier penetration. The selection of appropriate targeting ligands balances considerations of binding affinity, specificity, stability, and potential immunogenicity.

Intracellular targeting addresses the challenge of delivering drugs to specific subcellular compartments where their molecular targets reside. Cell-penetrating peptides facilitate cytoplasmic delivery by enhancing membrane translocation, while nuclear localization signals direct conjugated drugs or carriers to the nucleus for interaction with DNA or nuclear proteins. Mitochondrial targeting employs lipophilic cations such as triphenylphosphonium that accumulate within mitochondria due to the organelle's negative membrane potential, enabling delivery of antioxidants or pro-apoptotic agents to this critical metabolic center.

Chronotherapeutic approaches optimize drug delivery timing to align with circadian rhythms or disease progression patterns. These systems recognize that physiological processes and disease symptoms often show time-dependent variations, creating opportunities to enhance therapeutic effects or reduce adverse effects through appropriate timing. Programmable delivery systems using microelectronic controls, chronoprogrammed polymer systems, or biological rhythm-responsive elements enable synchronized drug release coordinated with these temporal patterns.

Biologics Delivery Systems

Protein and peptide delivery presents significant challenges due to the physicochemical properties and stability limitations of these molecules. Enzymatic degradation in the gastrointestinal tract largely precludes oral delivery of unprotected proteins, while their large molecular size and hydrophilicity limit membrane permeation. Advanced delivery systems for these biologics employ protective encapsulation, permeation enhancement, or alternative administration routes to overcome these barriers. Approaches include enteric microparticles that protect against gastric degradation, absorption enhancers that temporarily modify tight junction integrity, and conjugation with cell-penetrating peptides that facilitate cellular uptake.

Nucleic acid therapeutics including antisense oligonucleotides, small interfering RNA (siRNA), and mRNA require specialized delivery systems to reach their intracellular targets. These anionic macromolecules face multiple barriers including nuclease degradation, rapid renal clearance, limited cellular uptake, and endosomal entrapment. Lipid nanoparticles (LNPs) representing the most clinically advanced delivery platform for nucleic acids, combine ionizable lipids that condense nucleic acids through electrostatic interactions with helper lipids that enhance stability and facilitate endosomal escape. Alternative approaches include polymeric nanoparticles, conjugation with cell-targeting ligands, or physical methods such as electroporation that temporarily disrupt cell membranes.

Vaccine delivery systems aim to enhance immune response through optimized antigen presentation and adjuvant activity. Particulate systems including liposomes, polymeric nanoparticles, and virus-like particles improve antigen uptake by antigen-presenting cells while protecting against degradation. Adjuvant integration within delivery platforms can promote specific immune response patterns through modulation of innate immune activation. Advanced vaccine delivery technologies include microneedle arrays that enable painless transdermal administration, thermostable formulations that eliminate cold chain requirements, and controlled release systems that reduce the need for booster doses.

Cell-based delivery utilizes living cells as carriers for therapeutic agents, combining the targeting capabilities of the cell with the therapeutic effects of the cargo. Stem cells naturally migrate toward inflammation, injury, or tumor sites, making them attractive vehicles for targeted delivery. Immune cells including T cells and macrophages can be engineered to carry drugs or nanoparticles to disease sites, combining cellular immunotherapy with conventional pharmaceutical approaches. These sophisticated delivery strategies, while technically challenging, offer unprecedented precision for treating complex diseases resistant to conventional therapeutic approaches.

PHARMACEUTICAL EXCIPIENTS

Pharmaceutical excipients constitute the non-therapeutic components of drug formulations that perform essential functions in dosage form preparation, stability, and performance. Far from being inert fillers, modern excipients contribute actively to formulation functionality through carefully designed physicochemical properties and interactions with active ingredients and biological systems.

Functional Categories and Selection Criteria

Diluents provide bulk to formulations, enabling practical handling of potent drugs requiring small doses. Beyond this fundamental role, diluents influence multiple formulation properties including flow characteristics, compressibility, disintegration behavior, and compatibility with active ingredients. Common diluents include microcrystalline cellulose, which provides excellent compressibility and disintegration properties; lactose, offering good flow and compatibility with many drugs; and mannitol, providing sweet taste and non-hygroscopic properties valuable for moisture-sensitive formulations.

Binders hold particulate components together, providing mechanical strength to granules and tablets. These materials function through adhesive interactions, polymer chain entanglement, or solid bridge formation during drying or compression. Natural polymers including starch, gelatin, and acacia; semisynthetic derivatives such as hydroxypropyl methylcellulose; and synthetic polymers like polyvinylpyrrolidone offer different binding capacities, compatibility profiles, and processing characteristics suited to specific formulation requirements.

Disintegrants promote dosage form breakdown upon administration, facilitating drug release and dissolution. Traditional disintegrants like starch and microcrystalline cellulose operate primarily through swelling mechanisms, while superdisintegrants such as croscarmellose sodium, sodium starch glycolate, and crospovidone provide enhanced effectiveness through rapid and extensive swelling, wicking, or recovery of deformation after compression. The selection and concentration of disintegrants balance requirements for rapid disintegration against potential effects on formulation stability or premature drug release.

Lubricants reduce friction during tablet ejection from dies, preventing sticking to punch faces and reducing wear on tooling. These materials typically possess low shear strength crystal structures that create slip planes between moving surfaces. Magnesium stearate remains the most widely used lubricant due to its exceptional effectiveness, though concerns regarding its hydrophobicity and potential interference with dissolution have prompted investigation of alternatives including sodium stearyl fumarate, glyceryl behenate, and talc, each offering different performance characteristics and compatibility profiles.

Solubility and Dissolution Enhancers

Surfactants reduce interfacial tension between drug particles and dissolution media, facilitating wetting and enhancing dissolution rate. These amphiphilic molecules additionally form micelles above their critical micelle concentration, providing solubilization capacity for lipophilic drugs. Nonionic surfactants including polysorbates, polyoxyl castor oil derivatives, and sorbitan esters offer good compatibility and low toxicity, while anionic surfactants such as sodium lauryl sulfate provide greater solubilization capacity but higher irritation potential.

Cyclodextrins form inclusion complexes with lipophilic drug molecules, encapsulating them within hydrophobic central cavities while presenting hydrophilic exteriors to the aqueous environment. This molecular encapsulation enhances apparent aqueous solubility without chemical modification of the drug. Native cyclodextrins (α, β, and γ) offer different cavity sizes accommodating various molecular dimensions, while chemically modified derivatives provide enhanced solubility and safety profiles. The complexation efficiency depends on structural complementarity between the drug and cyclodextrin cavity, with appropriate molecular modeling and phase solubility studies guiding selection of optimal cyclodextrin types for specific compounds.

Co-solvents improve solubility by reducing solvent polarity and weakening hydrogen bonding networks that exclude lipophilic molecules from aqueous environments. Pharmaceutical co-solvents including propylene glycol, ethanol, glycerin, and polyethylene glycols combine reasonable solubilization capacity with acceptable safety profiles. These excipients typically demonstrate solubility enhancement proportional to concentration, though excessive concentrations may risk precipitation upon dilution in physiological fluids—a phenomenon termed "solvent death" that can significantly reduce bioavailability.

Solid dispersion technologies distribute drugs within hydrophilic carrier matrices at molecular levels, preventing crystallization and providing microenvironments that enhance dissolution. These sophisticated formulations employ carriers including polyvinylpyrrolidone, hydroxypropyl methylcellulose, polyethylene glycol, and recently developed polymers specifically designed for amorphous stabilization. Manufacturing methods including spray drying, hot melt extrusion, and co-precipitation create intimate drug-carrier mixtures that maintain drugs in high-energy states with enhanced dissolution characteristics.

Modified Release Excipients

Hydrophilic matrix formers including hydroxypropyl methylcellulose, sodium alginate, xanthan gum, and polyethylene oxide create gel layers upon hydration that control drug diffusion rates. These polymers exhibit different viscosity grades, substitution patterns, and molecular weights that influence hydration kinetics, gel strength, and erosion rates. The selection of appropriate polymer types and concentrations enables customization of release profiles ranging from first-order kinetics to near-zero-order release, depending on the balance between diffusion and erosion mechanisms.

Hydrophobic matrix materials including waxes, glycerides, and insoluble polymers create porous structures through which drugs diffuse or release through matrix erosion. These materials offer advantages for moisture-sensitive drugs and typically provide more robust performance across varying gastrointestinal conditions than hydrophilic matrices. Common examples include carnauba wax, glyceryl behenate, ethylcellulose, and ammonio-methacrylate copolymers, each providing different processing characteristics and release modification capacities.

Coating polymers for modified release include cellulosic derivatives (ethylcellulose, cellulose acetate), acrylic polymers (ammonio-methacrylate copolymers, methacrylic acid copolymers), and polyvinyl derivatives that form semipermeable or pH-dependent membranes around drug cores. These polymers vary in permeability characteristics, mechanical properties, and dissolution behavior in different physiological environments. Coating formulations typically include plasticizers that enhance film flexibility, pore-formers that modulate permeability, and sometimes anti-adherents that prevent agglomeration during processing.

Ion-exchange resins consist of insoluble polymer matrices containing functional groups capable of exchanging ions with the surrounding medium. These materials form insoluble drug-resin complexes that release the drug through ion exchange with counter-ions in gastrointestinal fluids. The release rate depends on resin cross-linking density, ionic strength of the release medium, and pKa relationships between the drug and resin functional groups. Common pharmaceutical ion-exchange resins include sulfonated polystyrene resins (cation exchangers) and quaternary ammonium functionalized resins (anion exchangers), each available in varying particle sizes and cross-linking densities for different release profiles.

Table 4.4: Pharmaceutical Excipients and Their Functions

Excipient Category	Function	Examples
Diluents/Fillers	Increase bulk volume	Lactose, MCC, starch
Binders	Hold ingredients together	PVP, HPMC, starch
Disintegrants	Promote tablet breakup	Croscarmellose, crospovidone
Lubricants	Reduce friction during compression	Magnesium stearate, talc
Glidants	Improve powder flow	Colloidal silica, talc
Wetting Agents	Enhance water penetration	SLS, polysorbates
Solubilizers	Increase drug solubility	Cyclodextrins, PEG
Preservatives	Prevent microbial growth	Parabens, benzalkonium chloride
Antioxidants	Prevent oxidation	BHT, ascorbic acid
Flavoring Agents	Improve taste	Menthol, sucralose
Coloring Agents	Aesthetics, identification	FD&C dyes, iron oxides
Coating Materials	Protection, appearance, release	HPMC, acrylic polymers
pH Adjusters	Maintain optimal pH	Citric acid, phosphates
Tonicity Agents	Match osmotic pressure	Sodium chloride, dextrose
Suspending Agents	Prevent settling	Xanthan gum, HPMC
Emulsifiers	Stabilize oil-water interfaces	Polysorbates, lecithin
Chelating Agents	Bind metal ions	EDTA, citric acid
Plasticizers	Increase polymer flexibility	Glycerin, PEG

Specialized Excipients

Bioadhesive polymers enhance residence time at application sites through interactions with biological surfaces. These materials, including carbomers, chitosan, hyaluronic acid, and various cellulose derivatives, adhere to mucosal surfaces through hydrogen bonding, ionic interactions, or physical entanglement with mucin glycoproteins. This prolonged contact increases local drug concentration gradients and extends absorption time, enhancing bioavailability particularly for drugs with absorption window limitations. The selection of appropriate bioadhesive polymers considers the target mucosal surface characteristics, required residence time, and compatibility with the active ingredient and other formulation components.

Penetration enhancers temporarily modify biological barriers to increase drug permeation. These compounds operate through various mechanisms including disruption of intercellular lipid organization, modification of protein domains within barriers, or alteration of mucus rheology. Fatty acids and their derivatives, surfactants, terpenes, and phospholipids represent common classes of penetration enhancers, each offering different enhancement mechanisms and tissue specificity. The selection of appropriate enhancers balances permeation improvement against potential irritation or damage to biological barriers, with preference for reversible effects that resolve after drug absorption.

Taste-masking excipients address palatability challenges for oral formulations, particularly important for pediatric medications and drugs with inherently aversive taste profiles.

Approaches include complexation with ion-exchange resins that reduce drug solubility in saliva, coating with polymeric films that delay dissolution until after swallowing, or incorporation of flavoring agents and sweeteners that compete with or mask aversive taste perceptions. Specialized taste-masking technologies such as lipid microencapsulation or cyclodextrin complexation provide molecular-level isolation of bitter compounds from taste receptors while maintaining appropriate release characteristics in gastrointestinal environments.

Preservatives prevent microbial contamination in liquid and semi-solid formulations, maintaining product safety throughout their intended shelf life. These compounds must demonstrate effectiveness against a spectrum of potential contaminants while exhibiting acceptable safety profiles for their intended routes of administration. Commonly used preservatives include parabens, which provide broad-spectrum activity but face increasing scrutiny regarding potential endocrine effects; benzalkonium chloride, particularly used in ophthalmic preparations; and newer alternatives such as sodium benzoate, potassium sorbate, and phenoxyethanol that address specific formulation requirements or consumer preferences for particular product types.

Table 4.5: Biopharmaceutics Classification System (BCS) and Formulation Strategies

BCS Class	Solubility	Permeability	Example Drugs
Class I	High	High	Metoprolol, propranolol
			Diltiazem, verapamil
			Acetaminophen, caffeine
			Lidocaine, prednisolone
Class II	Low	High	Ibuprofen, ketoprofen
			Carbamazepine, phenytoin
			Atorvastatin, cyclosporine
			Griseofulvin, danazol
Class III	High	Low	Ranitidine, metformin
			Cimetidine, acyclovir
			Atenolol, captopril
			Erythromycin, neomycin
Class IV	Low	Low	Hydrochlorothiazide
			Furosemide, chlorothiazide
			Taxol, amphotericin B
			Ganciclovir, topotecan

Summary

Pharmaceutics combines chemical and biological sciences to create optimal medication delivery systems meeting therapeutic needs while enhancing patient adherence. Dosage form design integrates physical-chemical properties of active ingredients with route-specific requirements, balancing stability, bioavailability, manufacturing feasibility, and patient acceptability factors. Each design addresses specific challenges—tablets require appropriate hardness and disintegration properties, injectables must maintain sterility and compatibility, while topical preparations need proper rheological characteristics for application and drug penetration. These properties directly influence drug absorption processes across biological membranes through passive diffusion, active transport, facilitated diffusion, and endocytosis mechanisms. Bioavailability—the rate and extent of active drug reaching systemic circulation—varies significantly between formulations and administration routes, affected by solubility limitations, first-pass metabolism, chemical instability, and various physiological barriers. Novel delivery systems extend beyond conventional approaches, employing controlled-release technologies including matrix systems, reservoir devices, osmotic pumps, and ion-exchange resins to maintain therapeutic concentrations over extended periods. Additional innovations include transdermal patches providing non-invasive delivery, liposomal encapsulation for targeted distribution, implantable devices for long-term release, and nanoparticle carriers enhancing solubility and tissue penetration. These advanced systems rely on carefully selected pharmaceutical excipients—non-therapeutic ingredients providing functional properties including binding, disintegration, lubrication, preservation, and stability enhancement. Through strategic formulation design integrating these elements, pharmaceutics optimizes medication delivery to maximize therapeutic outcomes while minimizing adverse effects across diverse patient populations and treatment scenarios.

Multiple Choice Questions

1. Which of the following dosage forms would be most appropriate for a drug that undergoes extensive first-pass metabolism?
   a) Oral tablet
   b) Transdermal patch
   c) Rectal suppository
   d) Intramuscular injection
2. A drug with a log P value of 3.5 would be expected to have which of the following characteristics?
   a) High water solubility
   b) Poor membrane permeability
   c) High lipophilicity
   d) Rapid renal elimination
3. According to the Biopharmaceutics Classification System (BCS), a drug with high solubility and low permeability would be classified as:
   a) Class I
   b) Class II
   c) Class III
   d) Class IV
4. Which of the following factors would most likely decrease the bioavailability of an orally administered drug?
   a) Micronization of drug particles
   b) Administration with a high-fat meal for a lipophilic drug
   c) Conversion to a more soluble salt form
   d) Significant first-pass metabolism
5. In a sustained-release matrix tablet, which of the following polymers would provide the slowest drug release rate?
   a) Hydroxypropyl methylcellulose with low viscosity
   b) Hydroxypropyl methylcellulose with high viscosity
   c) Sodium starch glycolate
   d) Croscarmellose sodium
6. Which of the following novel drug delivery systems would be most appropriate for targeting drugs specifically to the colon?
   a) Liposomes
   b) pH-dependent enteric coating
   c) Osmotic pump tablets
   d) Prodrugs activated by colonic bacteria
7. The primary function of a disintegrant in a tablet formulation is to:

a) Increase tablet hardness
b) Promote tablet break-up after administration
c) Improve powder flow during manufacturing
d) Enhance drug stability

8. Which pharmaceutical excipient would be most appropriate as a suspending agent in a liquid formulation?
a) Lactose
b) Magnesium stearate
c) Xanthan gum
d) Talc

9. The concept of "therapeutic equivalence" between two drug products requires:
a) Identical excipients in the same concentrations
b) Identical *in vitro* dissolution profiles
c) Pharmaceutical equivalence and bioequivalence
d) Identical manufacturing processes

10. Which of the following approaches would most effectively enhance the dissolution rate of a poorly water-soluble drug?
a) Formulating as a coated tablet
b) Preparation as a solid dispersion in a hydrophilic carrier
c) Using a higher compression force during tableting
d) Adding a lubricant such as magnesium stearate

Self-Assessment Questions

1. Analyze the physicochemical and physiological factors that must be considered when designing an oral controlled-release dosage form, explaining how specific formulation approaches address challenges in achieving consistent drug release over extended periods.
2. Describe the formulation considerations and manufacturing challenges associated with developing a stable injectable suspension, explaining how particle size, zeta potential, and rheological properties affect product performance and shelf life.
3. Compare and contrast the advantages and limitations of different tablet manufacturing methods analyzing how each process affects content uniformity, dissolution characteristics, and stability of the final product.
4. Explain how the physical-chemical properties of a drug (solubility, partition coefficient, pKa, molecular weight) influence its absorption across biological membranes, providing examples of how these properties might be modified to enhance bioavailability.
5. Describe how formulation approaches can overcome challenges related to solubility limitations, enzymatic degradation, and first-pass metabolism.
6. Describe the biopharmaceutical classification system (BCS) and explain how it guides formulation strategies for drugs with different solubility and permeability characteristics, providing specific examples for each BCS class.
7. Compare and contrast the mechanisms, advantages, and limitations of different novel drug delivery systems including liposomes, nanoparticles, transdermal patches, and implantable devices, providing examples of therapeutic applications for each.
8. Explain the principles of targeted drug delivery systems, describing how passive and active targeting strategies enhance therapeutic efficacy while reducing systemic exposure and associated adverse effects.
9. Analyze the functional roles of different pharmaceutical excipients in solid dosage formulations, explaining how inappropriate selection might compromise product performance.
10. Describe the specialized excipients used in parenteral formulations, explaining their purposes in ensuring stability, safety, and efficacy while analyzing potential compatibility issues and toxicity concerns.

Bibliography

1. Aulton ME, Taylor KMG. Aulton's pharmaceutics: The design and manufacture of medicines. 5th ed. Edinburgh: Elsevier; 2018.
2. Amidon GL, Lennernäs H, Shah VP, Crison JR. A theoretical basis for a biopharmaceutic drug classification: The correlation of *in vitro* drug product dissolution and *in vivo* bioavailability. Pharm Res. 1995;12(3):413-420.
3. Fasinu P, Pillay V, Ndesendo VM, du Toit LC, Choonara YE. Diverse approaches for the enhancement of oral drug bioavailability. Biopharm Drug Dispos. 2011;32(4):185-209.
4. Allen LV, Ansel HC. Ansel's pharmaceutical dosage forms and drug delivery systems. 11th ed. Philadelphia: Wolters Kluwer; 2018.
5. Liechty WB, Kryscio DR, Slaughter BV, Peppas NA. Polymers for drug delivery systems. Annu Rev Chem Biomol Eng. 2010;1:149-173.
6. Tibbitt MW, Dahlman JE, Langer R. Emerging frontiers in drug delivery. J Am Chem Soc. 2016;138(3):704-717.
7. Lam PL, Gambari R. Advanced progress of microencapsulation technologies: *In vivo* and *in vitro* models for studying oral and transdermal drug deliveries. J Control Release. 2014;178:25-45.
8. Rowe RC, Sheskey PJ, Quinn ME. Handbook of pharmaceutical excipients. 6th ed. London: Pharmaceutical Press; 2009.
9. Moreton RC. Excipient functionality. Pharm Technol. 2004;28(5):98-119.
10. Savjani KT, Gajjar AK, Savjani JK. Drug solubility: Importance and enhancement techniques. ISRN Pharm. 2012;2012:195727.

CHAPTER 5

PHARMACOLOGY FOUNDATIONS

Author

Dr. Ramesh Kumar Gupta, Associate Professor, Department of Pharmacology, Amity Institute of Pharmacy, Amity University, Lucknow, Uttar Pradesh, India

Abstract

Pharmacology explains how drugs produce therapeutic and adverse effects through their interactions with biological systems. Pharmacodynamics reveals the molecular mechanisms of drug action, with receptor theory explaining how medications interact with specific cellular targets through agonist, antagonist, and modulator relationships, producing dose-dependent responses that can be quantified through key parameters describing potency and efficacy. Pharmacokinetic processes of absorption, distribution, metabolism and excretion determine drug concentration at target sites, with mathematical models describing drug movement throughout the body, enabling prediction of appropriate dosing regimens and explaining variability in drug response across different patient populations. Drug-drug interactions occur through pharmacokinetic mechanisms altering drug concentrations or pharmacodynamic processes modifying responses without changing concentrations, with clinical significance determined by therapeutic index, interaction magnitude, and patient-specific risk factors requiring systematic management strategies. Adverse drug reactions range from predictable, dose-dependent extensions of pharmacological effects to unpredictable idiosyncratic responses, with detection, assessment, and preventive measures focusing on risk factor identification, monitoring programs, and reporting systems contributing to medication safety.

Keywords: *Receptor; Mechanisms; Drug Disposition; Therapeutic Response; Medication Safety; Physiological Effects*

Learning Objectives

After completion of the chapter, the learners should be able to:

- Differentiate between various receptor types and their signal transduction mechanisms in producing pharmacological effects.
- Calculate pharmacokinetic parameters including clearance, volume of distribution, half-life, and bioavailability from patient data.
- Predict the clinical significance of drug-drug interactions based on their mechanism, severity, and patient risk factors.
- Classify adverse drug reactions as Type A (augmented), Type B (bizarre), Type C (chronic), or Type D (delayed) with appropriate examples.
- Apply principles of pharmacogenomics to explain variations in drug response among different patient populations.
- Develop monitoring plans for medications with narrow therapeutic indices based on their pharmacokinetic and pharmacodynamic properties.

PHARMACODYNAMICS

Pharmacodynamics explores the biochemical and physiological effects of drugs on the body, examining the molecular mechanisms through which medications produce their therapeutic and adverse effects. This fundamental branch of pharmacology provides the theoretical framework for understanding how drugs interact with target structures to initiate cascades of biological events resulting in observable clinical responses. Comprehensive understanding of pharmacodynamic principles enables pharmacists to predict drug effects, explain variability in patient responses, optimize dosing regimens, and anticipate potential adverse reactions.

Receptor Theory and Drug-Receptor Interactions

Receptor theory provides the conceptual foundation for understanding how most drugs exert their effects through specific interactions with cellular targets. Receptors function as specialized protein structures located within cell membranes, cytoplasm, or nuclei that recognize and bind specific endogenous or exogenous molecules, triggering subsequent biological responses. The binding interaction between a drug and its receptor demonstrates remarkable molecular specificity, with complementary three-dimensional structures allowing precise molecular recognition similar to a lock-and-key relationship. This specificity explains why minor structural modifications in drug molecules can dramatically alter binding affinity and biological activity.

Table 5.1: Pharmacodynamic Parameters and Their Significance

Parameter	Definition	Clinical Significance	Examples
Potency	Dose required for effect	Affects dosing range	Fentanyl more potent than morphine
Efficacy	Maximum effect possible	Determines therapeutic potential	Full vs. partial agonists
EC50	Dose for 50% of max effect	Reflects drug sensitivity	Useful for dose-response curves
Emax	Maximum effect achievable	Reflects drug efficacy	Full vs. partial agonists
Affinity	Strength of drug-receptor binding	Influences potency	High affinity drugs act at lower doses
Intrinsic Activity	Ability to activate receptor	Determines if drug is agonist or antagonist	Full, partial, inverse agonists
Selectivity	Specificity for target	Affects side effect profile	β1 vs. non-selective β-blockers
Agonist	Activates receptor	Produces biological response	Albuterol at β2 receptors
Partial Agonist	Limited receptor activation	Ceiling effect, potential antagonism	Buprenorphine at μ-opioid receptors
Antagonist	Blocks receptor without activation	Inhibits agonist effects	Naloxone at opioid receptors
Inverse Agonist	Reduces constitutive activity	Opposite effect of agonist	Flumazenil at GABA receptors
Allosteric Modulator	Binds to secondary site	Modifies receptor function	Benzodiazepines at GABA receptors

Parameter	Definition	Clinical Significance	Examples
Spare Receptors	Excess receptors not needed for response	Allows for response at low occupancy	Insulin receptors
Desensitization	Reduced response with continued exposure	Tolerance development	Opioids, β-agonists
Therapeutic Index	LD50/ED50	Safety margin of drug	Digoxin has narrow therapeutic index

Drug-receptor binding typically involves non-covalent intermolecular forces including hydrogen bonding, ionic interactions, van der Waals forces, and hydrophobic interactions, creating reversible associations with binding strength determined by the number and type of these molecular connections. Receptor families encompass several major categories with distinct structural and functional characteristics. G protein-coupled receptors (GPCRs) represent the largest receptor family and serve as targets for approximately 30% of all marketed drugs. These transmembrane receptors activate intracellular G proteins upon ligand binding, initiating signal transduction cascades through secondary messengers such as cyclic AMP, diacylglycerol, and calcium. Ion channel receptors regulate ion flow across cell membranes, with ligand-gated channels opening in response to neurotransmitter binding and voltage-gated channels responding to membrane potential changes. Enzyme-linked receptors possess intrinsic enzymatic activity or associate directly with enzymes, commonly displaying kinase activity that phosphorylates target proteins. Nuclear receptors bind ligands that enable direct interaction with DNA, modulating gene transcription and protein synthesis with relatively slower onset but prolonged duration of action. Intracellular receptors located in the cytoplasm or nucleus interact with lipophilic molecules that can traverse cell membranes, forming complexes that regulate gene expression through various mechanisms.

Agonists, Antagonists, and Receptor Modulation

Drugs interacting with receptors can be classified based on their effects on receptor function, with distinct categories demonstrating characteristic influences on biological responses. Agonists bind to receptors and activate them, mimicking the action of endogenous ligands and producing similar biological effects. Full agonists generate maximal receptor activation at sufficient concentrations, producing a response indistinguishable from the endogenous ligand.

Table 5.2: Receptor Types and Signaling Mechanisms

Receptor Family	Mechanism	Examples	Drugs
G-Protein Coupled	Second messenger signaling	Adrenergic, muscarinic, opioid	Propranolol, atropine, morphine
Gs-coupled	↑ cAMP via adenylyl cyclase	β-adrenergic, H2, D1	Albuterol, famotidine, levodopa
Gi-coupled	↓ cAMP via adenylyl cyclase	α2-adrenergic, M2, D2	Clonidine, opioids, haloperidol
Gq-coupled	↑ IP3/DAG via phospholipase C	α1-adrenergic, M1, M3	Phenylephrine, bethanechol
Ion Channels	Direct ion flux regulation	nAChR, GABA, glutamate	Nicotine, benzodiazepines, ketamine
Ligand-gated	Channel opens with binding	GABA, nicotinic, 5HT3	Diazepam, succinylcholine, ondansetron
Voltage-gated	Potential-dependent opening	Na+, K+, Ca2+ channels	Lidocaine, nifedipine, phenytoin
Nuclear Receptors	Gene transcription regulation	Steroid, thyroid, vitamin D	Prednisone, levothyroxine, tamoxifen
Enzyme-linked	Enzymatic activity regulation	Insulin, growth factors	Insulin, monoclonal antibodies
Tyrosine Kinase	Protein phosphorylation	Insulin, EGF, PDGF	Insulin, erlotinib, imatinib
Guanylyl Cyclase	↑ cGMP	ANP, NO	Nitrates, sildenafil
Cytokine Receptors	JAK-STAT signaling	Interleukins, interferons	Adalimumab, interferon
Integrins	Cell adhesion regulation	Platelet glycoproteins	Abciximab, tirofiban

Partial agonists produce submaximal activation even at saturating concentrations, demonstrating lower efficacy while potentially maintaining high binding affinity.

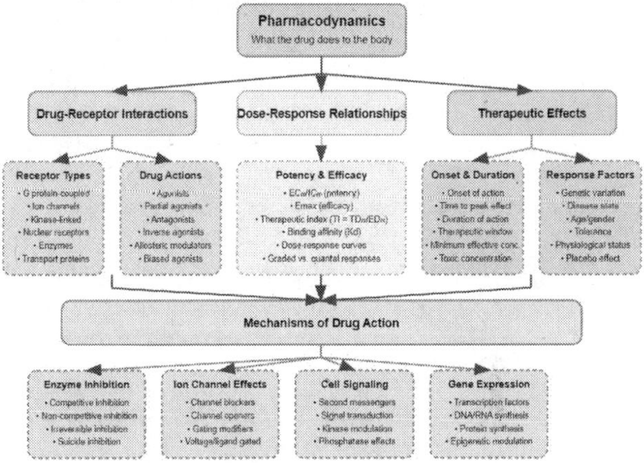

Figure 5.1: Principles of Pharmacodynamics

This property allows partial agonists to function as agonists in the absence of endogenous ligand while acting as functional antagonists in its presence by occupying receptors without producing full activation. Inverse agonists bind to receptors that exhibit constitutive activity and reduce this baseline signaling below normal levels, producing effects opposite to conventional agonists. Antagonists bind to receptors without activating them, preventing interaction with other ligands through various mechanisms. Competitive antagonists reversibly bind to the same receptor site as agonists, establishing concentration-dependent competition that can be overcome by increasing agonist concentration. Non-competitive antagonists bind to distinct sites on receptors or associated proteins, reducing receptor function through mechanisms that cannot be overcome by increasing agonist concentration. Irreversible antagonists form covalent bonds with receptor structures, permanently inactivating them until new receptors are synthesized. Allosteric modulators bind to sites distinct from the primary ligand binding location, inducing conformational changes that alter receptor function without directly activating or blocking the receptor. Positive allosteric modulators enhance receptor responsiveness to endogenous or exogenous ligands without activating the receptor independently. Negative allosteric modulators decrease receptor responsiveness by reducing binding affinity or coupling efficiency. Biased agonists selectively activate specific signal transduction pathways linked to a single receptor, potentially separating desired therapeutic effects from unwanted adverse effects mediated through alternative signaling pathways.

Dose-Response Relationships and Pharmacodynamic Parameters

Dose-response relationships characterize the fundamental connection between drug concentration and observed effect, providing quantitative frameworks for therapeutic decision-making. Graded dose-response curves plot the relationship between drug dose or concentration and the magnitude of biological response, typically displaying a sigmoidal shape with distinct phases: a threshold region where minimal effect occurs despite increasing concentration; a steep middle portion where response increases rapidly with small concentration changes; and an upper plateau representing maximal effect where further concentration increases produce no additional response. Quantal dose-response curves describe the relationship between drug dose and the proportion of a population exhibiting a specified effect, forming the basis for therapeutic index determination and population-based dosing recommendations. Mathematical models describing these relationships include the Hill equation (also called the sigmoid Emax model), which incorporates key pharmacodynamic parameters: maximum effect (Emax) representing the greatest possible response; potency (EC50) indicating the concentration producing 50% of maximal effect; and the Hill coefficient reflecting the steepness of the dose-response curve and providing insights into cooperative binding or complex response mechanisms. Efficacy describes a drug's ability to produce a maximal response, with high-efficacy drugs capable of generating the full spectrum of biological effects associated with receptor activation. Potency reflects the drug concentration required to produce a specific effect, with more potent drugs requiring lower concentrations to achieve the same response. While potency influences dosing requirements, efficacy more directly determines therapeutic potential, making high-efficacy, low-potency drugs generally preferable to high-potency, low-efficacy alternatives when maximal effect is desired. The therapeutic index (or therapeutic window) represents the ratio between the dose producing toxicity and the dose producing therapeutic effect, typically calculated as TD50/ED50 (toxic dose in 50% of population divided by effective dose in 50%). Drugs with narrow therapeutic indices require careful dosing and monitoring to maintain concentrations within the range producing desired effects while avoiding toxicity. Factors influencing the therapeutic index include the relationship between receptor systems mediating therapeutic and toxic effects, pharmacokinetic variables affecting drug disposition, and individual patient characteristics modifying drug response.

Pharmacodynamic Variability and Individualization

Pharmacodynamic variability represents a significant source of differential drug response among patients, necessitating individualized approaches to therapy. Genetic polymorphisms affecting receptor structure, expression, or associated signaling pathways contribute substantially to response variation. Pharmacogenomic factors include variations in β-adrenergic receptors influencing response to beta-blockers; vitamin K epoxide reductase polymorphisms affecting warfarin sensitivity; and serotonin receptor variations impacting antidepressant efficacy. Age-related changes significantly modify pharmacodynamic responses throughout the lifespan. Neonates and infants often demonstrate increased sensitivity to centrally acting medications due to immature blood-brain barrier function and receptor development. Elderly patients frequently exhibit enhanced responses to central nervous system depressants, anticoagulants, and cardiovascular medications due to changes in receptor density, signal transduction efficiency, and homeostatic mechanisms. Disease states directly alter pharmacodynamic responses through multiple mechanisms. Receptor up-regulation or down-regulation occurs in various conditions, such as increased beta-receptor sensitivity following chronic beta-blocker withdrawal or reduced insulin receptor responsiveness in type 2 diabetes. Altered signal transduction pathways are evident in heart failure with modified beta-adrenergic signaling and in various malignancies with dysregulated growth factor signaling. Impaired homeostatic mechanisms, particularly prominent in hepatic or renal dysfunction, reduce the body's ability to compensate for pharmacological effects, potentially amplifying drug responses. Drug-drug interactions at the pharmacodynamic level occur through several mechanisms distinct from pharmacokinetic interactions. Additive effects emerge when drugs acting through similar mechanisms are combined, producing a total effect equal to the sum of individual effects. Synergistic interactions generate combined effects greater than the mathematical sum of individual drug effects, as observed with certain antimicrobial combinations. Antagonistic interactions result in combined effects less than expected from individual agents, potentially reducing therapeutic efficacy when interacting drugs are coadministered. Physiological tolerance develops with repeated drug exposure, manifesting as progressively diminished response despite consistent dosing. Mechanisms include receptor desensitization through phosphorylation and internalization; compensatory regulation of receptor expression; and adaptation of downstream signaling pathways. Tolerance development often necessitates dose escalation to maintain therapeutic effect, particularly evident with opioid analgesics, benzodiazepines, and various cardiovascular medications.

PHARMACOKINETICS

Pharmacokinetics examines the mathematical description of drug movement throughout the body, encompassing the processes of absorption, distribution, metabolism, and excretion (ADME). This quantitative discipline provides the scientific foundation for understanding how the body handles medications, allowing prediction of drug concentrations at target sites, optimization of dosing regimens, and explanation of variability in drug response. Pharmacokinetic principles guide critical clinical decisions including route of administration selection, dosage adjustment for special populations, and management of drug interactions affecting medication disposition.

Absorption and Bioavailability

Drug absorption encompasses the processes by which medications enter the systemic circulation from the site of administration, with efficiency and rate determined by multiple pharmaceutical, physiological, and pathological factors.

Absorption mechanisms vary by route of administration and drug properties, with passive diffusion representing the predominant process for most drugs. This movement along concentration gradients occurs most efficiently for lipophilic, non-ionized compounds with molecular weights below 500 daltons. Active transport systems utilize specialized membrane carriers to move specific drugs against concentration gradients, requiring energy expenditure and demonstrating capacity limitations, substrate specificity, and potential for competitive inhibition. Facilitated diffusion employs carrier proteins enabling movement along concentration gradients without energy requirements. Oral drug absorption presents particular complexity due to variable gastrointestinal conditions and extensive presystemic elimination. Factors influencing oral absorption include gastrointestinal pH affecting drug ionization and subsequent membrane permeability; gastric emptying time determining small intestine delivery rate; intestinal transit time controlling residence at absorption sites; intestinal surface area with significant reduction in various malabsorption syndromes; gastrointestinal blood flow distributing absorbed drug into the systemic circulation; and formulation characteristics including dissolution rate, particle size, and excipient effects. Alternative administration routes offer distinct absorption characteristics and clinical advantages. Sublingual and buccal administration bypass hepatic first-pass metabolism through direct absorption into systemic circulation via the oral mucosa, providing rapid onset for selected medications while avoiding degradation by gastrointestinal enzymes or pH.

Table 5.3: Pharmacokinetic Parameters and Clinical Applications

Parameter	Definition	Units
Absorption (F)	Fraction of dose reaching systemic circulation	Fraction (0-1)
Distribution (Vd)	Apparent volume into which drug distributes	L or L/kg
Protein Binding	Fraction bound to plasma proteins	Percentage
Clearance (CL)	Volume of blood cleared of drug per time	L/hr or mL/min
Half-life ($t^{1/2}$)	Time for concentration to decrease by 50%	Hours
Area Under Curve (AUC)	Concentration vs. time integral	mg·h/L
Volume of Distribution	Apparent volume drug distributes into	L or L/kg
Bioavailability	Fraction of dose reaching circulation	Percentage
Time to Peak (Tmax)	Time to maximum concentration	Hours
Maximum Concentration (Cmax)	Highest concentration achieved	mg/L
Elimination Rate Constant (ke)	Fractional rate of elimination	hr^{-1}
Loading Dose	Initial dose to reach target quickly	mg
Maintenance Dose	Dose to maintain steady state	mg
Steady State	When input equals output	N/A

Transdermal delivery permits controlled, sustained absorption through the skin, minimizing peak-trough fluctuations while enabling continuous administration and avoiding first-pass metabolism. Intramuscular injection provides faster absorption than subcutaneous routes due to greater blood flow, though absorption rate varies with injection site vascularity and can be intentionally modified through formulation adjustments. Intravenous administration eliminates the absorption phase entirely, delivering medications directly into the systemic circulation with immediate and complete bioavailability. Bioavailability quantifies the fraction of administered drug reaching systemic circulation intact, with values ranging from 0-100% and intravenous administration representing complete (100%) bioavailability by definition.

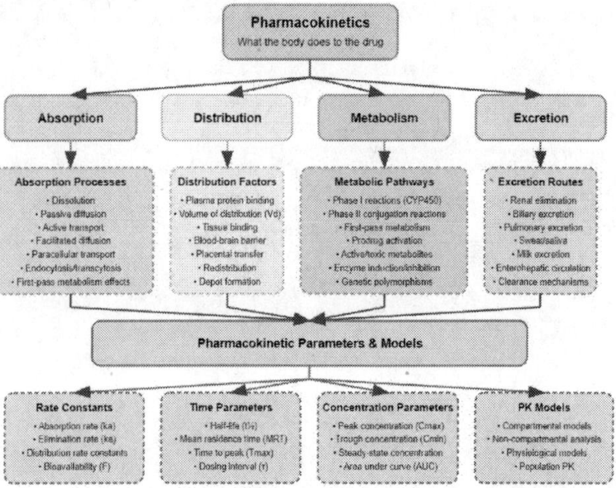

Figure 5.2: Pharmacokinetic Processes (ADME)

Absolute bioavailability compares systemic exposure from a specific route to intravenous administration, while relative bioavailability compares different formulations or routes without intravenous reference. First-pass metabolism significantly reduces bioavailability for many orally administered drugs through hepatic extraction following absorption into the portal circulation, with high-extraction drugs particularly susceptible to this effect. Bioequivalence assessment compares formulations based on rate and extent of absorption, with products considered bioequivalent when the 90% confidence intervals for key pharmacokinetic parameters (maximum concentration and area under the curve) fall within 80-125% of the reference product.

Drug Distribution and Protein Binding

Distribution describes the reversible transfer of drugs from the systemic circulation to peripheral tissues, determining medication concentrations at target and non-target sites throughout the body. Volume of distribution (Vd) represents a fundamental pharmacokinetic parameter relating the amount of drug in the body to measured plasma concentration. This theoretical volume, calculated as the ratio of drug dose to plasma concentration, does not correspond to an actual physiological space but provides valuable information about drug disposition characteristics. Small volumes (0.04-0.2 L/kg) typically indicate restriction to plasma compartment due to high protein binding or hydrophilicity limiting tissue penetration. Moderate volumes (0.2-0.7 L/kg) suggest distribution throughout total body water. Large volumes (>1 L/kg) indicate extensive tissue binding or sequestration, with extremely large values (>10 L/kg) typical of highly lipophilic drugs with extensive tissue accumulation. Physiological barriers significantly influence drug distribution patterns. The blood-brain barrier, composed of tight junctions between cerebral endothelial cells, restricts central nervous system penetration to highly lipophilic compounds or those utilizing specific transport systems. The placental barrier allows transfer of most lipophilic medications between maternal and fetal circulations, with fetal exposure influenced by placental blood flow, protein binding differences, and placental metabolism. The blood-testis barrier protects germinal epithelium from potentially harmful substances through tight junctions between Sertoli cells. Plasma protein binding temporarily renders medications pharmacologically inactive by preventing bound fraction from crossing cell membranes or interacting with target receptors. Albumin serves as the primary binding protein for acidic and neutral drugs, while alpha-1-acid glycoprotein preferentially binds basic compounds. The extent of protein binding, expressed as percentage bound, ranges from minimal (<30%) to extensive (>99%), with highly bound drugs demonstrating smaller volumes of distribution, longer elimination half-lives due to reduced clearance, and greater potential for displacement interactions. Clinical significance of protein binding depends on several factors including binding extent, therapeutic index, and clearance mechanisms. Highly bound drugs with narrow therapeutic indices are most susceptible to clinically significant displacement interactions, though compensatory clearance changes often moderate the impact of acute binding alterations. Displacement increases free drug concentration temporarily until elimination of unbound drug establishes a new steady state, potentially causing transient toxicity during this adjustment period. Pathophysiological conditions altering protein binding include hypoalbuminemia in hepatic dysfunction, nephrotic syndrome, or malnutrition; altered alpha-1-acid glycoprotein levels in acute inflammatory conditions; and uremia with accumulated endogenous binding competitors, all potentially necessitating dose adjustments for highly bound medications with narrow therapeutic indices.

Drug Metabolism and Biotransformation

Drug metabolism represents the enzymatic conversion of medications to more polar, water-soluble metabolites facilitating elimination through renal or biliary excretion pathways. This process typically renders lipophilic drugs more hydrophilic, though occasionally generates active metabolites with therapeutic or toxic properties distinct from the parent compound. Hepatic metabolism predominates for most medications, though significant biotransformation occurs in various extrahepatic sites including intestinal mucosa, lungs, kidneys, skin, and plasma. Phase I reactions introduce or expose polar functional groups through oxidation, reduction, or hydrolysis, modestly increasing water solubility while often generating reactive intermediates requiring further metabolism. Cytochrome P450 (CYP450) enzymes catalyze the majority of phase I oxidative reactions through a superfamily of heme-containing isoenzymes with distinct but overlapping substrate specificities. Major isoforms contributing to drug metabolism include CYP3A4/5 (involved in metabolism of approximately 50% of marketed drugs), CYP2D6, CYP2C9, CYP2C19, CYP1A2, and CYP2E1. Genetic polymorphisms significantly affect activity of several isoenzymes, creating distinct phenotypes including poor metabolizers lacking functional enzyme, intermediate metabolizers with reduced activity, extensive metabolizers with normal function, and ultrarapid metabolizers with multiple gene copies or enhanced expression. Phase II conjugation reactions attach endogenous substrates to drugs or phase I metabolites, dramatically increasing water solubility while typically inactivating pharmacological activity. Major conjugation pathways include glucuronidation catalyzed by UDP-glucuronosyltransferases; sulfation through sulfotransferases; acetylation via N-acetyltransferases demonstrating clinically significant genetic polymorphisms; glutathione conjugation particularly important for detoxifying reactive intermediates; and methylation through methyltransferases. Factors influencing metabolic capacity include genetic determinants creating interindividual variability in enzyme expression and function; age-related changes with reduced activity in neonates and modest decline in elderly patients; sex differences affecting specific isoenzyme expression; disease states particularly hepatic dysfunction directly reducing metabolic capacity; and enzyme induction or inhibition through drug interactions or environmental exposures. Enzyme induction results from increased protein synthesis following exposure to certain medications or environmental compounds, typically developing over several days and persisting for similar duration after inducer discontinuation. Common inducers include rifampin, phenytoin, carbamazepine, phenobarbital, and St. John's wort, predominantly affecting CYP3A4, CYP2C9, and CYP2C19 with potential for reduced efficacy of coadministered substrates.

Table 5.4: Drug Metabolism Pathways and Examples

Phase	Enzyme/Process	Reaction Type	Example Drugs
Phase I	CYP3A4	Oxidation	Midazolam, cyclosporine
Phase I	CYP2D6	Oxidation	Codeine, metoprolol
Phase I	CYP2C9	Oxidation	Warfarin, phenytoin
Phase I	CYP2C19	Oxidation	Omeprazole, clopidogrel
Phase I	CYP1A2	Oxidation	Theophylline, caffeine
Phase I	CYP2E1	Oxidation	Acetaminophen, ethanol
Phase I	Alcohol Dehydrogenase	Oxidation	Ethanol, methanol
Phase I	Esterases	Hydrolysis	Aspirin, enalapril
Phase I	Reduction	Reduction	Chloramphenicol, warfarin
Phase II	UGT	Glucuronidation	Morphine, acetaminophen
Phase II	SULT	Sulfation	Acetaminophen, minoxidil
Phase II	GST	Glutathione conjugation	Busulfan, ethacrynic acid
Phase II	NAT	Acetylation	Isoniazid, hydralazine
Phase II	COMT	Methylation	Levodopa, catecholamines
Phase II	TPMT	Methylation	6-mercaptopurine, azathioprine

Enzyme inhibition occurs through various mechanisms including competitive binding to active sites, formation of inactive complexes, and reduced enzyme synthesis, typically developing more rapidly than induction and resolving based on inhibitor elimination. Potent inhibitors include azole antifungals, macrolide antibiotics, protease inhibitors, and grapefruit juice components, with effects potentially causing toxicity from accumulated substrate drugs, particularly those with narrow therapeutic indices.

Drug Excretion and Clearance Concepts

Drug excretion encompasses the processes removing medications and their metabolites from the body, with renal elimination representing the predominant pathway for most water-soluble compounds and their metabolites. Renal drug excretion involves three distinct processes: glomerular filtration of unbound drug, dependent on molecular size and plasma protein binding; tubular secretion through active transport systems for selected compounds, independent of protein binding; and tubular reabsorption of lipophilic, non-ionized molecules following concentration in tubular filtrate. Net renal elimination reflects the combined effect of these processes, with clearance values potentially exceeding glomerular filtration rate when secretion contributes significantly. Biliary excretion provides an important alternative elimination pathway, particularly for high molecular weight compounds (>500 daltons) and extensively conjugated metabolites. This process involves active transport systems facilitating movement from hepatocytes into bile, with subsequent elimination through feces or potential reabsorption through enterohepatic circulation. This recycling process extends the presence of certain medications including oral contraceptives, digitoxin, and phenothiazines through intestinal hydrolysis of conjugates and reabsorption of parent compounds. Additional excretion pathways include pulmonary elimination significant primarily for volatile anesthetics and alcohols; secretion into breast milk creating potential for neonatal exposure; incorporation into hair and nails providing long-term detection markers; and exocrine gland secretion into sweat, saliva, and tears, generally contributing minimally to total elimination. Clearance represents the fundamental pharmacokinetic parameter quantifying the body's ability to eliminate drugs, defined as the volume of blood completely cleared of drug per unit time. Total body clearance reflects the combined contribution of all elimination pathways and directly determines drug concentration at steady state for any given dosing rate. Organ clearance depends on both blood flow delivering drug to the eliminating organ and the organ's extraction efficiency, with high-extraction drugs (>70% removed during single organ passage) demonstrating flow-limited clearance particularly sensitive to perfusion changes. Low-extraction drugs (<30% removed) exhibit capacity-limited clearance more dependent on enzymatic activity or transport function than blood flow. First-order kinetics characterize most drug elimination processes, with the rate of elimination directly proportional to concentration and constant fraction eliminated per unit time. This pattern produces exponential concentration decline with consistent half-life regardless of concentration. Zero-order kinetics occur when elimination mechanisms become saturated, resulting in constant amount eliminated per unit time independent of concentration, as observed with ethanol, phenytoin, and salicylates at higher concentrations. This pattern produces linear concentration decline and dose-dependent half-life prolongation. Special population considerations for drug elimination include pediatric patients with immature renal function at birth gradually developing adult capacity; elderly individuals experiencing age-related nephron loss with approximately 40% reduction in glomerular filtration by age 80; and patients with renal or hepatic dysfunction requiring careful dosage adjustment based on quantitative assessment of remaining organ function through creatinine clearance estimation or liver function classification.

DRUG-DRUG INTERACTIONS

Drug-drug interactions occur when the administration of one medication alters the clinical effect of another, potentially resulting in decreased therapeutic efficacy, enhanced toxicity, or occasionally beneficial effects. These interactions represent a significant source of preventable medication-related problems, with prevalence increasing exponentially with the number of concurrent medications. Understanding the mechanisms, clinical significance, and management strategies for drug interactions enables pharmacists to identify, predict, and mitigate potential adverse outcomes while optimizing therapeutic regimens for patients requiring multiple medications.

Pharmacokinetic Interaction Mechanisms

Pharmacokinetic interactions alter the concentration of medications at target sites by modifying absorption, distribution, metabolism, or excretion processes. Absorption interactions affect the rate or extent of gastrointestinal drug uptake through various mechanisms. Chelation and complex formation create nonabsorbable compounds, exemplified by tetracycline binding with calcium, aluminum, or iron resulting in significantly reduced antibiotic bioavailability. Gastric pH alterations by acid-suppressing medications can reduce absorption of drugs requiring acidic environments for dissolution (ketoconazole, itraconazole) while enhancing uptake of acid-labile compounds. Gastrointestinal motility changes influence drug transit time and absorption opportunity, with metoclopramide-accelerated emptying potentially reducing absorption of slowly dissolving formulations while anticholinergic-induced delay may enhance uptake.

Table 5.5: Common Drug-Drug Interactions and Their Mechanisms

Mechanism	Interacting Drugs	Effect
CYP3A4 Inhibition	Ketoconazole + midazolam	↑ midazolam levels, excessive sedation
CYP3A4 Induction	Rifampin + oral contraceptives	↓ contraceptive efficacy, pregnancy risk
CYP2D6 Inhibition	Fluoxetine + codeine	↓ codeine efficacy (blocks activation)
P-glycoprotein Inhibition	Verapamil + digoxin	↑ digoxin levels, toxicity risk
Protein Binding Displacement	Warfarin + sulfonamides	↑ free warfarin, bleeding risk
Absorption Impairment	Tetracycline + calcium	↓ tetracycline absorption, reduced efficacy
Pharmacodynamic Antagonism	β-blockers + β-agonists	Reduced efficacy of both
Pharmacodynamic Synergism	Warfarin + aspirin	↑ bleeding risk
QT Prolongation	Amiodarone + fluoroquinolones	↑ risk of Torsades de Pointes
Serotonin Syndrome	SSRIs + MAOIs	Potentially fatal serotonin excess
CNS Depression	Benzodiazepines + opioids	Respiratory depression, fatal overdose
Hyperkalemia	ACEIs + potassium-sparing diuretics	Dangerous potassium elevation
Nephrotoxicity	NSAIDs + aminoglycosides	Additive kidney damage
Lithium Toxicity	Lithium + thiazide diuretics	↑ lithium levels, toxicity
Digoxin Toxicity	Digoxin + amiodarone	↑ digoxin levels, toxicity

P-glycoprotein inhibition affects drugs subject to intestinal efflux, with inhibitors including verapamil, cyclosporine, and certain antiretrovirals increasing absorption of substrates such as digoxin, tacrolimus, and selected chemotherapeutics. Distribution interactions primarily involve displacement from plasma protein binding sites, with clinical significance limited to highly bound drugs (>90%) having narrow therapeutic indices and limited distribution volumes.

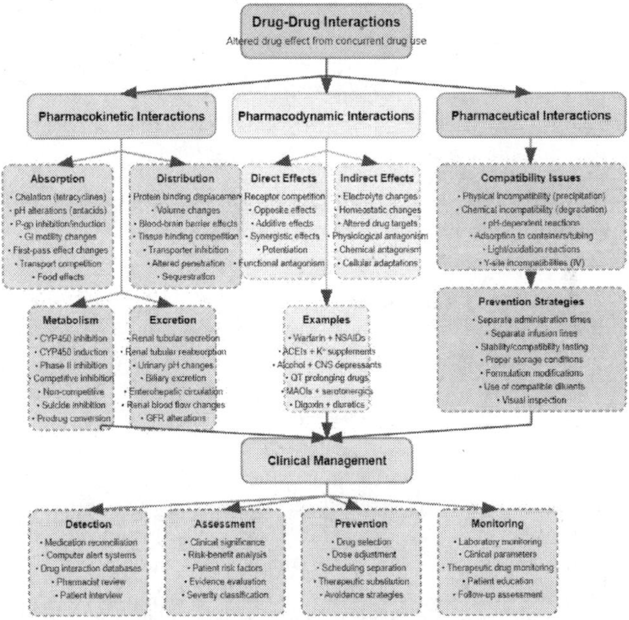

Figure 5.3: Drug-Drug Interaction Mechanisms

Warfarin displacement by sulfonamides, phenytoin, and valproic acid exemplifies this mechanism, potentially causing transient anticoagulation enhancement until hepatic clearance of increased free drug establishes new steady state. Metabolism interactions represent the most common and clinically significant pharmacokinetic interactions, predominantly involving cytochrome P450 enzymes. Enzyme inhibition occurs through competitive or non-competitive mechanisms, developing rapidly and persisting based on inhibitor elimination. Strong CYP3A4 inhibitors including ketoconazole, clarithromycin, and ritonavir can increase substrate concentrations by several-fold, creating significant toxicity risk for narrow therapeutic index medications. Enzyme induction develops more gradually through increased protein synthesis, typically requiring several days for maximal effect and similar duration for resolution following inducer discontinuation. Potent inducers including rifampin, carbamazepine, and phenytoin can substantially reduce concentrations of susceptible substrates, potentially causing therapeutic failure. Excretion interactions affect renal drug elimination through various mechanisms. Competition for active tubular secretion occurs with organic anion or cation transporters, exemplified by probenecid inhibition of penicillin secretion historically used to extend antibiotic effect. Urinary pH manipulation alters reabsorption of ionizable compounds, with alkalinization enhancing elimination of acidic drugs through ion trapping while accelerating reabsorption of basic compounds. Renal blood flow modifications by NSAIDs or ACE inhibitors can reduce drug filtration, potentially contributing to methotrexate toxicity or accumulation of renally eliminated medications.

Pharmacodynamic Interaction Mechanisms

Pharmacodynamic interactions involve altered drug effects at target sites without concentration changes, occurring through receptor-level modifications or physiological pathway interactions. Direct receptor interactions encompass several mechanisms producing altered responses. Receptor competition involves drugs targeting identical binding sites, exemplified by naloxone displacement of opioids from mu receptors, directly reversing analgesic and respiratory depressant effects. Receptor sensitization or desensitization alters response magnitude to concurrent or subsequent medications, as observed with tricyclic antidepressant enhancement of sympathomimetic effects through norepinephrine reuptake inhibition. Sequential block of compensatory responses occurs when medications interfere with physiological adaptations normally limiting drug effects, illustrated by beta-blocker prevention of reflex tachycardia typically compensating for nitrate-induced vasodilation, potentially causing severe hypotension. Physiological antagonism involves drugs producing opposing effects through different mechanisms, such as beta-agonist bronchodilation counteracting beta-blocker bronchoconstriction or benzodiazepine sedation opposing caffeine stimulation. Additive interactions produce combined effects approximately equal to the sum of individual drug effects when agents act through similar mechanisms or pathways. This pattern occurs with medications from the same therapeutic class (multiple benzodiazepines causing enhanced sedation) or different classes with similar physiological effects (combined antihypertensives from complementary classes producing additive blood pressure reduction). Synergistic interactions generate effects greater than the mathematical sum of individual drug actions, providing therapeutic benefit in controlled circumstances or unexpected toxicity in unintended combinations. Beneficial synergy underlies combination antimicrobial therapy with trimethoprim-sulfamethoxazole inhibiting sequential steps in bacterial folate synthesis, while dangerous synergy appears with combined serotonergic agents potentially precipitating serotonin syndrome. Potentiation occurs when one drug enhances another's effect without producing similar action independently, exemplified by clavulanic acid inhibition of beta-lactamase protecting concurrently administered beta-lactam antibiotics without direct antimicrobial activity. Organ system-specific interactions affect particular physiological systems through combined medication effects. Central nervous system interactions frequently involve additive or synergistic sedation with concurrent administration of alcohol, benzodiazepines, opioids, antihistamines, and numerous other centrally acting medications. Cardiovascular interactions include enhanced hypotension with multiple antihypertensives, phosphodiesterase inhibitors with nitrates, or QT interval-prolonging medications increasing arrhythmia risk when combined. Renal function interactions involve nephrotoxic potential enhancement when combining multiple agents affecting kidney perfusion, tubular function, or direct cellular toxicity, as observed with aminoglycosides, NSAIDs, and radiocontrast agents.

Clinical Significance Assessment and Management

Clinical significance assessment distinguishes interactions requiring intervention from theoretical concerns with minimal practical impact, guiding appropriate management decisions. Risk assessment incorporates multiple factors determining interaction consequence probability and severity. Pharmacokinetic interaction magnitude significantly influences clinical relevance, with concentration changes less than 50% rarely causing meaningful effects for most medications, while several-fold increases may produce toxicity even with wider therapeutic index drugs. Therapeutic index represents a critical determinant of interaction importance, with narrow index medications (warfarin, digoxin, antiseizure drugs, immunosuppressants) much more susceptible to clinically significant effects from moderate concentration changes. Concentration-response relationship steepness affects how pharmacokinetic changes translate to clinical effects, with steep curves (characteristic of many anticoagulants and antiarrhythmics) producing substantial response changes from modest concentration alterations. Patient specific factors modifying interaction significance include age-related elimination capacity changes; organ dysfunction affecting metabolic or excretion pathways; genetic polymorphisms influencing baseline metabolic capacity; and comorbidities potentially enhancing susceptibility to specific adverse effects. Documentation quality guides clinical decision-making through literature evaluation, considering study design strength, consistent findings across multiple reports, biological plausibility based on known mechanisms, and publication in peer-reviewed sources. Management strategies implement hierarchical approaches based on interaction severity and therapeutic alternatives. Avoidance represents the preferred strategy for severe, well-documented interactions when therapeutic alternatives exist, involving selection of non-interacting alternatives for either interacting medication based on therapeutic necessity. Separation of administration times effectively manages interactions involving physical or chemical incompatibility, chelation, or altered absorption, with separation interval determined by specific interaction mechanism and drug pharmacokinetics. Dose adjustment compensates for anticipated pharmacokinetic changes, either empirically based on typical interaction magnitude or through therapeutic drug monitoring when available, particularly valuable for narrow therapeutic index medications. Enhanced monitoring detects early signs of interaction consequences when complete avoidance proves impractical, with monitoring parameters and frequency determined by specific interaction effects and onset timing. Patient education regarding potential interaction manifestations, monitoring parameters, and reporting instructions provides an additional safety layer when patients receive potentially interacting combinations.

Significant Interaction Categories and Examples

Specific interaction categories demonstrate characteristic patterns requiring particular attention in pharmacy practice. Anticoagulant interactions represent frequent concerns due to narrow therapeutic indices and serious bleeding consequences from excessive anticoagulation. Warfarin demonstrates numerous significant interactions: potentiation through displacement from protein binding (sulfonamides); enhanced effect via CYP2C9 inhibition (amiodarone, fluconazole); reduced activity through enzyme induction (rifampin, carbamazepine); and altered vitamin K status affecting response (antibiotics disrupting gut flora). Direct oral anticoagulants interact primarily through P-glycoprotein transport pathways, with inhibitors including verapamil and dronedarone increasing concentrations and bleeding risk. Anti-infective interactions include several clinically significant patterns. Macrolide antibiotics (especially clarithromycin) and azole antifungals (particularly ketoconazole, itraconazole) potently inhibit CYP3A4, increasing concentrations of numerous substrates including statins (myopathy risk), benzodiazepines (excessive sedation), and immunosuppressants (toxicity potential). Rifamycins powerfully induce multiple CYP enzymes, dramatically reducing concentrations of hormonal contraceptives (contraceptive failure), antiretrovirals (virologic failure), and immunosuppressants (rejection risk). Fluoroquinolones form nonabsorbable complexes with multivalent cations, significantly reducing antibiotic effectiveness when administered with calcium, iron, or aluminum-containing products. Cardiovascular medication interactions include several clinically important combinations. Potassium-sparing diuretics with potassium supplements or ACE inhibitors create hyperkalemia risk through complementary mechanisms increasing serum potassium. Simvastatin undergoes extensive CYP3A4 metabolism with significantly increased myopathy risk when combined with inhibitors including certain calcium channel blockers (diltiazem, verapamil) and amiodarone, necessitating dose limitations or statin alternatives. Combined negative chronotropic agents (beta-blockers, non-dihydropyridine calcium channel blockers, digoxin) create additive effects potentially causing severe bradycardia or heart block. Central nervous system medication interactions frequently involve pharmacodynamic mechanisms with additive effects. Serotonin syndrome risk increases with combined serotonergic agents including SSRIs, SNRIs, tricyclic antidepressants, MAO inhibitors, triptans, and certain opioids (tramadol, meperidine), presenting with autonomic instability, neuromuscular abnormalities, and mental status changes. Neuroleptic malignant syndrome demonstrates similar presentation with combined dopamine antagonists or abrupt dopamine agonist withdrawal. Monoamine oxidase inhibitors create potentially fatal interactions with sympathomimetics and tyramine-containing foods through impaired catecholamine metabolism, producing hypertensive crisis, and with various antidepressants causing serotonin syndrome or hyperthermic crisis.

ADVERSE DRUG REACTIONS

Adverse drug reactions (ADRs) encompass noxious, unintended responses to medications occurring at doses normally used for prophylaxis, diagnosis, or treatment. These events represent a significant public health concern, contributing substantially to morbidity, mortality, and healthcare costs while potentially undermining medication adherence and therapeutic outcomes. Understanding ADR classification, predisposing factors, detection methods, and management strategies enables pharmacists to implement effective prevention programs, identify reactions promptly, and minimize associated harm through appropriate interventions.

Classification and Mechanisms of Adverse Drug Reactions

Adverse drug reactions can be classified through various frameworks providing complementary perspectives on their nature, predictability, and underlying mechanisms. The traditional classification distinguishes between Type A (augmented) and Type B (bizarre) reactions based on relationship to known pharmacology. Type A reactions represent extensions of known pharmacological effects, accounting for approximately 80% of all ADRs. These dose-dependent, predictable reactions typically demonstrate clear relationship to plasma concentration and respond to dose reduction. Examples include hypoglycemia with insulin, respiratory depression with opioids, and bleeding with anticoagulants. Type B reactions occur independently of known drug pharmacology, appearing unpredictably in susceptible individuals without clear dose-response relationship. These idiosyncratic reactions include immunologically mediated hypersensitivity and genetically determined abnormalities in drug metabolism or target structures. Examples include penicillin anaphylaxis, abacavir hypersensitivity, and malignant hyperthermia with anesthetic agents. Extended classification systems incorporate additional categories: Type C (chronic) reactions resulting from cumulative dose effects, such as hypothalamic-pituitary-adrenal axis suppression with corticosteroids; Type D (delayed) reactions appearing after prolonged latency periods, exemplified by teratogenesis and carcinogenesis; Type E (end-of-treatment) reactions occurring upon drug withdrawal, including adrenal insufficiency following steroid discontinuation and rebound hypertension after clonidine cessation; and Type F (failure) reactions representing unexpected therapeutic failures due to drug interactions or rapid metabolism.

Mechanistic classification provides insight into underlying processes causing adverse effects. Pharmacological ADRs directly result from primary or secondary pharmacological actions, including both therapeutic target effects at excessive levels and actions at non-target receptors producing predictable side effects. On-target adverse effects represent extension of intended mechanism beyond therapeutic needs, as with excessive blood pressure reduction causing symptomatic hypotension. Off-target effects result from drug actions at unintended receptors or pathways, exemplified by H_1-antihistamine binding to muscarinic receptors causing anticholinergic side effects. Immunological ADRs involve adaptive immune responses to drugs acting as immunogens or haptens when bound to carrier proteins. These reactions follow classic hypersensitivity patterns: Type I (IgE-mediated) reactions causing anaphylaxis and urticaria; Type II (cytotoxic) reactions involving antibody-dependent cell destruction as in drug-induced hemolytic anemia; Type III (immune complex) reactions such as serum sickness; and Type IV (delayed-type) hypersensitivity manifesting as contact dermatitis and certain drug rashes. Idiosyncratic ADRs occur through genetically determined mechanisms without immune system involvement, often resulting from metabolic pathway variations generating toxic intermediates or altered drug targets.

Table 5.6: Major Adverse Drug Reactions and Their Mechanisms

Reaction Type	Mechanism	Example Drugs
Type A (Augmented)	Exaggerated pharmacological effect	Opioids, anticoagulants
Type B (Bizarre)	Immunological/genetic	Penicillins, carbamazepine
Type C (Chronic)	Cumulative effect	Corticosteroids, NSAIDs
Type D (Delayed)	Carcinogenesis, teratogenesis	Thalidomide, isotretinoin
Type E (End of use)	Withdrawal	Benzodiazepines, opioids
Idiosyncratic	Unpredictable, genetic	Halothane, sulfonamides
Allergic	Immune-mediated	β-lactams, sulfonamides
Pseudoallergic	Non-immune histamine release	Vancomycin, opioids
Direct Toxicity	Cellular damage	Acetaminophen, cisplatin
Secondary Effects	Microbial resistance, imbalance	Antibiotics, immunosuppressants
Teratogenic	Fetal development disruption	Isotretinoin, thalidomide
Carcinogenic	DNA damage/mutation	Alkylating agents, estrogens
Organ-specific	Target organ damage	NSAIDs, aminoglycosides
Drug-disease Interactions	Disease alters drug response	β-blockers in asthma

Risk Factors and Predisposing Conditions

Multiple factors influence individual susceptibility to adverse drug reactions, with identification of high-risk patients enabling implementation of preventive strategies and enhanced monitoring. Age represents a significant risk factor across the lifespan. Pediatric patients demonstrate altered susceptibility due to developing metabolic pathways, different body composition, and age-specific vulnerability of certain organ systems, exemplified by sulfonamide displacement of bilirubin causing kernicterus in neonates. Geriatric patients experience increased ADR risk through multiple mechanisms including reduced renal and hepatic clearance, altered body composition affecting drug distribution, diminished physiological reserve limiting compensation for pharmacological effects, and increased regimen complexity creating interaction potential.

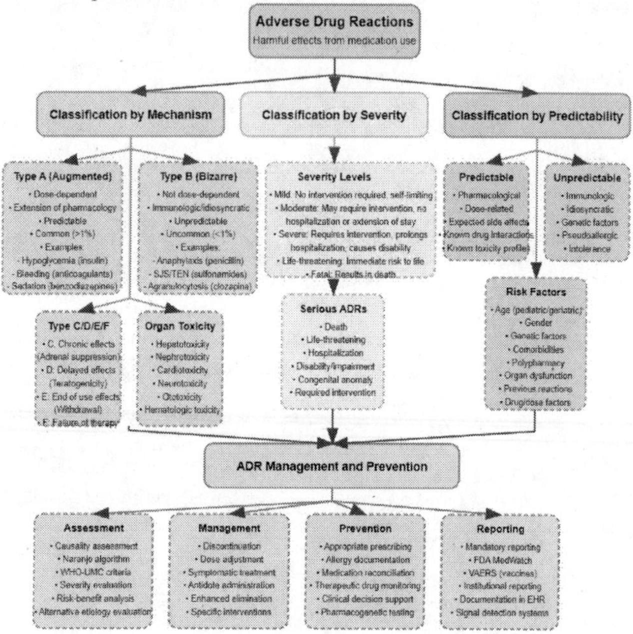

Figure 5.4: Adverse Drug Reaction Classification and Management

Sex differences influence ADR susceptibility through pharmacokinetic variations including generally lower body weight, higher body fat percentage, and hormonal influences on drug metabolism in females; and pharmacodynamic differences in receptor expression and sensitivity. Women experience approximately 1.5-1.7 times higher ADR incidence than men, with greater risk for dose-related reactions including torsades de pointes with QT-prolonging medications and hepatotoxicity with certain drugs. Genetic factors significantly impact ADR susceptibility through polymorphisms affecting pharmacokinetic and pharmacodynamic processes. Metabolic variations include ultrarapid CYP2D6 metabolism causing codeine toxicity through rapid morphine generation; CYP2C9 variants reducing warfarin clearance and increasing bleeding risk; and TPMT deficiency causing thiopurine-induced myelosuppression. Pharmacodynamic variations include malignant hyperthermia susceptibility with ryanodine receptor mutations and glucose-6-phosphate dehydrogenase deficiency predisposing to hemolysis with oxidizing medications. HLA associations with specific ADRs have been identified, including HLA-B57:01 with abacavir hypersensitivity, HLA-B15:02 with carbamazepine-induced Stevens-Johnson syndrome in Asian populations, and HLA-B*58:01 with allopurinol-induced severe cutaneous reactions. Concurrent disease states modify ADR risk through multiple mechanisms. Renal impairment increases toxicity risk for renally eliminated medications through reduced clearance, with aminoglycoside nephrotoxicity and metformin lactic acidosis representing notable examples requiring careful dosing adjustment. Hepatic dysfunction affects metabolism of numerous medications while reducing serum albumin and altering protein binding. Cardiovascular disease enhances susceptibility to hypotensive effects, QT prolongation, and fluid retention with various medications. Previous ADR history strongly predicts recurrence risk, particularly for immunologically mediated reactions demonstrating cross-reactivity within chemical classes. Polypharmacy represents perhaps the most significant modifiable risk factor, with ADR probability increasing exponentially rather than linearly with medication count due to complex interaction potential and additive toxicities.

Detection, Assessment, and Reporting

Detection, assessment, and reporting of adverse drug reactions require systematic approaches ensuring timely identification, accurate causality determination, and appropriate documentation to enhance patient safety and contribute to pharmacovigilance efforts. Detection methodologies encompass various strategies with complementary strengths. Direct patient assessment through structured questioning, physical examination, and laboratory monitoring provides real-time identification of potential ADRs during patient care encounters. Targeted monitoring applies heightened surveillance to high-risk medications, using standardized protocols tracking specific parameters: complete blood counts for myelosuppressive agents; liver function tests for hepatotoxic medications; QT interval monitoring for drugs prolonging cardiac repolarization; and renal function assessment for potentially nephrotoxic compounds. Computerized surveillance systems employ algorithms identifying laboratory abnormalities, medication patterns, or diagnostic codes suggesting potential ADRs, generating alerts for clinical evaluation. Signal detection methodologies analyze spontaneous reporting databases, electronic health records, or administrative claims data to identify disproportionate adverse event associations with specific medications compared to background rates. Causality assessment determines the probability of causal relationship between drug exposure and observed adverse event through structured evaluation frameworks. The Naranjo Algorithm quantifies causality probability through ten weighted questions addressing temporal relationship, dechallenge/rechallenge information, alternative explanations, plasma concentrations, dose-response relationship, previous reports, and placebo response, generating scores categorizing reactions as definite, probable, possible, or doubtful. The WHO-UMC system employs similar criteria without numerical scoring, classifying reactions based on temporal plausibility, alternative explanation likelihood, dechallenge/rechallenge information, and previous knowledge of the reaction. Bradford Hill criteria evaluate broader evidence for causal relationships, considering strength of association, consistency across reports, specificity, temporal relationship, biological gradient (dose-response), biological plausibility, coherence with existing knowledge, experimental evidence, and analogy with similar substances. Severity grading standardizes reaction classification using structured scales such as the Common Terminology Criteria for Adverse Events (CTCAE) ranging from Grade 1 (mild) through Grade 5 (death), facilitating consistent communication and appropriate intervention matching. Preventability assessment evaluates whether reactions were avoidable through optimal medication management, identifying opportunities for system improvement and error prevention. Reporting systems capture ADR information supporting both individual patient care and broader pharmacovigilance efforts. Institutional reporting utilizes standardized documentation within healthcare facilities, supporting quality improvement initiatives while facilitating communication among providers. Regulatory reporting through systems including the FDA's MedWatch program collects spontaneous reports from healthcare professionals and consumers, generating signals for further investigation. Manufacturers maintain pharmacovigilance departments collecting and analyzing adverse event reports, with regulatory obligations for serious reaction reporting within strict timeframes.

Management and Prevention Strategies

Management and prevention of adverse drug reactions require comprehensive approaches addressing both individual patient care and system-level interventions to reduce occurrence and minimize negative outcomes. Acute management principles depend on reaction type and severity while following general response frameworks. Severe or life-threatening reactions necessitate immediate drug discontinuation, focused symptomatic management, and consideration of specific antidotes or reversal agents when available. Anaphylaxis requires prompt epinephrine administration, airway management, and supportive care; cytochrome P450-mediated hepatotoxicity may benefit from N-acetylcysteine; heparin-induced thrombocytopenia requires alternative anticoagulation; and warfarin overanticoagulation can be reversed with vitamin K, prothrombin complex concentrates, or fresh frozen plasma depending on urgency. Less severe reactions permit more nuanced approaches, potentially including dose reduction, administration modification, prophylactic co-therapy addressing predictable side effects, or continued therapy with enhanced monitoring when benefits substantially outweigh risks. Non-immunological cutaneous reactions often resolve with continued therapy, while severe reactions including Stevens-Johnson syndrome require immediate discontinuation and specialized supportive care. Prevention strategies operate at multiple levels within healthcare systems. Medication selection optimization represents the foundation of prevention, considering patient-specific risk factors and selecting alternatives with more favorable safety profiles when appropriate. This process includes avoiding medications with known risk in susceptible populations, such as selecting non-thiazide diuretics in patients with gout history or avoiding QT-prolonging agents in those with congenital long QT syndrome. Dosing individualization addresses patient characteristics affecting pharmacokinetics and pharmacodynamics, including weight-based calculations; age-appropriate adjustments; organ function consideration for hepatically or renally eliminated drugs; and genetic information when available for medications with significant pharmacogenomic variability. Initial dose titration with "start low, go slow" approaches reduces ADR risk, particularly in elderly patients and those receiving medications with narrow therapeutic indices. Monitoring programs implement structured surveillance for specific ADRs, including baseline assessment establishing reference values; scheduled follow-up evaluations detecting changes from baseline; clearly defined parameters triggering intervention; and appropriate frequency balancing detection sensitivity against resource utilization. Patient education enhances safety through improved recognition and reporting of potential ADRs; understanding of monitoring requirements and follow-up schedules; knowledge of warning signs necessitating immediate medical attention; and adherence to administration instructions minimizing adverse effect risk. System-level interventions create organizational structures supporting ADR prevention. Computerized physician order entry with clinical decision support provides real-time alerts regarding potential drug interactions, duplicate therapy, contraindications, and dose appropriateness based on patient-specific factors. Medication reconciliation at transitions of care prevents unintended discrepancies creating ADR risk through duplication, omission, or interaction.

Summary

Pharmacology provides the scientific framework explaining how medications interact with biological systems to produce therapeutic and adverse effects. Pharmacodynamics examines drug-receptor interactions and subsequent biochemical responses, categorizing receptors into families including G-protein coupled receptors, ligand-gated ion channels, enzyme-linked receptors, and nuclear receptors. These interactions produce dose-response relationships characterized by potency, efficacy, therapeutic index, and receptor selectivity parameters. Receptor activation may trigger agonist (full or partial), antagonist, or inverse agonist effects, while allosteric modulators modify receptor function indirectly. Complementing these principles, pharmacokinetic processes govern medication movement throughout the body through four fundamental phases: absorption across biological membranes, distribution to tissues and binding to plasma proteins, metabolism via Phase I and II enzymatic transformations, and elimination through renal and biliary pathways. Mathematical models quantify these processes using parameters including bioavailability, volume of distribution, clearance, and half-life, allowing personalized dosing regimens accounting for patient-specific factors. Drug interactions represent a significant clinical consideration, occurring through pharmacokinetic mechanisms affecting absorption (chelation, pH alterations), distribution (protein binding displacement), metabolism (enzyme induction or inhibition), and elimination (competition for transporters), or through pharmacodynamic mechanisms involving receptor competition, signal transduction modification, or physiological antagonism. These interactions can produce therapeutic failures or toxicity requiring intervention. Adverse drug reactions manifest through predictable Type A reactions reflecting exaggerated pharmacological effects, unpredictable Type B idiosyncratic or immunological reactions, chronic Type C effects emerging with prolonged therapy, and delayed Type D responses including carcinogenesis and teratogenesis.

Multiple Choice Questions

1. Which of the following best describes a partial agonist?
   a) A drug that binds to a receptor but produces no response
   b) A drug that binds to a receptor and produces a submaximal response even at saturating concentrations
   c) A drug that binds to multiple receptor types with equal affinity
   d) A drug that produces an opposite effect to that of an agonist
2. A drug with a high therapeutic index would be characterized by:
   a) A narrow margin between effective and toxic doses
   b) A wide margin between effective and toxic doses
   c) High potency but low efficacy
   d) Rapid onset but short duration of action
3. The drug concentration that produces 50% of the maximum effect is known as:
   a) ED50
   b) LD50
   c) EC50
   d) TD50
4. A drug with significant protein binding would be expected to:
   a) Have a larger volume of distribution
   b) Be more readily filtered by the kidneys
   c) Have a longer elimination half-life
   d) Cross the blood-brain barrier more easily
5. Which of the following statements about first-pass metabolism is correct?
   a) It occurs primarily in the kidneys
   b) It reduces bioavailability of orally administered drugs
   c) It is more significant for drugs administered by the transdermal route
   d) It leads to increased drug concentrations in the systemic circulation
6. A pharmacokinetic drug interaction between warfarin and amiodarone would most likely result from:
   a) Displacement of warfarin from plasma protein binding sites
   b) Inhibition of warfarin metabolism by amiodarone
   c) Competition for active transport in the kidneys
   d) Altered gastric pH affecting warfarin absorption

7. Which of the following drug interactions represents a pharmacodynamic mechanism?
   a) Ciprofloxacin inhibiting the metabolism of theophylline
   b) Antacids reducing the absorption of tetracycline
   c) Alcohol enhancing the CNS depressant effects of benzodiazepines
   d) Rifampin inducing the metabolism of oral contraceptives
8. Type B adverse drug reactions are characterized by:
   a) Being dose-dependent and predictable
   b) Being dose-independent and unpredictable
   c) Occurring after prolonged drug administration
   d) Representing delayed therapeutic effects
9. A drug with a half-life of 12 hours would be expected to reach steady-state plasma concentration after approximately:
   a) 12 hours
   b) 24 hours
   c) 48 hours
   d) 60 hours
10. Which cytochrome P450 enzyme is responsible for metabolizing the greatest number of clinically used drugs?
    a) CYP1A2
    b) CYP2C9
    c) CYP2D6
    d) CYP3A4

Self-Assessment Questions

1. Explaining how concepts of affinity, efficacy, potency, and selectivity influence the therapeutic and adverse effect profiles of medications.
2. Compare and contrast the molecular mechanisms and clinical effects of full agonists, partial agonists, antagonists, and inverse agonists at G-protein coupled receptors, providing specific medication examples that illustrate each type of action.
3. Describing specific second messenger systems (cAMP, calcium, phosphoinositides) and analyzing how these mechanisms influence the onset, duration, and intensity of drug effects.
4. Analyze the factors affecting drug absorption from different administration routes (oral, parenteral, transdermal, inhalation), explaining how physiological conditions and formulation properties influence the rate and extent of bioavailability.
5. Describe the physiological determinants of drug distribution throughout the body, explaining how plasma protein binding, tissue affinity, and specialized barriers (blood-brain barrier, placenta) affect therapeutic concentrations at target sites.
6. Analyze the clinical significance of hepatic metabolism pathways (Phase I and Phase II reactions), explaining how genetic polymorphisms in metabolizing enzymes can lead to variability in drug response and potential for personalized therapy approaches.
7. Explain the concept of drug elimination half-life and its relationship to dosing interval selection, steady-state concentrations, and duration of effect, providing examples of how half-life differences guide clinical decision-making.
8. Describe the major mechanisms of pharmacokinetic drug interactions, analyzing their clinical significance and appropriate management strategies.
9. Explain how combinations affecting the same physiological system through different mechanisms can produce synergistic, additive, or antagonistic effects.
10. Explain the classification of adverse drug reactions (Type A, B, C, and D), describing their underlying mechanisms, predisposing factors, typical presentation patterns, and approaches to prevention and management.

Bibliography

1. Brunton LL, Hilal-Dandan R, Knollmann BC, editors. Goodman & Gilman's the pharmacological basis of therapeutics. 13th ed. New York: McGraw-Hill Education; 2018.
2. Benet LZ, Zia-Amirhosseini P. Basic principles of pharmacokinetics. Toxicol Pathol. 1995;23(2):115-123.
3. Rowland M, Tozer TN. Clinical pharmacokinetics and pharmacodynamics: Concepts and applications. 4th ed. Philadelphia: Lippincott Williams & Wilkins; 2011.
4. Leucuta SE, Vlase L. Pharmacokinetics and metabolic drug interactions. Curr Clin Pharmacol. 2006;1(1):5-20.
5. Hansten PD, Horn JR. Drug interactions analysis and management. St. Louis: Wolters Kluwer Health; 2014.
6. Edwards IR, Aronson JK. Adverse drug reactions: Definitions, diagnosis, and management. Lancet. 2000;356(9237):1255-1259.
7. Ritter JM, Flower R, Henderson G, Loke YK, MacEwan D, Rang HP. Rang & Dale's pharmacology. 9th ed. Edinburgh: Elsevier; 2020.
8. Katzung BG, Trevor AJ. Basic and clinical pharmacology. 14th ed. New York: McGraw-Hill Education; 2018.
9. Whirl-Carrillo M, McDonagh EM, Hebert JM, Gong L, Sangkuhl K, Thorn CF, et al. Pharmacogenomics knowledge for personalized medicine. Clin Pharmacol Ther. 2012;92(4):414-417.
10. Nebert DW, Russell DW. Clinical importance of the cytochromes P450. Lancet. 2002;360(9340):1155-1162.

CHAPTER 6

CLINICAL PHARMACY PRACTICE

Author

Dr. Ajmal Tariq Hussain, Assistant Professor,
Department of Pharmacy Practice, Amity Institute of Pharmacy,
Amity University, Lucknow, India

Abstract

Clinical pharmacy practice applies pharmaceutical science to optimize medication therapy outcomes through direct patient care activities across healthcare settings. Patient assessment establishes the foundation for clinical decision-making through systematic collection and interpretation of subjective information, physical findings, laboratory data, and medication histories, identifying drug-related problems requiring intervention. Therapeutic drug monitoring applies pharmacokinetic principles to medications with narrow therapeutic indices, using serum concentration measurements to guide individualized dosing adjustments that maximize efficacy while minimizing toxicity for agents including anticonvulsants, aminoglycosides, and immunosuppressants. Care plans translate assessment findings into structured interventions with clear, measurable goals addressing identified medication-related problems through evidence-based strategies, appropriate monitoring parameters, and follow-up timelines communicated across healthcare teams. Medication therapy management encompasses comprehensive services optimizing therapeutic outcomes through systematic medication review, identification of drug-related problems, development of personalized care plans, intervention implementation, and documentation, with particular focus on complex patients with multiple chronic conditions. The principles of clinical pharmacy practice improve patient outcomes by ensuring appropriate medication selection, optimizing dosing regimens, enhancing adherence, preventing adverse effects, and reducing healthcare costs through prevention of medication-related complications.

Keywords: *Medication Optimization; Clinical Decision-Making; Patient-Specific Therapy; Evidence-Based Practice; Therapeutic Outcomes*

Learning Objectives

After completion of the chapter, the learners should be able to:

- Conduct comprehensive patient interviews to gather essential medication, medical, and social history information for clinical decision-making.
- Interpret laboratory values and physical assessment findings to identify drug-related problems requiring pharmacist intervention.
- Design patient-specific therapeutic drug monitoring plans including appropriate sampling times, target concentrations, and dosage adjustment strategies.
- Develop SOAP-formatted care plans with specific, measurable, achievable, relevant, and time-bound therapeutic goals.
- Implement medication therapy management services addressing the five core elements: medication therapy review, personal medication record, medication-related action plan, intervention and referral, and documentation and follow-up.
- Apply evidence-based guidelines to prioritize interventions for patients with multiple medication-related problems.

PATIENT ASSESSMENT

Patient assessment forms the cornerstone of clinical pharmacy practice, providing the foundation for pharmaceutical care decisions and interventions. This systematic process involves gathering, organizing, and interpreting patient-specific information to identify medication-related problems and develop appropriate care plans. Comprehensive patient assessment enables pharmacists to optimize medication therapy, minimize adverse effects, and improve clinical outcomes through evidence-based, patient-centered care.

The patient interview represents the initial and often most valuable component of assessment, providing both objective information and subjective insights regarding the patient's medication experience. Effective interviewing requires a structured approach that balances comprehensive data collection with sensitivity to patient concerns and time constraints. Open-ended questions encourage patients to describe their medication experiences in their own words, often revealing problems not captured through closed-ended questioning. Specific questioning techniques such as the "brown bag review," where patients bring all their medications for discussion, help identify discrepancies between prescribed and actual medication regimens.

Cultural competence in patient assessment acknowledges how cultural backgrounds influence health beliefs, medication practices, and communication patterns. Culturally sensitive assessment adapts questioning approaches and interpretations to accommodate diverse health perspectives while avoiding stereotyping or assumptions. This may involve working with interpreters, recognizing culturally-specific descriptions of symptoms, or understanding cultural influences on medication adherence and healthcare engagement.

Table 6.1: Components of Patient Assessment

Assessment Component	Elements	Documentation Points
Chief Complaint	Patient's primary concern	Duration, severity, context
History of Present Illness	Timeline of current problem	Onset, quality, aggravating/relieving factors
Past Medical History	Previous diagnoses	Date of diagnosis, treatments, status
Medication History	Current and past medications	Name, dose, frequency, duration, adherence
Medication Allergies	Drug allergies and reactions	Specific reaction, timing, severity
Social History	Lifestyle factors	Tobacco, alcohol, illicit drugs, occupation
Family History	Diseases in blood relatives	Age of onset, relationship to patient
Review of Systems	Systematic body review	Positive and pertinent negative findings
Physical Examination	Relevant physical findings	Vital signs, organ-specific findings
Laboratory Data	Relevant test results	Current values, trends, reference ranges
Diagnostic Studies	Imaging, procedures	Results, clinical correlation
Medication Reconciliation	Comprehensive medication list	All prescription, OTC, supplements
Adherence Assessment	Evaluation of compliance	Barriers, missed doses, understanding
Functional Assessment	Activities of daily living	Independence level, need for assistance
Nutritional Assessment	Diet evaluation	Restrictions, supplements, interactions

Medication History and Reconciliation

Medication reconciliation involves comparing the patient's current medication regimen across transitions of care to identify and resolve discrepancies. This process addresses a significant source of medication errors, particularly during hospital admission, transfer between units, and discharge. Comprehensive medication histories include prescription medications, over-the-counter products, dietary supplements, and traditional or cultural remedies, with specific attention to dosage, frequency, duration, indication, and actual usage patterns that may differ from prescribed regimens.

The Best Possible Medication History (BPMH) concept emphasizes using multiple information sources to develop an accurate medication list, recognizing that no single source provides complete information. These sources include patient or caregiver interviews, inspection of medication containers, previous medical records, prescription databases, and communication with community pharmacies and prescribers. Research consistently demonstrates that comprehensive medication histories identify significantly more medications than routine admission histories, particularly for high-risk medications such as anticoagulants, insulin, and immunosuppressants.

Documentation of adverse drug reactions requires specific attention during medication history taking, with detailed characterization of the reaction's nature, timing, severity, and outcome. Distinguishing between allergic reactions mediated by immunologic mechanisms and adverse effects resulting from pharmacological properties enables appropriate avoidance strategies while preventing unnecessary restriction of therapeutic options. This differentiation proves particularly important for antimicrobial agents, where inaccurate "allergy" labels may lead to use of less effective or more toxic alternatives.

Physical Assessment Skills

Physical assessment skills enable pharmacists to gather objective data that complement the medication history and support clinical decision-making. These skills include measurement and interpretation of vital signs (blood pressure, heart rate, respiratory rate, temperature), which provide essential baseline information and may reveal medication effects or adverse reactions. For example, orthostatic blood pressure measurements help evaluate potential causes of dizziness, which might include antihypertensive overtreatment, autonomic neuropathy from diabetes, or volume depletion from diuretics.

Targeted cardiovascular assessment includes evaluation of peripheral edema, jugular venous pressure, and heart sounds, providing valuable information regarding heart failure management, fluid status, and potential medication effects. Respiratory assessment skills such as auscultation of lung sounds help distinguish between conditions requiring different medication approaches, such as asthma versus chronic obstructive pulmonary disease, or identify potential adverse effects such as medication-induced pulmonary edema or bronchospasm.

Neurological assessment focuses on elements relevant to medication therapy, including level of consciousness, cognitive function, cranial nerve function, motor strength, coordination, and reflexes. These assessments support evaluation of potential neurological medication effects, such as extrapyramidal symptoms from antipsychotics, cognitive impairment from anticholinergics, or neuropathy from certain chemotherapeutic agents. Standardized assessment tools including the Mini-Mental State Examination, Montreal Cognitive Assessment, or specific scales for Parkinson's symptoms or neuropathic pain provide objective, reproducible measures for monitoring medication effects over time.

Laboratory Data Interpretation

Laboratory data interpretation forms an essential component of pharmacist-conducted patient assessment, providing objective measures of organ function, disease control, medication effects, and potential toxicities. Pharmacists must understand normal ranges, clinical significance of abnormal values, and appropriate timing of laboratory monitoring for various medications and conditions. This knowledge enables detection of early signs of adverse drug effects, assessment of therapeutic effectiveness, and identification of necessary dosage adjustments.

Renal function assessment holds particular importance for medication management, as many drugs undergo renal elimination or require dosage adjustment in renal impairment. While serum creatinine provides a basic indicator of kidney function, estimated glomerular filtration rate (eGFR) calculated using equations such as the Cockcroft-Gault, MDRD, or CKD-EPI formulas offers more accurate assessment for dosing decisions. Interpretation must consider limitations of these estimation methods in certain populations, including the elderly, those with extremes of body size, or those with rapidly changing renal function.

Hepatic function evaluation guides medication selection and dosing for patients with liver disease, focusing on parameters that reflect synthetic function (albumin, prothrombin time), metabolic capacity (bilirubin), and cellular integrity (transaminases). Scoring systems such as Child-Pugh classification integrate multiple parameters to categorize severity of hepatic impairment, providing a framework for dosage adjustment recommendations. Pharmacists must recognize patterns of liver enzyme elevation that suggest medication-induced liver injury, distinguishing between hepatocellular, cholestatic, and mixed patterns that may indicate different pathophysiological mechanisms.

Therapeutic drug monitoring parameters extend beyond traditional serum drug concentrations to include biomarkers that reflect pharmacodynamic effects or early indicators of toxicity. For example, monitoring of HbA1c for diabetes medications, INR for warfarin, lipid profiles for antihyperlipidemic therapy, or neutrophil counts for clozapine provides information about therapeutic effectiveness or developing adverse effects. Integration of these parameters with clinical presentation and medication history enables comprehensive assessment of therapy appropriateness and effectiveness.

Risk Assessment Tools

Medication appropriateness criteria provide structured frameworks for evaluating prescribing quality, particularly in vulnerable populations. The Beers Criteria identify potentially inappropriate medications for older adults based on unfavorable risk-benefit ratios, while the STOPP/START criteria (Screening Tool of Older Person's Prescriptions/Screening Tool to Alert doctors to Right Treatment) address both inappropriate medications and potential prescribing omissions. Application of these tools during patient assessment identifies opportunities for deprescribing harmful or unnecessary medications and initiating beneficial therapies that may have been overlooked.

Fall risk assessment holds particular relevance for medication review, as numerous medication classes contribute to fall risk through effects on postural stability, cognition, blood pressure regulation, or vision. Validated assessment tools such as the Morse Fall Scale or STRATIFY (St. Thomas Risk Assessment Tool in Falling Elderly Inpatients) incorporate medication use alongside other risk factors to identify patients requiring intervention. Pharmacist-led assessments specifically evaluate medication contributions to fall risk, including anticholinergics, antipsychotics, benzodiazepines, antihypertensives, and hypoglycemic agents.

Cardiovascular risk assessment guides preventive pharmacotherapy decisions, particularly for antihypertensive, antihyperlipidemic, and antiplatelet therapies. Tools such as the Atherosclerotic Cardiovascular Disease (ASCVD) Risk Calculator integrate multiple risk factors to estimate 10-year risk, informing evidence-based decisions regarding statin therapy and blood pressure targets. Pharmacists apply these risk prediction tools during patient assessment to identify candidates for preventive therapies and educate patients regarding modifiable risk factors.

Adherence assessment identifies barriers to medication use as prescribed, distinguishing between intentional non-adherence (resulting from concerns about medications or lack of perceived need) and unintentional non-adherence (resulting from forgetfulness, complexity, cost, or physical limitations). Validated tools such as the Medication Adherence Rating Scale (MARS) or the Morisky Medication Adherence Scale provide standardized approaches to adherence evaluation. Comprehensive assessment explores specific adherence barriers including health literacy limitations, cultural beliefs, regimen complexity, adverse effects, and financial constraints, enabling targeted interventions to improve medication use.

THERAPEUTIC DRUG MONITORING

Therapeutic drug monitoring (TDM) involves the measurement and interpretation of drug concentrations in biological fluids to optimize dosage regimens for individual patients. This specialized aspect of clinical pharmacy practice applies pharmacokinetic principles to achieve desired therapeutic outcomes while minimizing toxicity risks, particularly for medications with narrow therapeutic indices or significant pharmacokinetic variability.

The fundamental premise of TDM rests on established relationships between plasma drug concentrations and both therapeutic and adverse effects. These concentration-effect relationships form the basis for therapeutic ranges—the concentration spans associated with optimal balance between efficacy and toxicity for specific indications. For many drugs, these relationships follow sigmoid Emax models, with efficacy increasing and plateauing at higher concentrations while toxicity risks rise continuously. The therapeutic range represents the concentration window where efficacy is adequate while toxicity remains acceptable.

Patient selection for TDM prioritizes clinical scenarios where measurement of drug concentrations provides meaningful guidance for therapy adjustment. These scenarios include: drugs with established concentration-effect relationships and narrow therapeutic indices; significant pharmacokinetic variability; difficulty in assessing clinical response; potential for serious toxicity; suspected non-adherence; potential drug interactions affecting pharmacokinetics; and special populations with altered pharmacokinetics such as pediatric patients, pregnant women, or those with organ dysfunction.

Pharmacokinetic Principles in TDM

Sample timing significantly influences interpretation of measured drug concentrations, requiring standardization relative to dosing times and achievement of steady state. Trough concentrations (collected immediately before the next scheduled dose) provide the most consistent basis for monitoring drugs with relatively short half-lives administered in multiple daily doses, as these concentrations exhibit less intra-individual variability than samples collected at other times. Peak concentrations (typically collected 0.5-2 hours after administration, depending on the specific drug) may be monitored when toxicity correlates with maximum concentration or when assessing absorption adequacy.

Table 6.2: Therapeutic Drug Monitoring Parameters

Drug	Therapeutic Range	Indications for Monitoring
Vancomycin	Trough: 10-15 mg/L 15-20 mg/L (severe)	Serious infections, renal dysfunction
Gentamicin	Peak: 5-10 mg/L Trough: <2 mg/L	Serious infections, renal dysfunction
Phenytoin	10-20 mg/L	Seizure control, toxicity concerns
Carbamazepine	4-12 mg/L	Seizure control, toxicity concerns
Valproic Acid	50-100 mg/L	Seizure control, toxicity concerns
Lithium	0.6-1.2 mEq/L	Bipolar disorder, toxicity concerns
Digoxin	0.8-2.0 ng/mL	Heart failure, arrhythmias
Theophylline	10-20 mg/L	Asthma, COPD
Cyclosporine	Varies by indication	Transplant, autoimmune conditions
Tacrolimus	Varies by indication	Transplant
Warfarin	INR 2-3 or 2.5-3.5	Anticoagulation
Phenobarbital	15-40 mg/L	Seizure control
Amikacin	Peak: 20-35 mg/L Trough: <5-10 mg/L	Serious infections
Methotrexate	Varies by protocol	Oncology, toxicity prevention

Steady state concepts hold particular importance in TDM, as

interpretation of drug concentrations differs significantly between steady and non-steady state conditions.

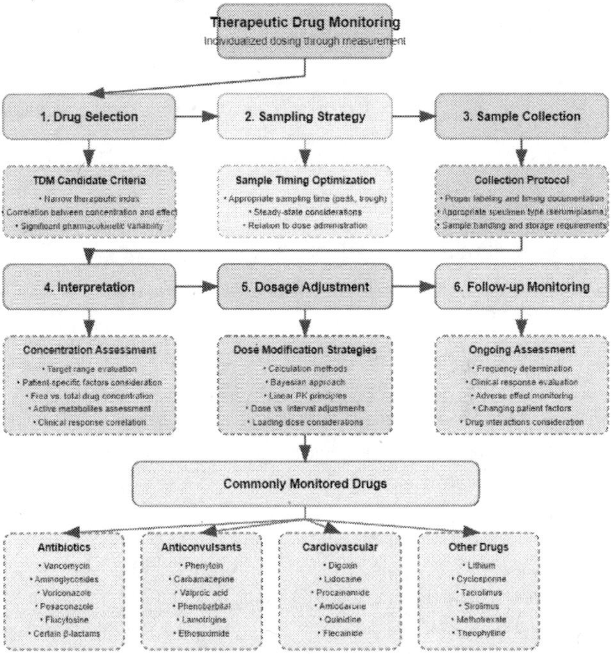

Figure 6.2: Therapeutic Drug Monitoring Process

Most therapeutic ranges are established for steady state conditions, reached after approximately 4-5 half-lives of consistent dosing. Premature concentration measurement before reaching steady state typically underestimates eventual steady state levels and may lead to inappropriate dosage increases. Exceptions include loading dose strategies that rapidly achieve therapeutic concentrations, or urgent situations where preliminary concentration data provide valuable guidance despite not reflecting eventual steady state.

Patient-specific factors influencing pharmacokinetics require consideration during TDM interpretation. Renal function affects elimination of many monitored drugs, with declining function typically requiring dosage reduction to avoid concentration-dependent toxicity. Hepatic impairment may reduce drug clearance through effects on metabolizing enzymes, plasma protein binding, or biliary excretion. Physiological changes in pregnancy alter drug disposition through changes in volume of distribution, protein binding, metabolism, and elimination. Critical illness introduces further complexities through alterations in tissue perfusion, capillary permeability, organ function, and plasma protein concentrations.

Monitoring of Specific Drug Classes

Antimicrobial TDM optimizes efficacy while preventing toxicity for agents including aminoglycosides, vancomycin, and antifungals. Aminoglycoside monitoring focuses on both peak concentrations (correlating with bactericidal efficacy) and trough concentrations (predicting nephrotoxicity and ototoxicity risks). Traditional multiple daily dosing regimens aim for peak:MIC ratios >8-10 while maintaining trough concentrations below toxicity thresholds. Extended-interval dosing (once-daily) strategies leverage concentration-dependent killing and post-antibiotic effect while minimizing toxicity through drug-free intervals, requiring different monitoring approaches focusing on area under the curve (AUC) estimation.

Vancomycin monitoring has evolved from simple trough concentration targeting to more sophisticated AUC-based approaches that better predict efficacy and nephrotoxicity risks. Current guidelines recommend AUC/MIC ratios ≥400 for serious MRSA infections, achieved through measurement of two concentrations (peak and trough) and Bayesian estimation methods or through validated estimation methods based on a single trough concentration. This shift reflects growing recognition that isolated trough concentrations correlate imperfectly with AUC and that excessive trough targeting may increase nephrotoxicity risks without improving outcomes.

Anticonvulsant monitoring addresses the challenges of highly variable pharmacokinetics, narrow therapeutic indices, and limited clinical markers of subtherapeutic dosing for drugs including phenytoin, carbamazepine, valproic acid, and newer agents like lamotrigine. Phenytoin presents particular complexity due to its nonlinear, capacity-limited metabolism, requiring consideration of both total and free (unbound) concentrations, especially in conditions affecting protein binding such as hypoalbuminemia, uremia, or pregnancy. The Michaelis-Menten kinetics of phenytoin necessitate specialized approaches to dosage adjustment, often employing the Sheiner-Tozer equation or similar methods to predict concentration changes resulting from dosage modifications.

Immunosuppressant monitoring balances rejection prevention against toxicity and infection risks for transplant patients receiving calcineurin inhibitors (cyclosporine, tacrolimus), mTOR inhibitors (sirolimus, everolimus), or antimetabolites (mycophenolate). These drugs exhibit significant inter- and intra-individual pharmacokinetic variability and narrow therapeutic indices, making TDM essential for optimizing outcomes. Monitoring approaches range from simple trough concentration measurement for tacrolimus to more complex limited sampling strategies estimating AUC for mycophenolate. Interpretation must consider time post-transplant (with higher target concentrations early after transplantation), concomitant immunosuppressants, infection risks, and rejection history.

Analytical Methods

Immunoassay techniques provide rapid turnaround time and widespread availability for many monitored drugs, using antibody-based detection methods that vary in specificity and precision. These methods include enzyme-multiplied immunoassay technique (EMIT), fluorescence polarization immunoassay (FPIA), and chemiluminescent microparticle immunoassay (CMIA). While convenient, immunoassays may suffer from cross-reactivity with metabolites or structurally similar compounds, potentially leading to falsely elevated results. This limitation proves particularly relevant for drugs like cyclosporine, where immunoassays detecting both parent drug and metabolites ("non-specific" assays) yield significantly higher values than more specific methods.

Chromatographic methods including high-performance liquid chromatography (HPLC) and liquid chromatography-tandem mass spectrometry (LC-MS/MS) offer superior specificity and often sensitivity compared to immunoassays. These techniques separate drugs from metabolites and potentially interfering substances based on physicochemical properties before detection, minimizing cross-reactivity concerns. LC-MS/MS has become the reference standard for many TDM applications due to its exceptional specificity, sensitivity, and ability to simultaneously measure multiple drugs or metabolites. However, these advantages come with higher instrumentation costs, greater technical complexity, and typically longer turnaround times compared to immunoassays.

Pre-analytical variables significantly influence measured drug concentrations and require standardization to ensure reliable results. These variables include sample timing relative to dose administration, sample type (serum versus plasma), collection tube additives, sample handling, and storage conditions. Inconsistency in these factors may introduce substantial variability unrelated to actual drug exposure. For example, collection in gel separator tubes may reduce measured concentrations of highly protein-bound drugs like phenytoin through adsorption to the gel barrier, while improper storage may accelerate degradation of unstable compounds such as mycophenolic acid.

Assay standardization and reference ranges relationship requires careful consideration when interpreting TDM results from different laboratories or comparing results to literature-derived therapeutic ranges. Method-dependent differences in measured concentrations necessitate method-specific reference ranges, particularly for drugs where immunoassays and chromatographic methods show systematic differences. Laboratory reports should clearly indicate the analytical method employed and the appropriate reference range for that specific method to prevent misinterpretation leading to inappropriate dosage adjustments.

Pharmacokinetic Dosage Adjustment

Population pharmacokinetic models provide starting points for dosage individualization by incorporating demographic and clinical factors known to influence drug disposition. These models, derived from pharmacokinetic studies in relevant patient populations, establish typical parameter values (clearance, volume of distribution) and their relationship to observable patient characteristics such as weight, age, renal function, or concomitant medications. Initial dosing recommendations based on these models provide rational starting points for subsequent individualization through measured concentrations and clinical response.

Bayesian forecasting represents the most sophisticated approach to TDM-guided dosage individualization, combining population pharmacokinetic priors with individual drug concentration measurements to estimate patient-specific pharmacokinetic parameters. This method optimally balances population-derived expectations with individual observations, giving greater weight to individual data as more measurements become available. Bayesian software tools enable precise prediction of concentration-time profiles resulting from various dosing regimens, supporting selection of optimal individualized regimens that achieve desired target concentrations.

Limited sampling strategies reduce the burden of multiple blood collections while maintaining accurate estimation of drug exposure. These approaches identify optimal sampling times and mathematical algorithms that predict AUC from a reduced number of strategically timed samples. For example, mycophenolate monitoring may employ three samples collected at 20 minutes, 1 hour, and 3 hours post-dose to accurately estimate total AUC with minimal patient inconvenience. These strategies prove particularly valuable for outpatient monitoring and pediatric patients where extensive sampling creates substantial practical challenges.

Integration of TDM with clinical response assessment ensures that concentration data inform rather than dictate therapeutic decisions. Drug concentrations represent surrogate markers rather than therapeutic endpoints themselves, requiring correlation with actual clinical outcomes including efficacy measures and adverse effect assessment. In some cases, clinical response may justify continuation of regimens producing concentrations outside typical target ranges, particularly when individual pharmacodynamic characteristics differ from population norms or when measured concentrations do not accurately reflect concentrations at effect sites.

CARE PLANS

Care plans translate patient assessment findings into systematic, patient-specific strategies for resolving medication-related problems and achieving therapeutic goals. These structured documents guide implementation of pharmaceutical care, facilitate interdisciplinary communication, and provide frameworks for monitoring and evaluating intervention outcomes. Effective care plans balance standardization for consistency with individualization to address unique patient needs and preferences.

The care planning process begins with problem identification based on comprehensive patient assessment. Medication-related problems may include untreated indications, inappropriate drug selection, subtherapeutic or excessive dosing, adverse drug reactions, interactions, nonadherence, or failures to receive indicated monitoring. Each identified problem undergoes prioritization based on urgency, severity, and patient concerns, recognizing that attempting to address all problems simultaneously may overwhelm both patients and providers.

Goal setting establishes specific, measurable objectives for each prioritized problem, providing clear targets for intervention and evaluation. These goals incorporate both clinical parameters (e.g., blood pressure <130/80 mmHg, HbA1c <7%) and patient-centered outcomes (e.g., improved functional status, symptom reduction, enhanced quality of life). Effective goal setting includes specific timeframes for achievement and involves patients in establishing priorities that reflect their values and preferences.

Problem Prioritization and Goal Setting

Clinical significance assessment guides prioritization of medication-related problems, distinguishing between issues requiring urgent intervention and those that can be addressed over longer timeframes. This assessment considers potential consequences of non-intervention, probability of adverse outcomes, timeframe for harm development, and availability of effective interventions. High-priority problems typically include potentially life-threatening drug interactions, severe adverse reactions, significant contraindications, or critical therapy omissions for serious conditions.

Patient preferences significantly influence problem prioritization and goal setting, reflecting the principle that care plans should address issues most important to patients rather than solely focusing on provider-defined priorities.

Table 6.3: Components of a Pharmaceutical Care Plan

Component	Description	Documentation Example
Patient Demographics	Basic identifying information	65-year-old male, hospital ID #12345
Medical Problem List	All active diagnoses	1. Hypertension (2010) 2. Type 2 diabetes (2015) 3. Osteoarthritis (2018)
Medication List	Current medications with details	1. Lisinopril 20 mg daily 2. Metformin 1000 mg twice daily 3. Acetaminophen 500 mg as needed
Allergies/ADRs	Known drug allergies/reactions	Penicillin (hives), Sulfa (rash)
Laboratory Values	Relevant lab results	SCr 1.2 mg/dL, HbA1c 7.8%, K+ 4.2 mEq/L
Drug Therapy Problems	Identified medication issues	1. Untreated indication (dyslipidemia) 2. Suboptimal dose (metformin)
Goals of Therapy	Desired outcomes with timeframes	1. BP <140/90 mmHg within 1 month 2. HbA1c <7% within 3 months
Interventions	Actions to resolve problems	1. Increase metformin to 1000 mg TID 2. Add atorvastatin 10 mg daily
Monitoring Parameters	What to monitor and when	1. BP weekly for 4 weeks 2. HbA1c in 3 months 3. LFTs in 6 weeks

Component	Description	Documentation Example
Patient Education	Information provided to patient	1. Hypoglycemia signs/symptoms 2. Home BP monitoring technique
Follow-up Plan	Timing and type of follow-up	Phone call in 2 weeks, clinic visit in 1 month
Resolution	Status of identified problems	Problem #1: Resolved 4/15/24 Problem #2: Partially resolved 5/1/24
Clinical Pharmacist	Provider identification	Jane Smith, PharmD, BCPS Date: 3/15/24
Rationale	Evidence/reasoning for decisions	1. ADA guidelines recommend intensifying therapy for HbA1c >7% 2. ASCVD risk score 7.8% indicates statin benefit
Alternative Plans	Other considered options	1. GLP-1 RA considered but cost prohibitive 2. Pravastatin alternative if myalgia develops

Exploration of patient perspectives regarding symptom burden, functional limitations, treatment concerns, and quality of life impacts reveals priorities that might differ substantially from those apparent through purely clinical assessment. This patient-centered approach enhances engagement with the care plan and improves adherence to recommended interventions.

Goal alignment across the healthcare team ensures coordinated efforts toward consistent objectives. This alignment requires communication with other providers regarding prioritized problems, established goals, and planned interventions. In settings with electronic health records, structured care plan documentation visible to all team members facilitates this coordination. Regular interdisciplinary care conferences provide forums for discussing complex cases, resolving potentially conflicting recommendations, and developing consensus approaches that optimize patient outcomes.

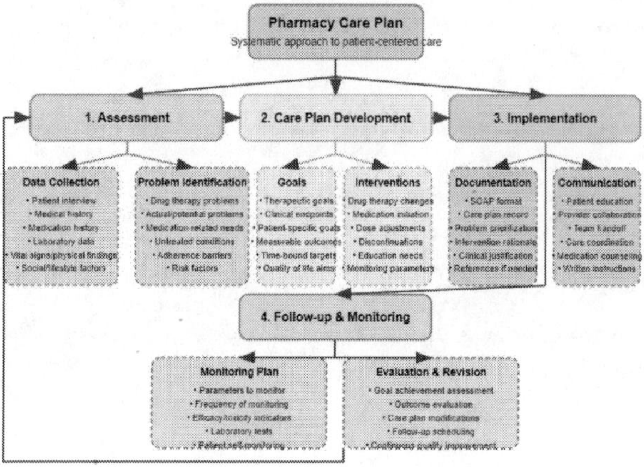

Figure 6.3: Process of Care Plan Development

Intervention Design

Pharmacological interventions address medication-related problems through modifications to drug therapy regimens. These modifications may include initiating new medications for untreated indications, discontinuing inappropriate or unnecessary medications, substituting safer or more effective alternatives, adjusting doses based on patient response or pharmacokinetic parameters, or modifying administration timing to enhance effectiveness or reduce adverse effects. Selection among intervention options considers evidence regarding efficacy, safety, cost, and patient-specific factors affecting acceptability and feasibility.

Non-pharmacological interventions complement medication adjustments to comprehensively address health needs. These interventions include lifestyle modifications (dietary changes, exercise recommendations, smoking cessation), physical modalities (compression therapy, positioning techniques), monitoring recommendations (home blood pressure or glucose monitoring), and referrals to other healthcare providers or community resources. Integration of these approaches with pharmacological interventions often produces synergistic benefits exceeding those achievable through medication optimization alone.

Educational interventions enhance patient understanding of their medications and health conditions, enabling informed decision-making and improved self-management. Effective educational approaches adapt content and delivery to individual learning preferences, health literacy levels, and specific knowledge gaps identified during assessment. Education extends beyond basic administration instructions to include purpose of medications, expected benefits, potential adverse effects, monitoring parameters, and appropriate actions for missed doses or developing problems. Teaching methods vary based on patient needs, potentially including verbal instruction, written materials, visual aids, demonstration, teach-back techniques, or digital resources.

Adherence support interventions address identified barriers to medication use as prescribed. These interventions range from practical approaches such as pill organizers, reminder systems, or simplified regimens to more complex behavioral interventions addressing motivation, health beliefs, or self-efficacy. Motivational interviewing techniques help patients explore ambivalence about medication use and develop personalized strategies for overcoming adherence challenges. For patients with cognitive or functional limitations affecting medication management, interventions might include caregiver education, specialized packaging, or coordination with community resources for medication administration assistance.

Documentation and Communication

SOAP format (Subjective, Objective, Assessment, Plan) provides a structured approach to care plan documentation that organizes patient information logically and facilitates clinical decision-making. The Subjective component captures patient-reported symptoms, concerns, and medication experiences. Objective information includes physical examination findings, laboratory results, and other measurable parameters. Assessment integrates subjective and objective data to identify problems and evaluate therapeutic progress. The Plan component details interventions addressing identified problems, including specific recommendations, rationale, monitoring parameters, and follow-up arrangements.

Care plan integration with electronic health records enhances accessibility to all healthcare team members, supporting coordination and continuity of care. Electronic documentation facilitates structured data capture that enables tracking of medication-related problems, interventions, and outcomes across patient populations. This capability supports quality improvement initiatives, identification of recurring medication safety issues, and evaluation of clinical pharmacy services impact. Advanced electronic systems may incorporate clinical decision support tools that suggest potential interventions based on documented problems or alert pharmacists to patients meeting criteria for specific pharmacy services.

Interdisciplinary communication of care plans ensures awareness of medication-related concerns and recommendations across the healthcare team. Effective communication strategies vary based on practice setting and urgency, ranging from formal consultation notes or care plan documentation to direct verbal communication for urgent issues. Clear articulation of assessment findings, clinical reasoning supporting recommendations, and specific follow-up responsibilities enhances recommendation acceptance and implementation. Communication with community pharmacies during care transitions proves particularly important for ensuring continuity of medication management plans established during institutional care episodes.

Patient communication of care plans employs patient-friendly language and formats that enhance understanding and engagement. Written medication lists with purpose, dosing instructions, and special considerations provide reference materials supporting adherence. Visual schedules using symbols or color coding may benefit patients with literacy limitations or language barriers. Personalized action plans for chronic conditions outline symptoms requiring medication adjustments or provider contact. These patient-directed materials complement verbal education, reinforcing key information and providing ongoing guidance between provider encounters.

Monitoring and Follow-up

Outcome monitoring assesses progress toward established goals through systematic collection of relevant clinical and patient-reported measures. This monitoring includes objective parameters such as laboratory values, vital signs, or physical examination findings alongside subjective measures including symptom burden, functional status, or quality of life assessments. Timing and frequency of monitoring depend on the condition's acuity, medication characteristics, and anticipated timeframe for observable therapeutic effects. Structured approaches to outcome documentation enable longitudinal tracking of response patterns and support evidence-based adjustments to the care plan when goals remain unmet.

Adverse effect monitoring focuses on early detection of medication-related problems through targeted assessment of parameters associated with common or serious adverse effects. This monitoring includes both objective measures (laboratory tests, physical findings) and systematic inquiry regarding subjective symptoms potentially attributable to medications. Proactive monitoring strategies for high-risk medications identify problems before they become severe, enabling intervention through dosage adjustment, supportive measures, or medication changes when necessary. Patient education regarding expected and concerning effects enhances this monitoring by enabling appropriate self-assessment and timely reporting.

Follow-up planning establishes specific arrangements for continued care after initial plan implementation, specifying timing, communication methods, and responsibilities for ongoing monitoring and plan refinement. These arrangements range from scheduled clinic appointments or telehealth encounters to asynchronous communication through patient portals, telephone check-ins, or home monitoring with remote reporting. Escalation pathways identify circumstances requiring more urgent follow-up than originally planned, with clear guidance for patients regarding concerning symptoms or findings warranting immediate contact.

Plan revision processes acknowledge the dynamic nature of patient needs and treatment responses, establishing systematic approaches for evaluating and modifying care plans over time. These processes include scheduled comprehensive plan reviews at intervals appropriate to the condition's stability and treatment complexity, alongside more focused reviews triggered by significant clinical changes, new information, or failure to achieve expected outcomes. Revision considerations include emerging evidence regarding treatment approaches, changes in patient circumstances or preferences, development of new problems requiring attention, and opportunities to simplify regimens as conditions stabilize.

MEDICATION THERAPY MANAGEMENT

Medication Therapy Management (MTM) encompasses a spectrum of patient-centered services that optimize therapeutic outcomes through improved medication use. These services extend beyond traditional dispensing functions to address the complex medication needs of patients with multiple chronic conditions, numerous medications, or high-risk therapies. MTM represents a systematic approach to identifying and resolving medication-related problems, enhancing therapeutic effectiveness, improving patient understanding, and optimizing health outcomes.

The core elements of MTM include medication therapy review, personal medication record development, medication-related action plan creation, intervention and referral, and documentation and follow-up. These elements provide a comprehensive framework for addressing medication-related needs while ensuring consistency across different practice settings and patient populations. Implementation adaptations accommodate various practice models, patient characteristics, and resource availability, while maintaining fidelity to these fundamental components.

Patient selection for MTM services typically employs criteria identifying individuals most likely to benefit from comprehensive medication management. These criteria commonly include multiple chronic conditions, complex medication regimens (often defined as use of multiple medications or high-risk drugs), recent hospitalizations, medication adherence challenges, or suboptimal disease control despite medication therapy. Risk stratification approaches prioritize patients with greatest need when resource constraints limit service availability, ensuring maximal impact of clinical pharmacy interventions.

Table 6.4: Medication-Related Problems and Resolution Strategies

Problem Category	Examples	Assessment
Unnecessary Therapy	Duplicate therapy, no indication	Review indications, duration
Need for Additional Therapy	Untreated indication, preventive therapy	Review guidelines, risk factors
Ineffective Drug	Poor response, resistance	Review efficacy markers, therapeutic alternatives
Dosage Too Low	Drug interaction	Check response, plasma levels
Adverse Drug Reaction	Side effects, allergic reactions	Assess causality, severity
Dosage Too High	Excessive dose, organ dysfunction	Check for toxicity, organ function
Nonadherence	Missing doses, improper administration	Assess barriers, understanding
Drug Interactions	Reduced efficacy, increased toxicity	Check interaction databases
Inappropriate Monitoring	Missing labs, inadequate follow-up	Review monitoring parameters
Cost Issues	Inability to afford medications	Discuss with patient
Improper Administration	Incorrect technique, timing	Observe, question patient
Formulary Issues	Non-formulary medications	Review formulary alternatives
Therapeutic Duplication	Multiple drugs in same class	Review medication list
Medication Errors	Wrong drug, dose, patient, time	Investigate cause

Comprehensive Medication Review

The comprehensive medication review (CMR) provides a systematic, in-depth assessment of all medications a patient is using, including prescription medications, over-the-counter products, dietary supplements, and complementary therapies. This holistic evaluation examines each medication's appropriateness, effectiveness, safety, and actual use patterns, identifying opportunities for regimen optimization. The CMR typically requires 30-60 minutes of direct patient interaction, allowing thorough exploration of medication experiences, concerns, and knowledge gaps that might not emerge during briefer encounters.

Therapeutic appropriateness assessment evaluates each medication against current evidence-based guidelines, considering indications, contraindications, potential alternatives, and alignment with patient-specific goals of care. This assessment identifies unnecessary medications without clear ongoing indications, potentially inappropriate medications for specific patient characteristics (e.g., applying Beer's criteria for older adults), therapeutic duplications across multiple prescribers, and untreated conditions that might benefit from pharmacotherapy. Integration of patient preferences and values ensures that appropriateness determinations reflect not only clinical guidelines but also individual priorities and acceptable risk-benefit tradeoffs.

Drug interaction screening extends beyond simple identification of potential interactions to include clinical relevance assessment and management strategy development. This process employs multiple information sources including electronic screening tools, laboratory parameters indicating interaction effects, and patient-reported symptoms potentially attributable to interactions. Assessment of interaction significance considers factors including evidence quality, mechanistic plausibility, temporal relationship to clinical findings, and availability of monitoring or management strategies. Management approaches range from increased monitoring to dose adjustments, spacing of administration times, or selection of alternative agents with lower interaction potential.

Therapy effectiveness evaluation determines whether medications are achieving intended therapeutic outcomes based on objective clinical parameters, subjective symptom assessment, and comparison with expected response timeframes. This evaluation identifies suboptimal responses potentially addressable through dosage adjustment, formulation changes, adherence support, or therapy modifications. For conditions with multiple treatment options, effectiveness assessment may reveal opportunities to transition from partially effective therapies to alternatives better suited to the individual patient's specific disease manifestations, comorbidities, or lifestyle factors.

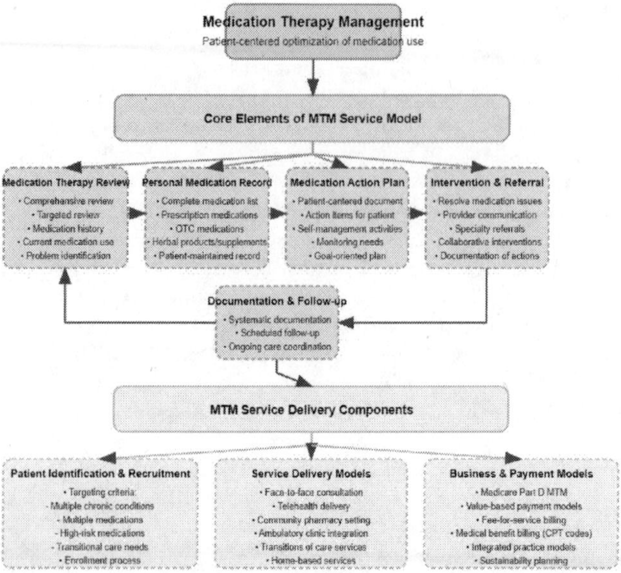

Figure 6.4: Medication Therapy Management

Targeted Medication Reviews

Focused problem-based reviews address specific medication-related concerns rather than comprehensively evaluating the entire medication regimen. These targeted reviews prove particularly valuable for addressing time-sensitive issues, follow-up of previously identified problems, or situations where resource constraints preclude comprehensive review. Common scenarios prompting targeted reviews include new symptoms potentially representing adverse drug effects, significant changes in clinical parameters such as renal function or electrolytes, addition of new medications with interaction potential, or specific medication adherence challenges identified by patients or other healthcare providers.

High-risk medication monitoring provides structured oversight for medications associated with significant toxicity risks or narrow therapeutic indices. These monitoring programs employ standardized protocols defining appropriate baseline assessment, ongoing monitoring parameters, acceptable result ranges, and intervention pathways for abnormal findings. Examples include anticoagulation management services tracking INR values for warfarin patients, clozapine monitoring programs ensuring appropriate neutrophil count assessment, or comprehensive monitoring of immunosuppressive regimens for transplant recipients. These focused services combine specialized pharmacist expertise with systematic tracking systems to ensure that critical monitoring occurs at appropriate intervals and that results receive timely evaluation.

Transition of care medication reconciliation addresses the substantial medication discrepancy and error risks that occur during transfers between care settings. These services systematically compare medication regimens across transitions, identifying unintentional discrepancies, duplicate therapies, omissions, or inappropriate continuations. Post-discharge medication reviews are particularly valuable, reconciling pre-admission medications with new hospital-initiated therapies and ensuring patients understand which medications to continue, which to discontinue, and how to take newly prescribed treatments. This reconciliation process significantly reduces adverse drug events and hospital readmissions related to medication discrepancies.

Disease-specific medication optimization focuses on evidence-based pharmacotherapy for particular chronic conditions, applying disease-specific guidelines and quality measures to identify opportunities for regimen enhancement. These targeted reviews ensure appropriate therapy selection, dosing optimization, and guideline adherence while addressing condition-specific adherence barriers and monitoring needs. Examples include heart failure medication optimization ensuring appropriate use of evidence-based therapies such as ACE inhibitors, beta-blockers, and aldosterone antagonists at target doses; diabetes medication management addressing glycemic control, cardiovascular risk reduction, and renal protection; or comprehensive asthma management evaluating controller medication appropriateness, inhaler technique, and action plan understanding.

Patient Education and Empowerment

Medication knowledge enhancement addresses specific understanding gaps identified during assessment, providing patients with essential information about their medications' purposes, administration requirements, expected effects, and monitoring needs. Effective education adapts content and delivery approaches to individual learning preferences, health literacy levels, and existing knowledge base. This personalized approach avoids overwhelming patients with excessive information while ensuring coverage of critical elements necessary for safe and effective medication use. Education extends beyond verbal instruction to include written materials, visual aids, demonstration, and teach-back techniques that verify understanding.

Table 6.5: Medication Therapy Management Core Elements

Core Element	Components	Documentation Requirements
Medication Therapy Review	Comprehensive review of medications	Complete medication list, identified problems
Personal Medication Record	Patient-centered medication list	All prescription, OTC, supplements
Medication-Related Action Plan	Patient-focused to-do list	Specific actions for patient to resolve problems
Intervention/Referral	Actions by pharmacist to resolve problems	Interventions made, communications with providers
Documentation and Follow-up	Record of services and outcomes	SOAP note, billing information, outcomes
Patient Selection	Identifying appropriate candidates	Risk factors, eligibility criteria
Patient Engagement	Involving patients in care	Communication strategies, motivational interviewing
Provider Communication	Sharing recommendations	Format, timing, content of communications
Measuring Outcomes	Evaluating service impact	Clinical, economic, humanistic measures
Quality Improvement	Continuous process improvement	Performance metrics, targets
Service Marketing	Promoting MTM services	Value proposition, target audiences
Integration with Care	Coordination with healthcare team	Role definition, workflow integration
Technology Utilization	Supporting MTM processes	Software selection, utilization

Self-management support enables patients to participate actively in their medication management through enhanced knowledge, skills, and confidence. This support includes practical medication management strategies such as organization systems, reminder techniques, or administration aids tailored to individual needs and preferences. For patients with chronic conditions requiring symptom monitoring or medication adjustments, self-management education includes recognition of significant changes requiring action, appropriate response protocols, and clear guidance regarding when to seek professional assistance. These approaches enhance patient autonomy while establishing safety parameters that prevent adverse outcomes from inappropriate self-management decisions.

Shared decision-making engages patients as active partners in treatment decisions by providing balanced information about options, eliciting personal preferences, and collaboratively developing plans that align with individual values and priorities. This approach proves particularly valuable when multiple reasonable treatment alternatives exist with different benefit-risk profiles or when patient adherence depends strongly on acceptance of therapy characteristics. Structured approaches to shared decision-making include presenting evidence regarding options in understandable formats, explicitly discussing uncertainty, exploring how various outcomes would affect the patient's life, and supporting preference-based choices even when they might differ from provider recommendations.

Health literacy accommodation recognizes the challenges many patients face in understanding and applying health information, adapting communication and materials to enhance comprehension regardless of literacy level. Strategies include using plain, non-technical language; focusing on key messages rather than exhaustive detail; employing visual aids that reduce reliance on text; organizing information in logical sequences with clear action steps; and creating a supportive environment where questions are encouraged. For patients with limited English proficiency, professionally trained interpreters provide accurate communication while materials in appropriate languages reinforce key information. These accommodations enhance understanding and enable informed participation in medication management decisions.

Summary

Clinical pharmacy practice applies pharmaceutical knowledge directly to patient care through structured assessment, monitoring, planning, and intervention processes. Patient assessment forms the cornerstone of clinical practice, employing comprehensive interviews to gather medication, medical, and social histories while incorporating physical assessment findings and laboratory data interpretation to identify medication-related problems. This holistic evaluation reveals issues including inappropriate therapy selection, dosing discrepancies, adverse effects, adherence barriers, and therapeutic duplications requiring pharmacist intervention. Therapeutic drug monitoring represents a specialized clinical function for medications with narrow therapeutic indices or significant variability in pharmacokinetic parameters, involving strategic sampling, concentration measurement, and dosage adjustment to maintain effective levels while avoiding toxicity. This process requires knowledge about distribution phases, elimination characteristics, and patient-specific factors affecting drug disposition. Care plans translate assessment findings into structured intervention frameworks, typically following SOAP (Subjective-Objective-Assessment-Plan) documentation format with clearly defined problems, specific therapeutic goals, interventions tailored to patient needs, and monitoring parameters for evaluating outcomes. These plans incorporate evidence-based guidelines while accounting for patient-specific factors including comorbidities, preferences, and socioeconomic considerations. Medication therapy management represents a comprehensive service model encompassing five core elements: medication therapy review identifying actual and potential problems, personal medication record documentation, medication-related action plan development, intervention implementation with appropriate referrals, and continuous follow-up evaluation. Through these systematic approaches to pharmaceutical care delivery, clinical pharmacists optimize medication regimens, resolve drug-related problems, prevent adverse events, and improve therapeutic outcomes while serving as essential members of interprofessional healthcare teams across diverse practice environments.

Multiple Choice Questions

1. Which of the following would be the most appropriate first step in conducting a comprehensive medication review?
   a) Reviewing the patient's laboratory values
   b) Obtaining a complete medication history
   c) Performing physical assessment measurements
   d) Checking insurance coverage for medications
2. A patient is receiving vancomycin for a MRSA infection. Which of the following would be the most appropriate time to obtain a trough level?
   a) 30 minutes after completion of the infusion
   b) 2 hours after completion of the infusion
   c) Midway through the dosing interval
   d) Within 30 minutes before the next scheduled dose
3. For which of the following medications is therapeutic drug monitoring most necessary?
   a) Atorvastatin
   b) Phenytoin
   c) Lisinopril
   d) Metformin
4. Which of the following best describes the "A" in the SOAP note format?
   a) Analysis of the patient's condition
   b) Assessment of drug therapy problems
   c) Allergies and adverse reactions
   d) Actions taken by the healthcare team
5. A pharmacist identifies that a patient with atrial fibrillation has a CHA_2DS_2-VASc score of 4 but is not currently receiving anticoagulation therapy. This finding would be documented in which section of the SOAP note?
   a) Subjective
   b) Objective
   c) Assessment
   d) Plan
6. Which of the following is a core element of Medication Therapy Management services as defined by the American Pharmacists Association?
   a) Dispensing of medications
   b) Medication therapy review
   c) Prescription counseling
   d) Insurance billing

7. A pharmacist is evaluating a patient's medication regimen and notices that the patient is taking omeprazole 20 mg daily but has no documented indication for acid suppression therapy. This would be classified as which type of drug therapy problem?
   a) Unnecessary drug therapy
   b) Needs additional drug therapy
   c) Dosage too low
   d) Adverse drug reaction
8. In pharmacokinetic drug monitoring, which parameter is most useful for determining the maintenance dose of a medication?
   a) Volume of distribution
   b) Clearance
   c) Absorption rate constant
   d) Time to maximum concentration
9. A comprehensive care plan for a patient with multiple chronic conditions should include:
   a) Only the highest priority medical conditions
   b) Only medication-related interventions
   c) Clearly defined goals for each identified problem
   d) Generic recommendations applicable to most patients with similar conditions
10. Which of the following best describes the purpose of a medication action plan provided to a patient during MTM services?
   a) A complete list of all medications for the prescriber's reference
   b) A patient-centered document with specific actions the patient should take
   c) A billing document for insurance reimbursement
   d) A legal record of counseling provided to the patient

Self-Assessment Questions

1. Describe the components of a comprehensive medication history, explaining how each element contributes to identifying medication-related problems and detailing specific questioning techniques that elicit accurate information from patients.
2. Explain how changes in renal function markers, liver enzymes, electrolytes, and hematological parameters might indicate medication effectiveness or toxicity.
3. Describe how factors such as distribution phases, protein binding, and elimination pathways affect the interpretation of measured drug concentrations.
4. Design an appropriate therapeutic drug monitoring plan for vancomycin therapy in a patient with fluctuating renal function, including optimal sampling times, target concentration ranges, and dosage adjustment strategies based on measured levels.
5. Compare and contrast the principles and applications of population pharmacokinetics versus patient-specific pharmacokinetic modeling in individualizing drug therapy, providing examples of clinical scenarios where each approach would be most valuable.
6. Develop a comprehensive SOAP note for a patient with uncontrolled type 2 diabetes, hypertension, and chronic kidney disease
7. Explain how competing guidelines, potential drug interactions, and patient-specific factors should be balanced when formulating recommendations.
8. Describe the core elements of medication therapy management services as defined by professional pharmacy organizations, explaining how each component contributes to improved patient outcomes and reduced healthcare costs.
9. Design a medication therapy management intervention for a patient taking multiple medications for chronic conditions, demonstrating how you would identify and resolve issues related to indication, effectiveness, safety, and adherence.
10. Analyze the documentation requirements for billable clinical pharmacy services, explaining the necessary elements for meeting reimbursement criteria while effectively communicating recommendations to other healthcare providers.

Bibliography

1. DiPiro JT, Talbert RL, Yee GC, Matzke GR, Wells BG, Posey LM, editors. Pharmacotherapy: A pathophysiologic approach. 11th ed. New York: McGraw-Hill Education; 2020.
2. Cipolle RJ, Strand LM, Morley PC. Pharmaceutical care practice: The patient-centered approach to medication management services. 3rd ed. New York: McGraw-Hill; 2012.
3. Murphy JE, editor. Clinical pharmacokinetics. 6th ed. Bethesda: American Society of Health-System Pharmacists; 2017.
4. Kang JS, Lee MH. Overview of therapeutic drug monitoring. Korean J Intern Med. 2009;24(1):1-10.
5. American College of Clinical Pharmacy. Standards of practice for clinical pharmacists. Pharmacotherapy. 2014;34(8):794-797.
6. Pestka DL, Frail CK, Palombi LC, Von Ruden J, Livet M, Sorensen TD. Strategies and steps fostering the success of medication management services in community pharmacies. J Am Pharm Assoc. 2016;56(5):504-512.e1.
7. Isetts BJ, Schondelmeyer SW, Artz MB, Lenarz LA, Heaton AH, Wadd WB, et al. Clinical and economic outcomes of medication therapy management services: The Minnesota experience. J Am Pharm Assoc. 2008;48(2):203-211.
8. Ramalho de Oliveira D, Brummel AR, Miller DB. Medication therapy management: 10 years of experience in a large integrated health care system. J Manag Care Pharm. 2010;16(3):185-195.
9. American Pharmacists Association; National Association of Chain Drug Stores Foundation. Medication therapy management in pharmacy practice: Core elements of an MTM service model (version 2.0). J Am Pharm Assoc. 2008;48(3):341-353.
10. Lee JK, Grace KA, Taylor AJ. Effect of a pharmacy care program on medication adherence and persistence, blood pressure, and low-density lipoprotein cholesterol: A randomized controlled trial. JAMA. 2006;296(21):2563-2571.

CHAPTER 7

PRESCRIPTION MANAGEMENT

Author

Dr. Amit Kumar, Associate Professor, Department of Pharmacy Practice, Amity Institute of Pharmacy, Amity University, Lucknow, India

Abstract

Prescription management encompasses the systematic processes ensuring accurate medication delivery from prescriber to patient while maintaining safety and regulatory compliance. Prescription processing follows a standardized workflow including receipt, verification, interpretation, entry, adjudication, preparation, and final verification, with each step incorporating critical safety checks and legal requirements including DEA regulations for controlled substances. Drug information resources support clinical decision-making through primary literature, tertiary references, electronic databases, and specialized compendia, with selection criteria including currency, authority, objectivity, and accessibility to answer medication questions from patients and healthcare providers. Medication safety practices prevent dispensing errors through system-level approaches including tall-man lettering, barcode verification, physical separation of look-alike products, standardized concentrations, and continuous quality improvement programs analyzing near-misses and actual errors to implement preventive strategies. Dispensing procedures ensure accurate medication preparation through standardized protocols for various dosage forms, with particular attention to specialized requirements for hazardous drugs, compounded preparations, and high-alert medications requiring independent double checks, while maintaining appropriate documentation, patient counseling, and follow-up monitoring. These protocols provide a system for medication provision that balances efficiency with the paramount priorities of accuracy, safety, legal compliance, and patient-centered care.

Keywords: *Workflow Management; Error Prevention; Information Evaluation; Regulatory Compliance; Patient Counseling*

Learning Objectives

After completion of the chapter, the learners should be able to:

- Evaluate prescriptions for legal requirements, therapeutic appropriateness, and potential errors before dispensing.
- Navigate primary, secondary, and tertiary drug information resources to efficiently answer medication-related questions.
- Implement medication safety practices including tall-man lettering, barcode verification, and separation of look-alike products.
- Develop workflows that incorporate safety checkpoints for high-alert medications requiring special handling.
- Apply principles of effective patient counseling tailored to specific medication types, dosage forms, and patient needs.
- Design quality assurance processes to detect, document, and prevent medication dispensing errors.

PRESCRIPTION PROCESSING

The prescription serves as the critical interface between prescriber, pharmacist, and patient in medication therapy. Prescription processing encompasses a series of methodical steps designed to ensure accurate, safe, and appropriate medication dispensing. Upon receiving a prescription, the pharmacist must conduct a thorough evaluation for authenticity, legality, and completeness. This initial assessment verifies the presence of essential elements: patient demographics, prescriber information, drug name, strength, dosage form, quantity, directions for use, refill information, and appropriate signatures. Incomplete or ambiguous prescriptions necessitate direct communication with the prescriber before proceeding.

Prescription Interpretation and Validation

Prescription interpretation demands precision and clinical judgment. The pharmacist must decipher prescriber handwriting when applicable, understand medical abbreviations, and correctly interpret dosing instructions. Validation extends beyond mere technical accuracy to clinical appropriateness. This involves evaluating whether the prescribed medication, dose, and regimen align with the patient's diagnosis, age, weight, allergies, comorbidities, and concurrent medications. Potential drug interactions, contraindications, and therapeutic duplications must be identified and resolved. Electronic prescribing systems have significantly reduced interpretation errors, yet vigilance remains essential even with digital prescriptions.

Table 7.1: Prescription Components and Requirements

Component	Description	Common Errors
Patient Information	Name, address, date of birth	Missing DOB, misspelled name
Prescriber Information	Name, address, phone, DEA (if controlled)	Missing DEA for controlled substances
Date	Date prescription was written	Expired prescription, illegible date
Medication Name	Generic or brand name	Look-alike/sound-alike confusion
Strength	Amount of active ingredient	Missing or incorrect strength
Dosage Form	Tablet, capsule, solution, etc.	Incompatible form for patient
Quantity	Amount to be dispensed	Unclear quantity, excessive amount
Directions for Use	How patient should take medication	Ambiguous directions, missing frequency
Refills	Number of authorized refills	Missing refill information
Substitution	Generic substitution instructions	DAW box not checked, unclear intent
Special Instructions	"Take with food," etc.	Contradictory instructions
Controlled Substance Schedule	II, III, IV, V classification	Missing schedule, improper format
Signature	Prescriber's handwritten signature	Missing signature, rubber stamp
Indication	Purpose of medication	Not included, irrelevant to prescribed drug
"Brand Necessary"	Indication that generic not allowed	Not properly indicated

Prescription Entry and Insurance Processing

Accurate data entry into the pharmacy management system creates the foundation for subsequent dispensing steps and patient record maintenance. Each prescription element must be meticulously entered, including appropriate translation of Latin abbreviations into patient-friendly instructions. Insurance processing involves navigating complex reimbursement systems to determine coverage, apply appropriate billing codes, calculate patient cost-sharing obligations, and resolve coverage issues. Prior authorization requirements frequently necessitate additional documentation and communication with prescribers and insurers. The pharmacist must maintain awareness of formulary alternatives when medication costs present barriers to patient adherence.

Prescription Labeling and Documentation

Prescription labels serve as the patient's primary reference for medication use. Labels must adhere to regulatory requirements while presenting information in a clear, accessible format. Essential elements include patient name, prescription number, prescriber information, dispensing date, medication name, strength, quantity, expiration date, directions for use, and refill status.

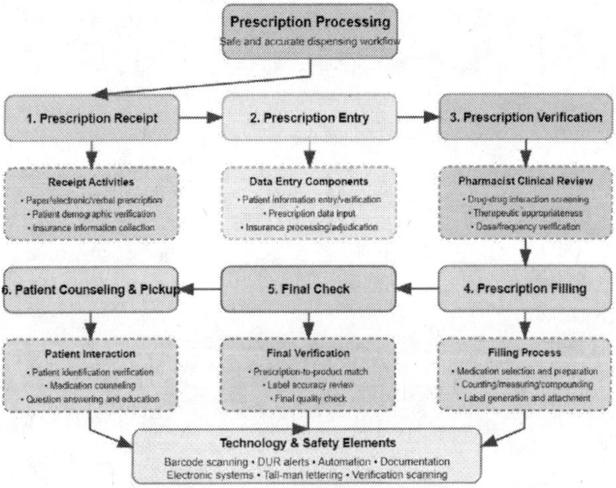

Figure 7.1: Prescription Processing

Auxiliary labels communicate critical warnings regarding administration, storage, or potential side effects. Comprehensive documentation in the pharmacy system maintains the medication profile for future reference, supports continuity of care, and satisfies legal requirements for prescription record retention.

Table 7.2: Prescription Processing Workflow

Step	Actions	Documentation
Receipt	Accept prescription, verify completeness	Time received, receiving personnel
Patient Intake	Gather patient information, insurance	Insurance information, patient profile
Insurance Processing	Submit claim, resolve rejections	Claim number, rejection codes
Prescription Entry	Enter into pharmacy system	Entry pharmacist, time entered
DUR Screening	Check for interactions, duplications	Resolution of alerts, pharmacist initials
Prescription Filling	Select product, measure/count, package	Lot number, expiration date
Pharmacist Verification	Final check of filled prescription	Verifying pharmacist, time
Patient Counseling	Offer counseling, provide information	Counseling provided/refused
Prescription Release	Verify patient identity, collect payment	Signature for pickup, payment collected
Documentation	Record all required information	Storage of original, filing records
Refill Processing	Verify refill authorization	Refill number, date processed
Transfer Processing	Send/receive prescription information	Transfer pharmacist, date/time
Controlled Substance Handling	Additional verification steps	DEA Form requirements, perpetual inventory
Prescription Filing	Organize and store records	Filing method, retention period

DRUG INFORMATION RESOURCES

Effective pharmacy practice demands access to and proficient use of authoritative drug information resources. These resources support evidence-based clinical decisions, verify medication properties, resolve therapeutic questions, and provide patient education materials. Primary literature encompasses original research published in peer-reviewed journals, representing the most current but often highly specialized knowledge. Secondary literature, including review articles, meta-analyses, and systematic reviews, synthesizes primary research for practical application. Tertiary resources compile established information in accessible formats for efficient clinical reference.

Table 7.3: Drug Information Resources and Their Applications

Resource Type	Examples	Best Uses	Limitations
Tertiary References	Micromedex, Lexicomp, Facts & Comparisons	Quick answers, general information	May not include latest research
Pharmacopeia	USP/NF, BP, JP	Standards for drug quality, identity	Limited clinical information
Clinical Guidelines	AHA, ADA, IDSA, NCCN	Evidence-based treatment recommendations	May not address unusual cases
Drug Package Inserts	FDA-approved labeling	FDA-approved information, legal reference	May not include off-label uses
Primary Literature	NEJM, JAMA, Lancet, BMJ	Latest research, clinical trials	Requires critical analysis skills
Drug Interaction Checkers	Micromedex, Lexicomp, Epocrates	Quick screening for interactions	Varying levels of clinical

Resource Type	Examples	Best Uses	Limitations
			significance
Pharmacokinetic References	Applied Pharmacokinetics, DiPiro	Detailed PK parameters, calculations	Complex information, limited drugs
Toxicology Resources	Poisindex, Toxnet	Management of overdoses, exposures	Emergency focus, limited general info
Complementary Medicine	Natural Medicines Database, Herbs & Supplements	Evidence for alternative therapies	Limited research available
Pediatric Dosing	Pediatric Dosage Handbook, Lexicomp	Age-specific dosing, pediatric formulations	Limited drugs with pediatric data
Pregnancy/Lactation	Medications & Mother's Milk, Briggs	Safety data for pregnant/nursing women	Limited research available
Patient Education	MedlinePlus, FDA patient materials	Patient-friendly information	May oversimplify complex issues
Drug Identification	Identidex, Pills.com	Visual identification of unknown medications	Limited to U.S. products, visual only
Pharmacy Law	State pharmacy laws, DEA manuals	Regulatory requirements	State-specific variations

Core Reference Resources

Pharmacists rely on several foundational references in daily practice. Pharmacopoeias, such as the United States Pharmacopeia-National Formulary (USP-NF), establish official standards for drug substances, dosage forms, and compounded preparations. Drug compendia, exemplified by the American Hospital Formulary Service Drug Information and Martindale: The Complete Drug Reference, provide comprehensive monographs on medication properties, indications, and clinical considerations. Drug interaction databases enable rapid identification of potential interactions, their clinical significance, and recommended management strategies. Therapeutic guidelines from professional organizations offer evidence-based recommendations for specific conditions, helping pharmacists evaluate prescription appropriateness against current standards of care.

Digital and Electronic Resources

The contemporary pharmacy landscape increasingly relies on digital resources that offer enhanced searchability, integration with pharmacy systems, and frequent updates. Clinical decision support software incorporates drug information within workflow, generating alerts for potential problems during prescription processing. Mobile applications provide point-of-care access to drug information, dosing calculators, and clinical tools. Subscription databases compile multiple resources within unified platforms, facilitating efficient information retrieval. When selecting electronic resources, pharmacists must evaluate factors including comprehensiveness, update frequency, evidence quality, usability, and integration capabilities with existing systems.

Evaluating Information Quality

The proliferation of drug information sources necessitates critical evaluation skills. Pharmacists must assess resource reliability by examining publisher reputation, author credentials, citation of primary literature, recency of information, and disclosure of potential conflicts of interest. Information currency holds particular importance given the rapid evolution of pharmaceutical knowledge and therapeutic recommendations. When counseling patients, pharmacists often translate complex information into accessible language while preserving accuracy. Maintaining a systematic approach to information retrieval—defining the question precisely, selecting appropriate resources, and synthesizing findings—enhances efficiency and effectiveness in addressing drug information queries.

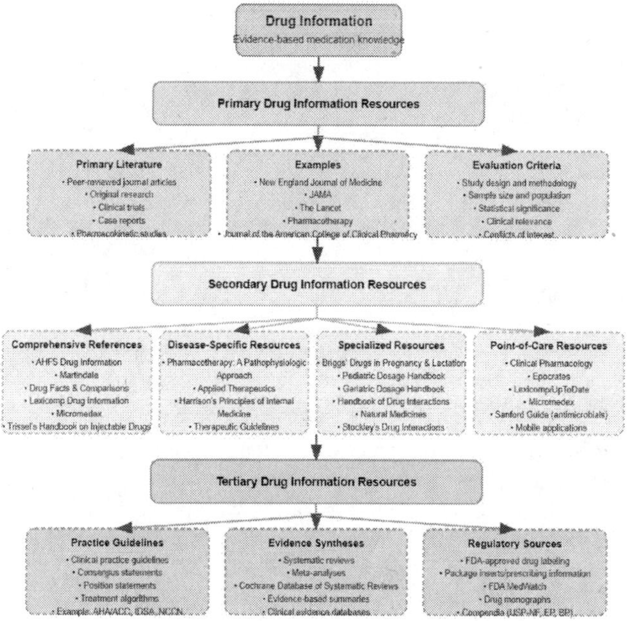

Figure 7.2: Drug Information Resources

MEDICATION SAFETY

Medication safety constitutes a foundational element of pharmacy practice, encompassing strategies to prevent, identify, and mitigate medication errors throughout the medication use process. The Institute of Medicine's landmark report "To Err Is Human" highlighted the prevalence and consequences of medication errors, catalyzing systematic approaches to enhancing safety. Medication errors may occur at any stage—prescribing, transcribing, dispensing, administering, or monitoring—with varying potential for patient harm. The pharmacist serves as a critical safeguard, implementing multiple verification systems and safety protocols to protect patients from preventable adverse events.

Error Prevention Strategies

Proactive error prevention incorporates both system-level and individual practices. Standardization of processes reduces variation and associated error opportunities. Tall-man lettering distinguishes look-alike drug names (e.g., hydrOXYzine vs. hydrALAzine), while physical separation of sound-alike or look-alike medications minimizes selection errors.

Table 7.4: Medication Safety Systems and Strategies

Safety System	Description	Potential Pitfalls
Tall Man Lettering	Capitalization of dissimilar letters	Inconsistent application
Bar Code Scanning	Verification via product bar codes	Technical failures, workarounds
Clinical Decision Support	Computerized alerts and reminders	Alert fatigue, excessive overrides
Automated Dispensing Cabinets	Computerized medication storage	Override abuse, restocking errors
Independent Double Checks	Second person verification	Time constraints, familiarity bias
Standardized Concentrations	Limiting available concentrations	Special needs patients, resistance to change
Fail-Safe Systems	Preventing connection errors	Implementation costs, transition periods
Medication Reconciliation	Comprehensive medication review	Incomplete information, time constraints
Root Cause Analysis	Systematic error investigation	Focus on individuals vs. systems
Forcing Functions	Physical barriers to prevent errors	Workarounds, implementation challenges
High-Alert Medication Protocols	Special procedures for risky drugs	Compliance issues, workflow disruption
Error Reporting Systems	Systems to report and track errors	Underreporting, lack of follow-up
Look-Alike/Sound-Alike Strategies	Preventing name confusion	Limited effectiveness without multiple strategies
Unit-Dose Packaging	Individual dose packaging	Cost, environmental concerns
Smart Infusion Pumps	Programmable limits on infusion rates	Programming errors, library updates

Bar-code verification technology confirms medication identity at multiple points in the dispensing process. Independent double-checks require two qualified individuals to separately verify critical aspects of high-risk medications. Eliminating error-prone abbreviations, symbols, and dose designations reduces misinterpretation risk. Environmental factors, including adequate lighting, minimal distractions, and appropriate workload management, support accurate performance of pharmacy tasks.

Safety Monitoring and Reporting

Continuous safety monitoring enables identification of potential and actual medication errors, near-misses, and adverse drug events. Internal reporting systems document incidents within the pharmacy, supporting analysis of error patterns and implementation of targeted improvements. External reporting to organizations such as the Institute for Safe Medication Practices (ISMP) and the FDA's MedWatch program contributes to national safety surveillance and dissemination of alerts regarding emerging risks. Root cause analysis explores systemic factors contributing to significant errors, moving beyond individual blame to address underlying process vulnerabilities. Safety culture encourages transparent reporting, interdisciplinary collaboration, and organizational learning from error events.

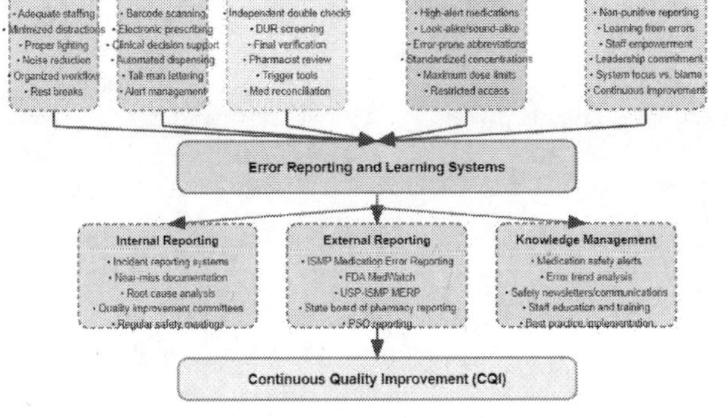

Figure 7.3: Medication Safety Systems

High-Alert Medications

Certain medications carry heightened risk of causing significant patient harm when used in error. These high-alert medications, including anticoagulants, insulins, opioids, concentrated electrolytes, and chemotherapeutic agents, warrant enhanced safeguards. Specialized protocols might include restricted access, enhanced documentation requirements, standardized order sets, auxiliary warnings, and comprehensive independent verification processes. Patient education regarding high-alert medications emphasizes proper administration techniques, recognition of adverse effects, and monitoring parameters. Pharmacy oversight of high-alert medications extends beyond dispensing to include monitoring of laboratory values, therapeutic responses, and potential complications throughout the course of therapy.

DISPENSING PROCEDURES

Dispensing procedures transform the theoretical prescription into the physical medication package delivered to the patient. This process integrates scientific knowledge, technical precision, regulatory compliance, and patient-centered care. Rigorous adherence to established workflows and verification protocols ensures that the right patient receives the right medication in the right dose, form, and quantity with the right information at the right time. While technology increasingly supports dispensing activities, the pharmacist's professional judgment and final verification remain indispensable safeguards.

Medication Preparation and Packaging

Medication preparation begins with proper product selection, confirming the correct medication, strength, and dosage form against the prescription. The pharmacist must verify product integrity, checking expiration dates and examining for signs of tampering or deterioration. Medication counting, measuring, or preparation requires clean technique and appropriate equipment maintenance. Packaging considerations include child-resistant containers (with documented exceptions for patients unable to manipulate such packaging), light-protective amber vials for photosensitive medications, and specialized packaging systems for patients with adherence challenges. Unit-dose packaging, blister packs, and medication organizers support accurate administration, particularly for complex regimens or patients with cognitive limitations.

Table 7.5: Dispensing Procedures for Special Drug Categories

Drug Category	Special Handling	Documentation
Schedule II	Secure storage, perpetual inventory	File separate from other Rx, 2 years
Schedule III-V	Secure storage	File separate from other Rx, 2 years
Refrigerated Items	Cold chain maintenance, insulated packaging	Temperature logs
Hazardous Drugs	PPE for handling, special containment	Exposure records, training documentation
Compounded Sterile Products	Aseptic technique, beyond-use dating	Master formulation record, lot tracking
Non-sterile Compounds	Appropriate equipment, beyond-use dating	Master formulation record
Partial Fills	Balance tracking	Remaining quantity, date
Emergency Supply	Limited quantity	Reason for emergency supply
Reconstituted Products	Beyond-use dating	Lot numbers, expiration
Insulin Products	Temperature control	Proper device selection
Narrow Therapeutic Index	Additional verification	Therapeutic monitoring records
Biologics	Temperature control, handling	Lot number tracking
Investigational Drugs	Blinding maintenance	Study-specific documentation
Opioid Antagonists	Multiple formulation options	State-specific documentation

Final Verification and Quality Assurance

Final verification represents the pharmacist's ultimate responsibility in the dispensing process. This comprehensive check encompasses verification of the correct medication, strength, dosage form, quantity, and instructions against the original prescription. The pharmacist examines label accuracy, auxiliary warnings, and appropriate documentation. Quality assurance extends beyond individual prescriptions to encompass system-level measures: routine equipment calibration, temperature monitoring for refrigerated products, proper inventory rotation, and regular assessment of error rates and near-misses. Continuous quality improvement initiatives analyze workflow efficiency, identify potential failure points, and implement refinements to enhance dispensing accuracy and safety.

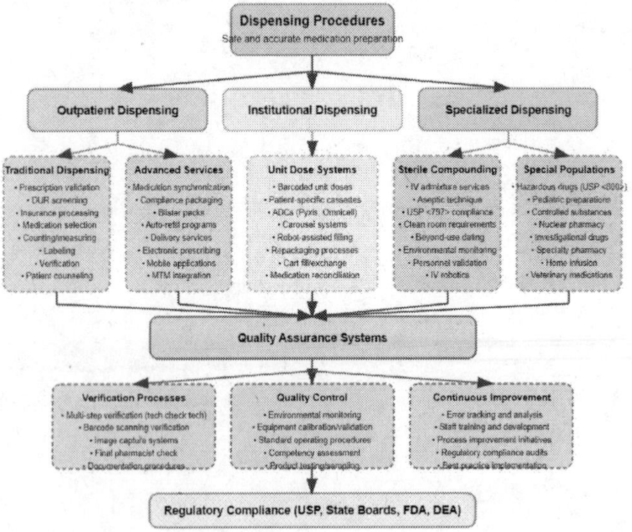

Figure 7.4: Medication Dispensing Procedures

Patient Counseling and Education

The dispensing process culminates in patient counseling, transforming the physical medication into therapeutic benefit through appropriate use. Effective counseling addresses medication purpose, administration technique, expected benefits, potential adverse effects, storage requirements, and important precautions. Demonstration devices support proper use of complex delivery systems such as inhalers, injections, or transdermal applications. The pharmacist must assess patient understanding through teach-back methods, asking patients to restate key information in their own words. Cultural competence and health literacy awareness guide communication approaches, ensuring information accessibility regardless of language barriers, educational background, or cognitive status.

Summary

Prescription management encompasses multistage processes ensuring medications reach patients safely, accurately, and appropriately. Prescription processing begins with receipt verification examining legal requirements including prescriber credentials, patient identifiers, medication specifications, and controlled substance compliance. Clinical screening follows, evaluating therapeutic appropriateness through allergy assessment, dosage verification, duplicate therapy checks, and drug interaction analysis before securing insurance authorization. Drug information resources support these clinical decisions, organized as primary literature presenting original research, secondary resources offering critical evaluations of primary findings, and tertiary compilations providing synthesized recommendations. Electronic databases, monographs, guidelines, and specialized references offer comprehensive medication data regarding indications, contraindications, dosing, adverse effects, and monitoring parameters. Medication safety principles minimize error risks through high-leverage strategies including fail-safe systems preventing incorrect medications, forcing functions requiring action completion, constraint approaches limiting access to high-risk medications, and standardization reducing variability. Additional safety practices include tall-man lettering differentiating similar names, barcode verification confirming product selection, and separated storage for look-alike products. Dispensing procedures translate approved prescriptions into accurately prepared medications through methodical workflows starting with product selection, continuing through preparation of appropriate quantities and auxiliary labeling, and culminating in final verification before patient release. This helps in effective counseling addressing administration techniques, expected effects, potential adverse reactions, and proper storage conditions.

Multiple Choice Questions

1. Which of the following is required on a prescription for a Schedule II controlled substance?
   a) Prescriber's NPI number only
   b) Prescriber's DEA number and signature
   c) Patient's driver's license number
   d) Insurance ID number
2. A prescription for a non-controlled substance is valid for:
   a) 6 months from the date written, in all states
   b) 12 months from the date written, in all states
   c) Varies by state law, typically 6-12 months
   d) 3 refills or 6 months, whichever comes first
3. Which of the following would be classified as a primary drug information resource?
   a) Lexicomp
   b) Original research article in a peer-reviewed journal
   c) Pharmacotherapy: A Pathophysiologic Approach
   d) UpToDate
4. A pharmacy receives a prescription for "Metoprolol 50 mg daily." Without additional clarification, this prescription is problematic because:
   a) The dose is too high for initial therapy
   b) The prescriber didn't specify tartrate or succinate salt form
   c) Metoprolol requires twice-daily dosing
   d) The duration of therapy is missing
5. In the prescription verification process, which of the following checks would be most appropriate to perform during clinical screening?
   a) Verifying that the correct NDC was selected
   b) Checking for drug interactions with the patient's medication profile
   c) Ensuring the label is affixed to the correct container
   d) Confirming the prescription was entered with the correct quantity
6. Which of the following strategies is most effective in preventing dispensing errors?
   a) Having the same pharmacist perform order entry and final verification
   b) Implementing barcode scanning during dispensing and verification

c) Dispensing all medications in identical packaging

d) Relying on patient counseling to catch errors

7. A patient brings in a prescription for "hydrocortisone cream." When implementing best practices for prescription clarification, the pharmacist should:

   a) Dispense 1% hydrocortisone cream as it's the most commonly used strength

   b) Contact the prescriber to clarify the strength, amount, and application instructions

   c) Ask the patient what strength they've used previously and dispense that

   d) Dispense all available strengths so the patient can choose

8. When counseling a patient on a newly prescribed inhaled corticosteroid, which of the following is most important to address?

   a) The potential for immediate symptom relief

   b) Proper inhalation technique and device usage

   c) The need to taper the medication when discontinuing

   d) That the medication can be used as needed for symptoms

9. Which drug information resource would be most appropriate for quickly checking if a medication is safe to use during pregnancy?

   a) Basic & Clinical Pharmacology textbook

   b) Package insert

   c) Briggs' Drugs in Pregnancy and Lactation

   d) The Merck Manual

10. A patient is prescribed ciprofloxacin and regularly takes a calcium supplement. The most appropriate intervention would be to:

    a) Recommend taking the medications at the same time to improve adherence

    b) Advise taking the calcium supplement 2 hours before or 6 hours after ciprofloxacin

    c) Recommend discontinuing the calcium supplement while on ciprofloxacin

    d) Suggest switching to a different antibiotic

Self-Assessment Questions

1. Explain how prescription verification processes differ for controlled substances versus non-controlled medications.
2. Describe the clinical screening process for new prescriptions, detailing the specific elements reviewed and explaining how electronic systems and professional judgment complement each other in identifying potential problems.
3. Evaluate the insurance verification and prior authorization process, explaining potential barriers to medication access and strategies pharmacists can employ to resolve coverage issues while minimizing treatment delays.
4. Compare and contrast primary, secondary, and tertiary drug information resources, providing specific examples of each type and explaining when each would be most appropriate for answering different categories of clinical questions.
5. Analyze the strengths and limitations of commonly used drug information databases and compendia, explaining how critical evaluation skills should be applied when using these resources to make clinical decisions.
6. Describe a systematic approach to literature evaluation when answering drug information questions, explaining how study design, methodology, statistical analysis, and potential biases affect the application of research findings to patient care.
7. Analyze the systems approach to medication safety, explaining how high-reliability principles including redundancy, standardization, forcing functions, and constraints can be implemented in pharmacy workflows to prevent errors.
8. Describe the process of root cause analysis following a medication error, explaining how contributing factors are identified across multiple system levels and how effective corrective actions can prevent similar errors.
9. Explain the critical quality checkpoints in the dispensing process from prescription receipt through patient counseling, analyzing how each verification step contributes to error prevention and medication safety.
10. Develop a comprehensive patient counseling plan for a newly prescribed medication with complex administration requirements and significant safety concerns, detailing specific information, demonstration techniques, and verification methods to ensure proper use.

Bibliography

1. Cohen MR. Medication errors. 2nd ed. Washington, DC: American Pharmacists Association; 2007.
2. American Society of Health-System Pharmacists. ASHP guidelines on preventing medication errors in hospitals. Am J Health Syst Pharm. 2018;75(19):1493-1517.
3. Institute for Safe Medication Practices. ISMP list of high-alert medications in community/ambulatory healthcâre. Horsham (PA): ISMP; 2021.
4. American Society of Health-System Pharmacists. ASHP guidelines on the pharmacist's role in providing drug information. Am J Health Syst Pharm. 2015;72(7):573-577.
5. Leape LL, Bates DW, Cullen DJ, Cooper J, Demonaco HJ, Gallivan T, et al. Systems analysis of adverse drug events. JAMA. 1995;274(1):35-43.
6. Flynn EA, Barker KN, Carnahan BJ. National observational study of prescription dispensing accuracy and safety in 50 pharmacies. J Am Pharm Assoc. 2003;43(2):191-200.
7. Kohn LT, Corrigan JM, Donaldson MS, editors. To err is human: Building a safer health system. Washington, DC: National Academy Press; 2000.
8. Wheeler AJ, Scahill S, Hopcroft D, Stapleton H. Reducing medication errors at transitions of care is everyone's business. Aust Prescr. 2018;41(3):73-77.
9. Schiff GD, Klinger E, Salazar A, Bates DW, Biondolillo M, Goldmann D. Screening for adverse drug events: A randomized trial of automated calls coupled with phone-based pharmacist counseling. J Gen Intern Med. 2019;34(2):285-292.
10. Phansalkar S, Desai AA, Bell D, Yoshida E, Doole J, Czochanski M, et al. High-priority drug-drug interactions for use in electronic health records. J Am Med Inform Assoc. 2012;19(5):735-743.

CHAPTER 8

MAJOR DRUG CLASSES I

Author

Mrs. Vinny Therissa Mangam, Assistant Professor, Department of Pharmaceutical Analysis, Aditya College of Pharmacy, Aditya University, Surampalem, Andhra Pradesh, India

Abstract

Major drug classes involving cardiovascular, respiratory, gastrointestinal, and endocrine conditions represent cornerstone therapies for prevalent chronic diseases. Cardiovascular medications comprises of antihypertensives acting through distinct mechanisms (ACE inhibitors, ARBs, calcium channel blockers, diuretics, beta-blockers), antiarrhythmics classified by electrophysiologic effects, lipid-lowering agents including statins and newer targeted therapies, anticoagulants spanning vitamin K antagonists and direct oral agents, and heart failure medications including beta-blockers, sacubitril/valsartan, and SGLT2 inhibitors demonstrating mortality benefits. Respiratory drugs target bronchospasm through beta-agonists with varying onset and duration profiles; reduce inflammation through inhaled corticosteroids and biological agents targeting specific inflammatory pathways; address allergic responses with antihistamines, leukotriene modifiers, and mast cell stabilizers; and treat pulmonary infections with diverse antimicrobial classes, each requiring specific administration techniques and monitoring parameters. Gastrointestinal agents include acid-suppressing medications (proton pump inhibitors, H2-antagonists), antiemetics targeting central and peripheral pathways, laxatives with mechanical and stimulant mechanisms, antidiarrheals, pancreatic enzymes, and newer biologics for inflammatory bowel disease targeting specific immune pathways. Endocrine medications consist of diabetes therapies including insulins with distinct pharmacokinetic profiles, oral agents with varied mechanisms, and newer injectable therapies; thyroid replacements requiring narrow therapeutic monitoring; reproductive hormones used in contraception and hormone replacement; and osteoporosis treatments spanning bisphosphonates, RANK ligand inhibitors, and anabolic agents, each with specific administration requirements and monitoring needs.

Keywords: *Chronic Disease; Mechanism of Action; Therapeutic Selection; Drug Administration; Monitoring Parameters*

Learning Objectives

After completion of the chapter, the learners should be able to:

- Compare and contrast the mechanisms of action, indications, contraindications, and monitoring parameters for major classes of cardiovascular medications.
- Select appropriate respiratory medications based on specific airway disease pathophysiology, patient factors, and device considerations.
- Recommend appropriate gastrointestinal agents for specific conditions based on mechanism of action, onset of effect, and adverse effect profiles.
- Design monitoring plans for patients on endocrine therapies that address both efficacy markers and potential adverse effects.
- Develop patient education strategies for complex medication regimens used in chronic disease management.
- Identify and manage clinically significant drug interactions associated with common cardiovascular, respiratory, gastrointestinal, and endocrine medications.

CARDIOVASCULAR SYSTEM

Cardiovascular medications constitute a cornerstone of modern pharmacotherapy, addressing the leading causes of morbidity and mortality worldwide. These agents target multiple physiological pathways to manage hypertension, dyslipidemia, thrombotic disorders, heart failure, and arrhythmias. Treatment approaches typically involve combination therapy addressing different pathophysiological mechanisms to achieve optimal outcomes. The pharmacist's role extends beyond dispensing to include monitoring therapeutic efficacy, identifying adverse effects, ensuring medication adherence, and facilitating appropriate lifestyle modifications that complement pharmacological interventions.

Antihypertensive Agents

Hypertension management employs several complementary drug classes targeting different mechanisms of blood pressure regulation. Thiazide diuretics reduce blood pressure through modest sodium and water excretion, with subsequent vasodilation from decreased peripheral vascular resistance. These agents remain first-line therapy for many patients due to their efficacy, safety profile, and cost-effectiveness, though electrolyte abnormalities necessitate periodic monitoring. Angiotensin-converting enzyme inhibitors (ACEIs) prevent the formation of angiotensin II, reducing vasoconstriction and aldosterone release while potentially offering cardiorenal protective effects independent of blood pressure reduction.

Table 8.1: Antihypertensive Medications

Drug Class	Examples	Mechanism of Action
ACE Inhibitors	Lisinopril Enalapril Ramipril	Block angiotensin II production
ARBs	Losartan Valsartan Candesartan	Block angiotensin II receptors
Calcium Channel Blockers (Dihydropyridines)	Amlodipine Nifedipine Felodipine	Block calcium entry into vascular smooth muscle
Calcium Channel Blockers (Non-dihydropyridines)	Diltiazem Verapamil	Block calcium entry into cardiac cells
Thiazide Diuretics	Hydrochlorothiazide Chlorthalidone Indapamide	Inhibit Na+/Cl- reabsorption in distal tubule
Loop Diuretics	Furosemide Bumetanide Torsemide	Inhibit Na+/K+/2Cl- reabsorption in loop of Henle
Potassium-Sparing Diuretics	Spironolactone Eplerenone Amiloride	Block aldosterone or ENaC
Beta Blockers	Metoprolol Carvedilol Bisoprolol	Block beta-adrenergic receptors
Alpha Blockers	Doxazosin Terazosin Prazosin	Block alpha-adrenergic receptors
Central Alpha-2 Agonists	Clonidine Methyldopa	Stimulate central alpha-2 receptors
Direct Vasodilators	Hydralazine Minoxidil	Relax vascular smooth muscle
Direct Renin Inhibitors	Aliskiren	Inhibit renin activity

The characteristic dry cough results from bradykinin accumulation and may necessitate transition to angiotensin II receptor blockers (ARBs), which provide similar benefits without affecting bradykinin metabolism. Calcium channel blockers induce vasodilation through inhibition of calcium influx into vascular smooth muscle cells, with dihydropyridines (e.g., amlodipine) demonstrating greater vascular selectivity compared to non-dihydropyridines (e.g., diltiazem, verapamil), which exert additional effects on cardiac conduction. Beta-adrenergic blockers reduce cardiac output and renin release, with newer vasodilatory agents offering more favorable metabolic profiles than traditional non-selective compounds.

Lipid-Modifying Medications

Dyslipidemia management focuses primarily on reducing atherosclerotic cardiovascular risk through targeting specific lipid fractions. Statins (HMG-CoA reductase inhibitors) remain the foundation of therapy, reducing low-density lipoprotein cholesterol (LDL-C) through inhibition of hepatic cholesterol synthesis and upregulation of LDL receptors. The demonstrated mortality benefit extends beyond lipid effects to include plaque stabilization and anti-inflammatory properties. Myalgias represent the most common adverse effect, with true myopathy and rhabdomyolysis occurring rarely but requiring vigilant monitoring. Ezetimibe selectively inhibits intestinal cholesterol absorption, providing modest LDL-C reduction as monotherapy but substantial additive effects when combined with statins. PCSK9 inhibitors, administered as subcutaneous injections, dramatically reduce LDL-C by preventing degradation of LDL receptors, offering therapeutic options for patients with familial hypercholesterolemia or statin intolerance. Fibrates primarily reduce triglycerides and modestly increase high-density lipoprotein cholesterol (HDL-C) through activation of peroxisome proliferator-activated receptor-alpha (PPAR-α), though their role has diminished with evidence suggesting limited cardiovascular outcome benefits beyond statin therapy.

Anticoagulants and Antiplatelets

Thrombotic disorder management employs agents targeting the coagulation cascade or platelet function. Traditional anticoagulation with warfarin inhibits vitamin K-dependent clotting factors (II, VII, IX, X), requiring close monitoring through International Normalized Ratio (INR) testing due to numerous food and drug interactions affecting its metabolism. Direct oral anticoagulants (DOACs) offer targeted inhibition of specific coagulation factors—either thrombin (dabigatran) or factor Xa (rivaroxaban, apixaban, edoxaban)—with predictable pharmacokinetics enabling fixed dosing without routine monitoring. However, renal function assessment remains essential for appropriate dose selection. Antiplatelet agents prevent thrombotic events through various mechanisms: aspirin irreversibly inhibits cyclooxygenase-1 (COX-1), reducing thromboxane A2 production; P2Y12 inhibitors (clopidogrel, prasugrel, ticagrelor) prevent ADP-mediated platelet activation; and glycoprotein IIb/IIIa inhibitors block the final common pathway of platelet aggregation in acute coronary syndromes. Dual antiplatelet therapy balances enhanced antithrombotic efficacy against increased bleeding risk, with duration tailored to specific clinical scenarios.

Heart Failure Medications

Heart failure pharmacotherapy aims to reduce symptoms, improve quality of life, and decrease mortality through targeting neurohormonal activation and hemodynamic derangements. Angiotensin-converting enzyme inhibitors (ACEIs) and angiotensin receptor blockers (ARBs) counteract the detrimental effects of renin-angiotensin-aldosterone system activation, reducing afterload and preventing pathologic remodeling. Beta-adrenergic blockers, once contraindicated in heart failure, now represent foundational therapy through attenuation of sympathetic nervous system hyperactivation, with carvedilol, metoprolol succinate, and bisoprolol demonstrating mortality benefits in landmark trials. Mineralocorticoid receptor antagonists (spironolactone, eplerenone) provide additional neurohormonal modulation while reducing potassium wasting, though hyperkalemia risk necessitates careful monitoring, particularly when combined with ACEIs or ARBs. The angiotensin receptor-neprilysin inhibitor sacubitril/valsartan represents a therapeutic advancement by simultaneously blocking angiotensin II effects while preventing degradation of beneficial natriuretic peptides. Loop diuretics manage congestion without mortality benefit, requiring careful dose titration to balance symptom relief against electrolyte disturbances and renal dysfunction. Sodium-glucose cotransporter-2 (SGLT2) inhibitors have emerged as a novel therapeutic class with demonstrated benefits in heart failure with reduced ejection fraction, even in non-diabetic patients, potentially through multiple mechanisms including improved cardiac energetics and reduced cardiac preload.

Table 8.2: Cardiovascular Medications

Drug Class	Examples	Mechanism of Action
HMG-CoA Reductase Inhibitors (Statins)	Atorvastatin Rosuvastatin Simvastatin	Inhibit cholesterol synthesis
PCSK9 Inhibitors	Alirocumab Evolocumab	Decrease LDL receptor degradation
Bile Acid Sequestrants	Cholestyramine Colesevelam	Bind bile acids in intestine
Fibric Acid Derivatives	Fenofibrate Gemfibrozil	Activate PPAR-α
Niacin	Niacin/Nicotinic acid	Multiple lipid effects
Cardiac Glycosides	Digoxin	Inhibit Na+/K+ ATPase
Antiarrhythmics Class I	Flecainide Propafenone Procainamide	Sodium channel blockers
Antiarrhythmics Class III	Amiodarone Sotalol Dofetilide	Potassium channel blockers
Antiplatelet Agents	Aspirin Clopidogrel Ticagrelor	Inhibit platelet aggregation
Anticoagulants - Vitamin K Antagonists	Warfarin	Inhibit vitamin K-dependent clotting factors
Anticoagulants - Direct Oral	Apixaban Rivaroxaban Dabigatran	Target specific clotting factors
Nitrates	Nitroglycerin Isosorbide mononitrate	Increase nitric oxide, vasodilation
Inotropes	Milrinone Dobutamine	Increase cardiac contractility

RESPIRATORY SYSTEM

Respiratory pharmacotherapy addresses both acute and chronic conditions affecting the airways and lung parenchyma. These medications target bronchoconstriction, inflammation, mucus hypersecretion, and infectious processes to restore respiratory function and improve quality of life. Delivery methods significantly influence therapeutic efficacy, with inhalation routes providing direct delivery to the target tissues while minimizing systemic exposure. Proper inhaler technique remains critical for therapeutic success, necessitating thorough patient education and periodic reassessment by pharmacists.

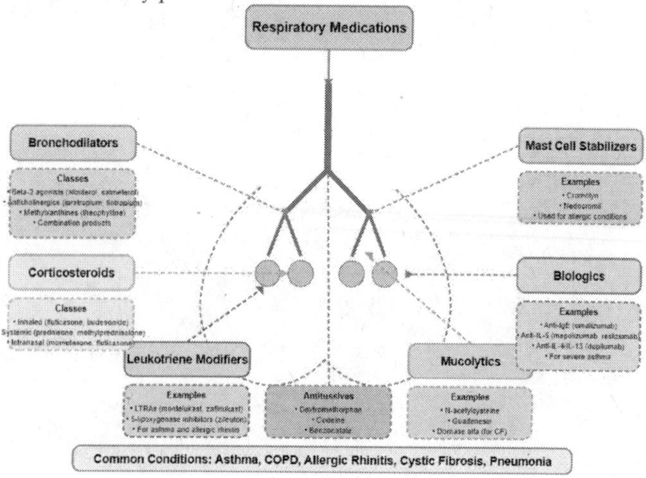

Figure 8.1: Drugs acting on Respiratory System

Bronchodilators

Bronchodilators relieve airflow limitation through relaxation of airway smooth muscle via different mechanisms. Beta2-adrenergic agonists stimulate adenylyl cyclase, increasing intracellular cyclic adenosine monophosphate (cAMP) and producing bronchodilation. Short-acting agents (salbutamol, terbutaline) provide rapid symptom relief within minutes but with brief duration, serving primarily as rescue medication. Long-acting formulations (salmeterol, formoterol, indacaterol) maintain bronchodilation over 12-24 hours, supporting maintenance therapy in asthma and chronic obstructive pulmonary disease (COPD). Potential adverse effects include tremor, tachycardia, and hypokalemia, particularly with excessive use. Anticholinergic bronchodilators block muscarinic receptors, inhibiting acetylcholine-mediated bronchoconstriction. Short-acting compounds (ipratropium) demonstrate efficacy primarily in COPD, while long-acting agents (tiotropium, umeclidinium, glycopyrronium) provide sustained bronchodilation with once-daily dosing and potential reduction in exacerbation frequency. Dry mouth represents the most common adverse effect, with urinary retention and glaucoma exacerbation occurring rarely. Methylxanthines (theophylline) offer modest bronchodilation through phosphodiesterase inhibition and adenosine antagonism, but their narrow therapeutic index and numerous drug interactions have relegated them to third-line therapy in contemporary practice.

Anti-inflammatory Respiratory Medications

Airway inflammation represents a central pathophysiological feature in chronic respiratory diseases, necessitating targeted anti-inflammatory therapy. Inhaled corticosteroids (ICS) reduce airway inflammation through multiple mechanisms, including inhibition of inflammatory cytokine production, reduction of inflammatory cell recruitment, and downregulation of inflammatory mediators.

Table 8.3: Drugs acting on Respiratory System

Drug Class	Generic Examples	Mechanism of Action	Indications
Short-Acting Beta-2 Agonists (SABAs)	Albuterol Levalbuterol	Stimulate beta-2 receptors in airways	Acute bronchospasm Exercise-induced bronchospasm
Long-Acting Beta-2 Agonists (LABAs)	Salmeterol Formoterol Olodaterol	Stimulate beta-2 receptors with extended duration	Asthma (with ICS) COPD maintenance
Short-Acting Muscarinic Antagonists (SAMAs)	Ipratropium	Block muscarinic receptors in airways	COPD Asthma exacerbations

Drug Class	Generic Examples	Mechanism of Action	Indications
Long-Acting Muscarinic Antagonists (LAMAs)	Tiotropium Umeclidinium Aclidinium	Block muscarinic receptors with extended duration	COPD maintenance Severe asthma
Inhaled Corticosteroids (ICS)	Fluticasone Budesonide Beclomethasone	Reduce airway inflammation	Asthma control COPD with exacerbations
Leukotriene Modifiers	Montelukast Zafirlukast Zileuton	Block leukotriene effects or synthesis	Asthma Allergic rhinitis
Mast Cell Stabilizers	Cromolyn Nedocromil	Prevent mast cell degranulation	Mild asthma Exercise-induced bronchospasm
Methylxanthines	Theophylline	Phosphodiesterase inhibition	Asthma COPD
Combination Inhalers (ICS/LABA)	Fluticasone/salmeterol Budesonide/formoterol	Combined anti-inflammatory and bronchodilator	Asthma control COPD with exacerbations
Combination Inhalers (LAMA/LABA)	Umeclidinium/vilanterol Tiotropium/olodaterol	Combined bronchodilator effects	COPD maintenance
Oral Corticosteroids	Prednisone Methylprednisolone	Systemic anti-inflammatory	Asthma, COPD exacerbations

Drug Class	Generic Examples	Mechanism of Action	Indications
Biologics for Asthma	Omalizumab Mepolizumab Benralizumab	Target specific inflammatory mediators	Severe asthma Specific phenotypes
Antitussives	Dextromethorphan Codeine	Suppress cough reflex	Dry, non-productive cough
Expectorants	Guaifenesin	Increase respiratory tract fluid	Productive cough

These agents serve as cornerstone therapy for persistent asthma but demonstrate more selective utility in COPD, primarily for patients with eosinophilic inflammation or frequent exacerbations. Local adverse effects include oropharyngeal candidiasis and dysphonia, which can be mitigated through proper inhaler technique and post-administration mouth rinsing. Leukotriene modifiers (montelukast, zafirlukast) inhibit inflammatory pathways mediated by leukotrienes, providing modest bronchodilation and inflammation reduction, particularly in exercise-induced and aspirin-exacerbated respiratory disease. Biologic therapies have revolutionized management of severe eosinophilic and allergic respiratory diseases through targeted inhibition of specific inflammatory pathways: anti-IgE therapy (omalizumab) for allergic asthma; anti-IL-5 agents (mepolizumab, reslizumab) and anti-IL-5 receptor antibodies (benralizumab) for eosinophilic inflammation; and anti-IL-4 receptor antibodies (dupilumab) blocking both IL-4 and IL-13 signaling in type 2 inflammation.

Combination Therapy and Delivery Devices

Respiratory disease management frequently employs combination therapy targeting complementary pathophysiological mechanisms. Fixed-dose combination inhalers improve adherence through simplified regimens while leveraging potential synergistic effects between drug classes. Inhaled corticosteroid/long-acting beta2-agonist (ICS/LABA) combinations serve as maintenance therapy in asthma and selected COPD phenotypes. Triple therapy incorporating long-acting anticholinergics with ICS/LABA offers additional benefit for frequent exacerbators. Delivery devices significantly influence medication effectiveness through determining lung deposition patterns and patient usability. Pressurized metered-dose inhalers (pMDIs) require coordinated actuation and inhalation, often necessitating spacer devices for optimal delivery, particularly in pediatric and geriatric populations. Dry powder inhalers (DPIs) eliminate coordination challenges but require sufficient inspiratory flow for proper dispersion and delivery. Nebulizers accommodate patients unable to use handheld inhalers effectively but require longer administration times and more complex maintenance. Soft mist inhalers represent an emerging technology generating a slow-moving aerosol cloud, potentially enhancing lung deposition while requiring minimal inspiratory effort. Device selection must consider patient-specific factors including age, cognitive status, manual dexterity, inspiratory capacity, and personal preference.

Respiratory Infections and Special Conditions

Additional respiratory medications address specific conditions beyond obstructive airway diseases. Mucolytics (N-acetylcysteine, dornase alfa) reduce mucus viscosity through disruption of mucin polymers, facilitating clearance in conditions with abnormal secretions, including cystic fibrosis and bronchiectasis. Antitussives target persistent cough through central mechanisms (codeine, dextromethorphan) or peripheral pathways (benzonatate), though limited evidence supports their efficacy in chronic cough syndromes. Inhaled antibiotics (tobramycin, aztreonam, colistin) provide targeted therapy for chronic airway infections in cystic fibrosis and bronchiectasis, achieving high local concentrations while minimizing systemic toxicity. Pulmonary arterial hypertension therapies include endothelin receptor antagonists (bosentan, ambrisentan, macitentan), phosphodiesterase-5 inhibitors (sildenafil, tadalafil), soluble guanylate cyclase stimulators (riociguat), and prostacyclin pathway agents (epoprostenol, treprostinil, selexipag), targeting different aspects of the pathophysiological cascade. Idiopathic pulmonary fibrosis management employs antifibrotic agents (pirfenidone, nintedanib) that slow disease progression through multiple mechanisms including inhibition of transforming growth factor-beta and fibroblast growth factor receptor signaling.

GASTROINTESTINAL AGENTS

Gastrointestinal pharmacotherapy addresses disorders affecting digestive function, acid secretion, motility, and mucosal integrity. These medications alleviate symptoms, promote healing, and prevent complications in conditions ranging from common functional disorders to inflammatory and malignant diseases. Treatment approaches balance efficacy against potential risks, particularly with long-term therapy, necessitating periodic reassessment of continued indication and appropriate duration.

Acid-Suppressing Medications

Acid-suppressing agents represent among the most frequently prescribed medications worldwide for management of acid-related disorders. Proton pump inhibitors (PPIs) provide potent acid suppression through irreversible inhibition of the H+/K+-ATPase enzyme in gastric parietal cells. These agents effectively treat gastroesophageal reflux disease (GERD), peptic ulcer disease, and Helicobacter pylori infections when combined with antibiotics. Despite their favorable short-term safety profile, prolonged PPI therapy has been associated with potential adverse effects including increased risk of Clostridium difficile infection, community-acquired pneumonia, nutrient malabsorption (vitamin B12, magnesium, calcium), and chronic kidney disease, though causal relationships remain controversial. Histamine-2 receptor antagonists (H2RAs) provide less potent but still significant acid suppression through competitive inhibition of histamine at parietal cell H2 receptors. These agents offer advantages in on-demand therapy for intermittent symptoms and may confer reduced risk of long-term complications compared to PPIs. Antacids neutralize gastric acid directly, providing rapid but short-duration symptom relief for occasional heartburn. These agents contain various combinations of aluminum, magnesium, and calcium salts, each with specific considerations regarding constipation or diarrhea potential and drug interaction profiles through altered gastric pH or chelation effects.

Table 8.4: Drugs Acting on Gastrointestinal System

Drug Class	Generic Examples	Mechanism of Action	Indications
Proton Pump Inhibitors	Omeprazole Esomeprazole Pantoprazole	Inhibit H+/K+ ATPase pump	GERD PUD H. pylori eradication NSAID prophylaxis
H2 Receptor Antagonists	Famotidine Ranitidine Cimetidine	Block histamine H2 receptors	GERD PUD Heartburn
Antacids	Aluminum/Magnesium hydroxide Calcium carbonate	Neutralize gastric acid	Heartburn Indigestion
Sucralfate	Sucralfate	Forms protective barrier on ulcers	PUD GERD
Misoprostol	Misoprostol	Prostaglandin analog	NSAID prophylaxis Abortion Labor induction
Promotility Agents	Metoclopramide Erythromycin	Increase GI motility	Gastroparesis GERD Post-operative ileus
5-HT3 Antagonists	Ondansetron Granisetron Palonosetron	Block serotonin receptors	Chemotherapy-induced nausea Postoperative nausea Radiation-induced nausea

Drug Class	Generic Examples	Mechanism of Action	Indications
NK1 Receptor Antagonists	Aprepitant Fosaprepitant Rolapitant	Block substance P receptors	Chemotherapy-induced nausea Postoperative nausea
Laxatives - Bulk Forming	Psyllium Methylcellulose Polycarbophil	Increase stool bulk	Constipation IBS-C
Laxatives - Osmotic	Polyethylene glycol Magnesium citrate Lactulose	Draw water into intestine	Constipation Bowel prep Hepatic encephalopathy
Laxatives - Stimulant	Bisacodyl Senna Cascara	Increase intestinal motility	Constipation Bowel prep
Laxatives - Lubricant	Mineral oil	Lubricates intestinal contents	Constipation
Antidiarrheals	Loperamide Diphenoxylate/atropine	Decrease intestinal motility	Acute diarrhea Chronic diarrhea
IBS Agents	Linaclotide Plecanatide Eluxadoline	Varies by agent	IBS-C IBS-D Chronic idiopathic constipation
Inflammatory Bowel Disease Agents	Mesalamine Sulfasalazine Balsalazide	Anti-inflammatory in GI tract	Ulcerative colitis Crohn's disease
Antiemetics - Others	Prochlorperazine Promethazine Scopolamine	Various mechanisms	Nausea and vomiting Motion sickness

Agents for Motility Disorders

Gastrointestinal motility disorders involve abnormal coordination or propulsion of intestinal contents, manifesting as dyspepsia, gastroparesis, constipation, or diarrhea. Prokinetic agents enhance gastrointestinal motility through various mechanisms. Metoclopramide stimulates upper gastrointestinal motility via dopamine D2 receptor antagonism and 5-HT4 receptor agonism, though extrapyramidal adverse effects limit long-term use, particularly in elderly patients. Erythromycin enhances motility through motilin receptor agonism, with tachyphylaxis limiting sustained efficacy. Laxatives address constipation through diverse mechanisms: osmotic agents (polyethylene glycol, lactulose, magnesium salts) draw water into the intestinal lumen; stimulant laxatives (bisacodyl, senna) directly stimulate intestinal peristalsis; stool softeners (docusate) reduce surface tension of the stool-water interface; and newer secretagogues (lubiprostone, linaclotide) enhance intestinal fluid secretion through chloride channel activation or guanylate cyclase-C stimulation. Antidiarrheal agents include opioid receptor agonists (loperamide) reducing intestinal motility and secretion, bile acid sequestrants (cholestyramine) for bile acid diarrhea, and adsorbents (bismuth subsalicylate) binding toxins and providing antimicrobial effects.

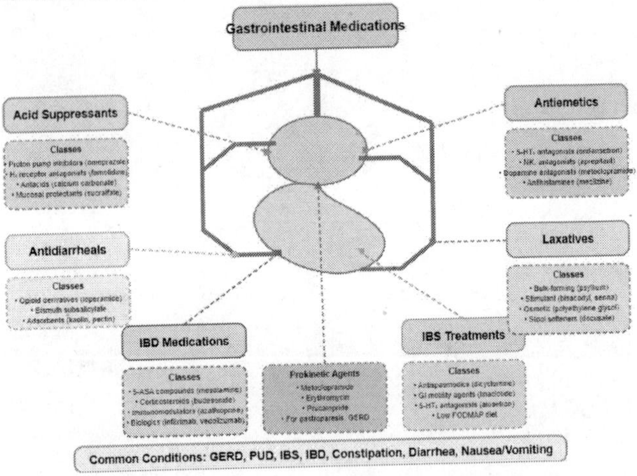

Figure 8.2: Gastrointestinal Agents and Their Sites of Action

Anti-inflammatory and Immunomodulatory Gastrointestinal Medications

Inflammatory bowel diseases (IBD) require targeted anti-inflammatory and immunomodulatory therapy addressing underlying immune dysregulation. Aminosalicylates (mesalamine, sulfasalazine) provide topical anti-inflammatory effects through multiple mechanisms including inhibition of prostaglandin synthesis and nuclear factor-kappa B (NF-κB) activation, serving as first-line therapy for mild-to-moderate ulcerative colitis but with limited efficacy in Crohn's disease. Corticosteroids (prednisone, budesonide) offer potent anti-inflammatory effects for acute disease flares but are unsuitable for maintenance therapy due to significant adverse effects with prolonged use. Immunomodulators including thiopurines (azathioprine, 6-mercaptopurine) and methotrexate enable steroid-sparing maintenance therapy through suppression of T-cell activation and proliferation, though their delayed onset of action precludes use in acute exacerbations. Biologic therapies have transformed IBD management through targeted inhibition of specific inflammatory pathways: anti-tumor necrosis factor agents (infliximab, adalimumab, golimumab, certolizumab pegol); anti-integrin therapies (vedolizumab) selectively blocking gut-homing lymphocytes; anti-IL-12/23 antibodies (ustekinumab) inhibiting multiple inflammatory cytokine pathways; and Janus kinase inhibitors (tofacitinib) blocking intracellular signal transduction. Treatment selection balances efficacy against safety considerations including infection risk, malignancy potential, and paradoxical immune-mediated adverse effects.

Antiemetics and Other Specialized Gastrointestinal Agents

Nausea and vomiting management employs agents targeting different neurotransmitter pathways in the emetic reflex arc. Serotonin (5-HT3) receptor antagonists (ondansetron, granisetron, palonosetron) effectively prevent chemotherapy-induced and postoperative nausea and vomiting through inhibition of serotonin action in the chemoreceptor trigger zone and gastrointestinal tract. Neurokinin-1 (NK1) receptor antagonists (aprepitant, fosaprepitant) block substance P effects in the central nervous system, providing additive benefit in highly emetogenic chemotherapy regimens. Dopamine antagonists (prochlorperazine, metoclopramide) address various forms of nausea through central and peripheral mechanisms. Antihistamines (dimenhydrinate, meclizine) primarily target motion sickness through vestibular system effects. Cannabinoids (dronabinol, nabilone) offer alternative options for refractory cases, particularly in chemotherapy-induced nausea. Specialized gastrointestinal agents include pancreatic enzyme replacements (pancrelipase) for exocrine pancreatic insufficiency, containing lipase, amylase, and protease in enteric-coated formulations to prevent gastric degradation. Antispasmodics (dicyclomine, hyoscyamine) reduce smooth muscle contractility in irritable bowel syndrome and other functional gastrointestinal disorders through antimuscarinic effects. Probiotics provide potential benefit in selected conditions including antibiotic-associated diarrhea, though specific strain selection and quality control significantly influence outcomes.

ENDOCRINE SYSTEM

Endocrine pharmacotherapy addresses disorders involving hormone production, secretion, and receptor function. These medications replace deficient hormones, suppress excessive production, or modify hormone action to restore physiological function. Endocrine disorders frequently require lifelong therapy with careful monitoring to balance efficacy against potential adverse effects from under or over-replacement.

Diabetes Medications

Diabetes management employs multiple pharmacological classes targeting different aspects of glucose regulation. Insulin therapy provides direct replacement in type 1 diabetes and advanced type 2 diabetes when endogenous production becomes insufficient. Modern insulin formulations include rapid-acting analogs (lispro, aspart, glulisine) for mealtime coverage; long-acting basal insulins (glargine, detemir, degludec) providing steady background insulin levels; and intermediate-acting preparations (NPH) with properties between these extremes. Insulin delivery options include multiple daily injections or continuous subcutaneous insulin infusion through insulin pumps, with emerging closed-loop systems integrating continuous glucose monitoring for automated dosing adjustments. Among oral antihyperglycemic agents, metformin remains the preferred initial therapy for type 2 diabetes through multiple mechanisms including reduced hepatic glucose production and enhanced peripheral insulin sensitivity, with minimal hypoglycemia risk and potential cardiometabolic benefits beyond glycemic control. Sulfonylureas (glimepiride, glipizide, glyburide) stimulate pancreatic insulin secretion through ATP-sensitive potassium channel closure in beta cells, providing potent glucose lowering but with significant hypoglycemia and weight gain potential. Dipeptidyl peptidase-4 (DPP-4) inhibitors (sitagliptin, saxagliptin, linagliptin) prevent degradation of incretin hormones, enhancing glucose-dependent insulin secretion with weight-neutral effects and minimal hypoglycemia risk. Sodium-glucose cotransporter-2 (SGLT2) inhibitors (empagliflozin, canagliflozin, dapagliflozin) provide insulin-independent glucose lowering through inhibition of renal glucose reabsorption, with demonstrated cardiovascular and renal benefits extending beyond glycemic control. Injectable incretin-based therapies include glucagon-like peptide-1 (GLP-1) receptor agonists (liraglutide, semaglutide, dulaglutide) that enhance glucose-dependent insulin secretion while suppressing glucagon, slowing gastric emptying, and promoting satiety, resulting in significant weight reduction alongside glycemic improvement.

Thyroid Medications

Thyroid disorders represent common endocrine conditions requiring precise medication management. Hypothyroidism treatment primarily employs levothyroxine (T4), providing the prohormone subsequently converted to the active triiodothyronine (T3) in peripheral tissues. This approach mimics physiological hormone regulation while avoiding the fluctuations associated with direct T3 administration. Optimal absorption requires consistent administration timing relative to food and potentially interacting medications, including calcium supplements, iron preparations, and acid-suppressing agents. Therapeutic monitoring utilizes thyroid-stimulating hormone (TSH) as the primary marker, with dose adjustments targeting the reference range or specific goals based on patient characteristics including age and comorbidities.

Table 8.5: Drugs Acting on Endocrine System

Drug Class	Generic Examples	Mechanism of Action	Indications
Insulins - Rapid-Acting	Lispro Aspart Glulisine	Glucose uptake, glycogenesis	Type 1 DM Type 2 DM DKA
Insulins - Short-Acting	Regular insulin	Glucose uptake, glycogenesis	Type 1 DM Type 2 DM DKA Hyperkalemia
Insulins - Intermediate-Acting	NPH insulin	Glucose uptake, glycogenesis	Type 1 DM Type 2 DM
Insulins - Long-Acting	Glargine Detemir Degludec	Glucose uptake, glycogenesis	Type 1 DM Type 2 DM

Drug Class	Generic Examples	Mechanism of Action	Indications
Sulfonylureas	Glipizide Glyburide Glimepiride	Increase insulin secretion	Type 2 DM
Meglitinides	Repaglinide Nateglinide	Increase insulin secretion	Type 2 DM
Biguanides	Metformin	Decrease hepatic glucose production	Type 2 DM Prediabetes PCOS
Thiazolidinediones	Pioglitazone Rosiglitazone	Improve insulin sensitivity	Type 2 DM
DPP-4 Inhibitors	Sitagliptin Saxagliptin Linagliptin	Increase incretins	Type 2 DM
GLP-1 Receptor Agonists	Semaglutide Dulaglutide Liraglutide	Increase insulin, decrease glucagon	Type 2 DM Weight management Cardiovascular risk reduction
SGLT-2 Inhibitors	Empagliflozin Dapagliflozin Canagliflozin	Block glucose reabsorption in kidney	Type 2 DM Heart failure CKD
Amylin Analogs	Pramlintide	Slow gastric emptying, suppress glucagon	Type 1 DM Type 2 DM
Thyroid Hormones	Levothyroxine Liothyronine	Replace/supplement thyroid hormone	Hypothyroidism Myxedema coma
Antithyroid Drugs	Methimazole Propylthiouracil	Inhibit thyroid hormone synthesis	Hyperthyroidism Thyroid storm

Drug Class	Generic Examples	Mechanism of Action	Indications
Corticosteroids	Prednisone Dexamethasone Hydrocortisone	Multiple anti-inflammatory and metabolic effects	Inflammatory conditions Autoimmune disorders Adrenal insufficiency
Sex Hormones - Estrogens	Estradiol Conjugated estrogens	Bind estrogen receptors	Menopausal symptoms Contraception Hormone replacement

Hyperthyroidism management includes thionamides (methimazole, propylthiouracil) inhibiting thyroid hormone synthesis through blockade of the thyroid peroxidase enzyme and interruption of iodotyrosine coupling. These agents serve as primary therapy for Graves' disease or as preparation for definitive treatment with radioactive iodine or surgery. Potential adverse effects range from minor rashes to serious complications including agranulocytosis and hepatotoxicity, necessitating vigilant monitoring. Adjunctive symptomatic management employs beta-blockers to control adrenergic manifestations including tachycardia, tremor, and anxiety during the interval before thionamides achieve hormonal control.

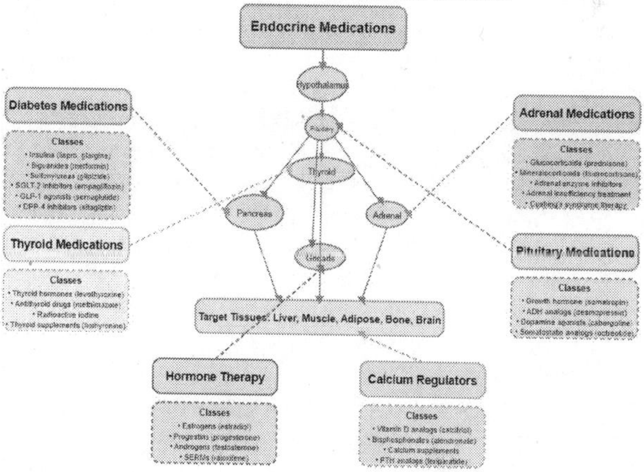

Figure 8.3: Endocrine Medications and Target Pathways

Adrenal and Gonadal Hormone Medications

Adrenal hormone therapy encompasses both glucocorticoid and mineralocorticoid replacement or suppression. Glucocorticoid replacement in adrenal insufficiency employs hydrocortisone, prednisone, or dexamethasone in regimens mimicking physiological cortisol patterns while preventing symptoms of deficiency. Conversely, pharmacological glucocorticoid therapy for inflammatory and autoimmune conditions requires careful consideration of potential adverse effects including hyperglycemia, osteoporosis, adrenal suppression, and increased infection susceptibility. Mineralocorticoid replacement with fludrocortisone addresses aldosterone deficiency, maintaining sodium-potassium balance and preventing orthostatic hypotension. Gonadal hormone therapy includes estrogen preparations for female hypogonadism, menopausal hormone therapy, and contraception. Estrogen formulations vary in composition (estradiol, conjugated equine estrogens), delivery route (oral, transdermal, vaginal), and combination with progestins to protect endometrial integrity. Testosterone replacement addresses male hypogonadism through various formulations including transdermal gels, intramuscular injections, and subcutaneous pellets, with monitoring for potential adverse effects including polycythemia, exacerbation of obstructive sleep apnea, and effects on prostate health.

Medications for Bone Metabolism and Other Endocrine Disorders

Bone metabolism disorders require agents targeting osteoclast-mediated bone resorption or osteoblast-driven bone formation. Antiresorptive therapies include bisphosphonates (alendronate, risedronate, zoledronic acid) that bind hydroxyapatite and inhibit osteoclast function, providing the foundation of osteoporosis management but requiring specific administration protocols to enhance absorption and minimize esophageal irritation. Receptor activator of nuclear factor kappa-B ligand (RANKL) inhibitors (denosumab) prevent osteoclast formation and activation through blockade of this essential signaling pathway, offering alternatives for patients unable to tolerate bisphosphonates. Anabolic agents including parathyroid hormone analogs (teriparatide, abaloparatide) and sclerostin inhibitors (romosozumab) stimulate new bone formation, particularly beneficial in severe osteoporosis with prevalent fractures. Calcium and vitamin D supplementation support bone health as adjunctive therapy, with doses tailored to dietary intake and measured serum levels. Other specialized endocrine medications include somatostatin analogs (octreotide, lanreotide) for acromegaly and neuroendocrine tumors; vasopressin analogs (desmopressin) for diabetes insipidus; and growth hormone therapy for growth hormone deficiency and specific genetic disorders affecting growth. Medications for pituitary disorders include dopamine agonists (cabergoline, bromocriptine) for prolactinomas and pegvisomant for growth hormone receptor blockade in refractory acromegaly.

Summary

Cardiovascular medications combat the leading causes of morbidity and mortality through diverse mechanisms targeting various physiological pathways. Antihypertensives include ACE inhibitors and angiotensin receptor blockers modulating the renin-angiotensin-aldosterone system, calcium channel blockers reducing vascular tone, diuretics affecting fluid balance, and beta-blockers reducing cardiac output—each selected based on comorbidities, demographic factors, and tolerability profiles. Antiarrhythmics regulate cardiac conduction and rhythm through sodium, potassium, and calcium channel modulation, while anticoagulants including warfarin, direct oral anticoagulants, and antiplatelets prevent thromboembolic events. Hyperlipidemia agents—statins, ezetimibe, PCSK9 inhibitors, and fibrates—reduce atherosclerotic risk through various lipid-modifying mechanisms. Respiratory medications target bronchoconstrictive and inflammatory pathways in asthma and COPD, with short-acting bronchodilators providing rescue relief, long-acting agents maintaining airway patency, inhaled corticosteroids suppressing inflammation, and biological therapies addressing severe, refractory disease. Inhalation device selection significantly impacts therapeutic efficacy, requiring patient-specific considerations regarding coordination abilities and inspiratory capacity. Gastrointestinal agents address diverse conditions including acid-related disorders through proton pump inhibitors and H2 antagonists, motility disturbances using prokinetics and antispasmodics, and inflammatory conditions with aminosalicylates and immunomodulators. Antiemetics target various neurotransmitter pathways including dopamine, serotonin, and histamine receptors based on emesis etiology. Endocrine medications regulate hormonal systems including diabetes therapies (insulins, GLP-1 agonists, SGLT2 inhibitors, and other agents addressing glucose regulation through complementary mechanisms), thyroid replacement hormones requiring precise titration, and reproductive hormones used for contraception, hormone replacement, and fertility management. These medication classes require individualized selection, careful monitoring for efficacy and toxicity, and ongoing adjustment to optimize therapeutic outcomes.

Multiple Choice Questions

1. Which of the following antihypertensive medications would be most appropriate for initial therapy in a patient with heart failure with reduced ejection fraction?
   a) Diltiazem
   b) Lisinopril
   c) Amlodipine
   d) Hydrochlorothiazide
2. A patient with stable angina is currently taking metoprolol. Which of the following would be the most appropriate add-on therapy if the patient continues to have symptoms?
   a) Propranolol
   b) Isosorbide mononitrate
   c) Digoxin
   d) Spironolactone
3. A patient with atrial fibrillation has a CHA_2DS_2-VASc score of 3. Which of the following would be the most appropriate anticoagulation strategy?
   a) No anticoagulation needed
   b) Aspirin 81 mg daily
   c) Direct oral anticoagulant or warfarin
   d) Dual antiplatelet therapy
4. Which of the following statins has the highest potency in lowering LDL cholesterol at standard doses?
   a) Pravastatin
   b) Atorvastatin
   c) Fluvastatin
   d) Lovastatin
5. A patient with asthma uses an albuterol inhaler multiple times daily for symptom control. According to current guidelines, which of the following would be the most appropriate next step in therapy?
   a) Add a long-acting beta agonist (LABA) alone
   b) Add an inhaled corticosteroid
   c) Add a leukotriene receptor antagonist
   d) Switch to a combination LABA/anticholinergic inhaler
6. Which of the following medications would be most appropriate for maintenance therapy in a patient with COPD who has an FEV_1 of 45% predicted and frequent exacerbations?
   a) Albuterol as needed

b) Montelukast daily
c) Tiotropium daily
d) Prednisone daily

7. A patient with gastroesophageal reflux disease (GERD) has been taking omeprazole 20 mg daily for 8 weeks without symptom improvement. Which of the following would be the most appropriate next step?
a) Switch to famotidine
b) Increase omeprazole to 40 mg daily
c) Add metoclopramide
d) Recommend surgical intervention

8. Which of the following medications would be most appropriate for a patient with diarrhea-predominant irritable bowel syndrome?
a) Polyethylene glycol
b) Metoclopramide
c) Loperamide
d) Lubiprostone

9. A patient with type 2 diabetes has an A1C of 8.2% despite maximum tolerated metformin therapy. The patient has established atherosclerotic cardiovascular disease. Which of the following would be the most appropriate add-on medication?
a) Glipizide
b) Sitagliptin
c) Empagliflozin
d) Pioglitazone

10. A patient with hypothyroidism is taking levothyroxine 100 mcg daily. Recent thyroid function tests show: TSH 0.1 mIU/L (normal 0.5-5.0) and free T4 1.3 ng/dL (normal 0.7-1.8). The most appropriate recommendation would be to:
a) Increase the dose to 112 mcg daily
b) Decrease the dose to 88 mcg daily
c) Add liothyronine (T3) therapy
d) Maintain the current dose and recheck levels in 4-6 weeks

Self-Assessment Questions

1. Compare and contrast the mechanisms of action, clinical indications, adverse effects, and monitoring parameters of major antihypertensive classes
2. Explain how medications targeting different pathophysiological mechanisms complement each other and how therapy should be sequenced and monitored.
3. Evaluate the anticoagulant options (warfarin, direct oral anticoagulants, parenteral agents) for various thromboembolic conditions, explaining how factors including renal function, drug interactions, monitoring requirements, and reversal options influence therapeutic selection.
4. Describe the lipid-lowering approaches for a patient with atherosclerotic cardiovascular disease and statin intolerance, analyzing the evidence supporting alternative agents and combination therapies while considering efficacy, safety, and cost considerations.
5. Compare and contrast the pharmacological management of asthma versus chronic obstructive pulmonary disease, explaining how differences in underlying pathophysiology influence medication selection, device choices, and therapeutic goals.
6. Analyze the appropriate selection of inhaler devices based on patient factors including age, cognitive status, inspiratory capacity, and coordination abilities, explaining how device mismatching affects therapeutic outcomes.
7. Evaluate the step-wise approach to gastroesophageal reflux disease management, comparing the mechanisms, efficacy, safety profiles, and appropriate use of different acid-suppressing therapies while addressing concerns about long-term proton pump inhibitor use.
8. Explain how medication selection is influenced by disease location, severity, complication risks, and treatment goals.
9. Explain how different medication classes address various pathophysiological defects and how combination therapy should be optimized.
10. Explain factors affecting dosing requirements, potential interactions affecting absorption or metabolism, appropriate laboratory monitoring, and clinical assessment of treatment adequacy.

Bibliography

1. Whelton PK, Carey RM, Aronow WS, Casey DE Jr, Collins KJ, Dennison Himmelfarb C, et al. 2017 ACC/AHA/AAPA/ABC/ACPM/AGS/APhA/ASH/ASPC/NMA/PCNA Guideline for the prevention, detection, evaluation, and management of high blood pressure in adults: A report of the American College of Cardiology/American Heart Association Task Force on Clinical Practice Guidelines. Hypertension. 2018;71(6):e13-e115.
2. Arnett DK, Blumenthal RS, Albert MA, Buroker AB, Goldberger ZD, Hahn EJ, et al. 2019 ACC/AHA Guideline on the primary prevention of cardiovascular disease: A report of the American College of Cardiology/American Heart Association Task Force on Clinical Practice Guidelines. Circulation. 2019;140(11):e596-e646.
3. Global Initiative for Asthma. Global strategy for asthma management and prevention, 2021. Available from: www.ginasthma.org
4. Global Initiative for Chronic Obstructive Lung Disease. Global strategy for the diagnosis, management, and prevention of chronic obstructive pulmonary disease, 2021 report. Available from: www.goldcopd.org
5. Chey WD, Leontiadis GI, Howden CW, Moss SF. ACG Clinical Guideline: Treatment of Helicobacter pylori infection. Am J Gastroenterol. 2017;112(2):212-239.
6. American Diabetes Association. Standards of medical care in diabetes—2021. Diabetes Care. 2021;44(Suppl 1):S1-S232.
7. Lacy BE, Mearin F, Chang L, Chey WD, Lembo AJ, Simren M, et al. Bowel disorders. Gastroenterology. 2016;150(6):1393-1407.e5.
8. Garber JR, Cobin RH, Gharib H, Hennessey JV, Klein I, Mechanick JI, et al. Clinical practice guidelines for hypothyroidism in adults: Cosponsored by the American Association of Clinical Endocrinologists and the American Thyroid Association. Endocr Pract. 2012;18(6):988-1028.
9. Grundy SM, Stone NJ, Bailey AL, Beam C, Birtcher KK, Blumenthal RS, et al. 2018 AHA/ACC/AACVPR/AAPA/ABC/ACPM/ADA/AGS/APhA/ASPC/NLA/PCNA Guideline on the management of blood cholesterol: A report of the American College of Cardiology/American Heart Association Task Force on Clinical Practice Guidelines. Circulation. 2019;139(25):e1082-e1143.
10. January CT, Wann LS, Calkins H, Chen LY, Cigarroa JE, Cleveland JC Jr, et al. 2019 AHA/ACC/HRS focused update of the 2014 AHA/ACC/HRS Guideline for the management of patients with atrial fibrillation: A report of the American College of Cardiology/American Heart Association Task Force on Clinical Practice Guidelines and the Heart Rhythm Society. J Am Coll Cardiol. 2019;74(1):104-132

CHAPTER 9

MAJOR DRUG CLASSES II

Author

Mr. Prakash Nathaniel Kumar Sarella, Associate Professor, Department of Pharmaceutics, Aditya College of Pharmacy, Aditya University, Surampalem, Andhra Pradesh, India

Abstract

Major drug classes involving infectious diseases, neurological conditions, pain, and cancer represent critical therapies for acute and chronic conditions requiring specialized knowledge. Antimicrobial agents include antibacterials classified by mechanism (cell wall inhibitors, protein synthesis inhibitors, DNA/RNA disruptors) and spectrum; antivirals targeting specific viral replication steps for HIV, hepatitis, herpes, and respiratory infections; antifungals addressing superficial and systemic mycoses; and antiparasitics, with selection guided by microbial identification, susceptibility, pharmacokinetic considerations, and antimicrobial stewardship principles preventing resistance development. Central nervous system drugs include antidepressants spanning multiple mechanisms (SSRIs, SNRIs, atypical agents); antipsychotics divided into conventional and atypical classes with varying receptor profiles; mood stabilizers for bipolar disorder; anxiolytics with particular attention to dependence potential; and anticonvulsants categorized by seizure type indication and molecular targets, each requiring specific monitoring for efficacy and unique adverse effect profiles. Pain management medications range from non-opioid analgesics (acetaminophen, NSAIDs) to opioids with varying potency, duration, and formulations; adjuvant agents including anticonvulsants and antidepressants for neuropathic pain; and topical analgesics, with therapy selection balancing efficacy against adverse effects, tolerance, and abuse potential through multimodal approaches. Oncology drugs include traditional cytotoxic agents classified by mechanism (alkylating agents, antimetabolites, microtubule inhibitors); targeted therapies addressing specific molecular pathways; immunotherapies enhancing anti-tumor immune responses; hormone therapies for receptor-positive cancers; and supportive care medications managing treatment side effects, each requiring specialized handling, complex administration protocols, and comprehensive monitoring for potentially severe adverse reactions.

Keywords: *Pathogen-Specific Therapy; Neurotransmitter; Receptor Modulation; Multimodal Analgesia; Targeted Treatment; Drug Resistance*

Learning Objectives

After completion of the chapter, the learners should be able to:

- Apply antimicrobial stewardship principles to select appropriate agents based on suspected pathogens, site of infection, and local resistance patterns.
- Differentiate between the mechanisms, indications, and adverse effect profiles of various classes of central nervous system medications.
- Design multimodal pain management approaches incorporating opioid and non-opioid analgesics based on pain type, intensity, and patient-specific factors.
- Develop supportive care strategies to manage common adverse effects associated with chemotherapy and targeted cancer therapies.
- Recommend appropriate monitoring parameters for antimicrobials, CNS agents, pain medications, and oncology drugs based on efficacy and safety considerations.
- Implement risk mitigation strategies for medications with significant abuse potential or narrow therapeutic indices.

ANTIMICROBIAL AGENTS

Antimicrobial agents represent a diverse array of compounds targeting pathogenic microorganisms through various mechanisms of action. Proper selection requires consideration of the likely pathogen, infection site, patient characteristics, and local resistance patterns. The principle of antimicrobial stewardship guides judicious use to maximize therapeutic efficacy while minimizing adverse effects, resistance development, and collateral ecological damage. Pharmacists play a critical role in optimizing antimicrobial therapy through ensuring appropriate agent selection, dosing, duration, and monitoring.

Beta-Lactam Antibiotics

Beta-lactam antibiotics share a common structural element—the beta-lactam ring—and exert bactericidal effects through inhibition of cell wall synthesis. Penicillins bind to penicillin-binding proteins (PBPs), disrupting peptidoglycan cross-linking essential for bacterial cell wall integrity. Natural penicillins (penicillin G, penicillin V) demonstrate narrow-spectrum activity against gram-positive cocci and select anaerobes. Aminopenicillins (ampicillin, amoxicillin) expand coverage to include some gram-negative organisms. Antipseudomonal penicillins (piperacillin, ticarcillin) provide activity against Pseudomonas aeruginosa and other resistant gram-negative bacilli.

Table 9.1: Antimicrobial Classes and Characteristics

Antibiotic Class	Generic Examples	Mechanism of Action	Spectrum
Penicillins	Amoxicillin Penicillin V Piperacillin	Inhibit cell wall synthesis	Gram-positive Some gram-negative
Cephalosporins - 1st Gen	Cefazolin Cephalexin	Inhibit cell wall synthesis	Gram-positive Limited gram-negative
Cephalosporins - 2nd Gen	Cefuroxime Cefaclor	Inhibit cell wall synthesis	Improved gram-negative
Cephalosporins - 3rd Gen	Ceftriaxone Cefdinir Cefpodoxime	Inhibit cell wall synthesis	Broad gram-negative Variable gram-positive
Cephalosporins - 4th/5th Gen	Cefepime Ceftaroline	Inhibit cell wall synthesis	Extended gram-negative MRSA (ceftaroline)
Carbapenems	Meropenem Ertapenem Imipenem	Inhibit cell wall synthesis	Very broad spectrum Including ESBL
Monobactams	Aztreonam	Inhibit cell wall synthesis	Aerobic gram-negative
Fluoroquinolones	Ciprofloxacin Levofloxacin Moxifloxacin	Inhibit DNA gyrase	Broad spectrum
Macrolides	Azithromycin Clarithromycin Erythromycin	Inhibit protein synthesis	Gram-positive Atypicals
Tetracyclines	Doxycycline Minocycline Tetracycline	Inhibit protein synthesis	Broad spectrum Atypicals

Antibiotic Class	Generic Examples	Mechanism of Action	Spectrum
Aminoglycosides	Gentamicin Tobramycin Amikacin	Inhibit protein synthesis	Aerobic gram-negative
Sulfonamides	Sulfamethoxazole Sulfadiazine	Inhibit folate synthesis	Variable gram-positive/negative
Oxazolidinones	Linezolid Tedizolid	Inhibit protein synthesis	Resistant gram-positive MRSA, VRE
Glycopeptides	Vancomycin Telavancin	Inhibit cell wall synthesis	Gram-positive MRSA
Lipopeptides	Daptomycin	Disrupt cell membrane	Resistant gram-positive
Antifungals - Azoles	Fluconazole Voriconazole Ketoconazole	Inhibit ergosterol synthesis	Candida Various fungi
Antifungals - Echinocandins	Caspofungin Micafungin	Inhibit cell wall synthesis	Candida Some Aspergillus
Antifungals - Polyenes	Amphotericin B Nystatin	Bind ergosterol	Broad antifungal
Antivirals - Neuraminidase Inhibitors	Oseltamivir Zanamivir	Inhibit viral release	Influenza A and B

Beta-lactamase inhibitor combinations (amoxicillin-clavulanate, piperacillin-tazobactam) overcome resistance mediated by certain bacterial enzymes that hydrolyze the beta-lactam ring. Cephalosporins, classified by generations reflecting their antimicrobial spectrum, provide increasingly broad gram-negative coverage in higher generations while often sacrificing gram-positive activity. First-generation agents (cefazolin, cephalexin) target primarily gram-positive cocci; second-generation compounds (cefuroxime, cefoxitin) offer improved gram-negative coverage; third-generation cephalosporins (ceftriaxone, cefotaxime) provide enhanced gram-negative activity including some extended-spectrum beta-lactamase (ESBL) producers;

and fourth-generation (cefepime) and fifth-generation (ceftaroline, ceftolozane) agents address specific resistance mechanisms while maintaining broad-spectrum efficacy. Carbapenems (meropenem, imipenem, ertapenem) represent the broadest-spectrum beta-lactams, reserved for multidrug-resistant infections due to their stability against most beta-lactamases. Monobactams (aztreonam) provide focused activity against aerobic gram-negative organisms without cross-reactivity in patients with penicillin allergy.

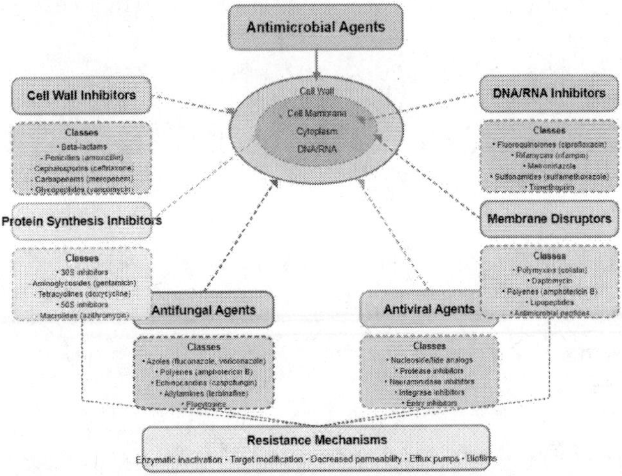

Figure 9.1: Antimicrobial Agents Classification and Mechanisms

Non-Beta-Lactam Antibiotics

Non-beta-lactam antibiotics encompass multiple structural classes with diverse mechanisms of action. Aminoglycosides (gentamicin, tobramycin, amikacin) irreversibly bind bacterial ribosomes, disrupting protein synthesis. These agents demonstrate concentration-dependent bactericidal activity against aerobic gram-negative bacilli, with enhanced efficacy through once-daily dosing regimens that maximize peak concentrations while minimizing nephrotoxicity and ototoxicity through extended drug-free intervals. Therapeutic drug monitoring guides dose optimization, particularly in patients with fluctuating renal function. Tetracyclines (doxycycline, minocycline, tigecycline) inhibit protein synthesis through reversible binding to the 30S ribosomal subunit, providing broad-spectrum activity including atypical pathogens. Newer glycylcycline derivatives overcome specific resistance mechanisms while maintaining activity against multidrug-resistant organisms. Macrolides (erythromycin, azithromycin, clarithromycin) bind the 50S ribosomal subunit, inhibiting protein synthesis in susceptible organisms including atypical respiratory pathogens. These agents demonstrate immunomodulatory properties independent of antimicrobial effects, contributing to their utility in chronic inflammatory respiratory conditions. Quinolones, particularly fluoroquinolones (ciprofloxacin, levofloxacin, moxifloxacin), inhibit bacterial DNA gyrase and topoisomerase IV, disrupting DNA replication. Their broad spectrum, excellent tissue penetration, and oral bioavailability support utility across diverse infections, though emerging safety concerns including tendinopathy, dysglycemia, and neurotoxicity have prompted more restrictive use. Oxazolidinones (linezolid, tedizolid) inhibit protein synthesis through a unique mechanism preventing formation of the initiation complex, providing activity against resistant gram-positive organisms including methicillin-resistant Staphylococcus aureus (MRSA) and vancomycin-resistant enterococci (VRE).

Antiviral Medications

Antiviral medications target specific stages of viral replication cycles, offering therapeutic options for various viral infections. HIV treatment employs combination antiretroviral therapy (cART) incorporating multiple drug classes to suppress viral replication and prevent resistance development. Nucleoside/nucleotide reverse transcriptase inhibitors (NRTIs) provide the backbone of many regimens through competitive inhibition of viral reverse transcriptase and chain termination of viral DNA synthesis. Non-nucleoside reverse transcriptase inhibitors (NNRTIs) bind directly to reverse transcriptase, inducing conformational changes that inhibit enzymatic activity. Protease inhibitors prevent cleavage of viral polyproteins essential for production of functional viral particles. Integrase strand transfer inhibitors (INSTIs) block integration of viral DNA into the host genome, offering potent viral suppression with favorable tolerability. Entry inhibitors, including CCR5 antagonists and fusion inhibitors, prevent viral access to target cells. Hepatitis C virus (HCV) treatment has evolved dramatically with direct-acting antivirals targeting specific viral proteins including NS3/4A protease, NS5A, and NS5B polymerase, enabling interferon-free regimens with cure rates exceeding 95% across most genotypes. Influenza antivirals include neuraminidase inhibitors (oseltamivir, zanamivir) preventing viral particle release from infected cells, and polymerase inhibitors (baloxavir) disrupting viral mRNA synthesis. Herpesvirus infections utilize nucleoside analogs (acyclovir, valacyclovir, famciclovir) that undergo phosphorylation by viral thymidine kinase before inhibiting viral DNA polymerase, providing targeted activity in infected cells. Cytomegalovirus treatment employs specialized agents (ganciclovir, valganciclovir, foscarnet) with enhanced activity against this challenging pathogen.

Antifungal and Antiparasitic Agents

Antifungal therapy addresses superficial and invasive fungal infections through targeting unique components of fungal cells. Azole antifungals (fluconazole, itraconazole, voriconazole, posaconazole) inhibit ergosterol synthesis through blocking the cytochrome P450-dependent enzyme 14-alpha-demethylase, disrupting fungal cell membrane integrity. These agents demonstrate variable spectrums of activity, with newer compounds offering enhanced coverage of molds and resistant yeasts. Significant drug interactions occur through inhibition of cytochrome P450 enzymes, necessitating careful medication reconciliation. Echinocandins (caspofungin, micafungin, anidulafungin) inhibit beta-(1,3)-D-glucan synthase, disrupting fungal cell wall synthesis. This distinct mechanism provides efficacy against resistant Candida species with favorable safety profiles due to the absence of beta-glucan in mammalian cells. Polyenes (amphotericin B) bind ergosterol directly, creating transmembrane channels that increase permeability and lead to cell death. Lipid formulations mitigate the substantial nephrotoxicity associated with conventional amphotericin B while maintaining antifungal efficacy. Antiparasitic agents address protozoal and helminthic infections through diverse mechanisms. Antimalarials include multiple classes: quinolines (chloroquine, hydroxychloroquine) preventing heme detoxification; artemisinin derivatives disrupting parasite membranes through free radical generation; and antifolates inhibiting nucleic acid synthesis. Antiprotozoal agents for intestinal and tissue infections include nitroimidazoles (metronidazole, tinidazole), quinolines, and various antiparasitic compounds with specific indications for amebiasis, giardiasis, trichomoniasis, and leishmaniasis. Antihelminthic treatment employs benzimidazoles (albendazole, mebendazole) disrupting microtubule formation, macrocyclic lactones (ivermectin) enhancing inhibitory neurotransmission, and praziquantel inducing calcium influx and paralysis in susceptible organisms.

CENTRAL NERVOUS SYSTEM DRUGS

Central nervous system (CNS) medications address neurological and psychiatric disorders through modulation of neurotransmitter systems, receptor function, and neuronal excitability. These agents navigate the considerable challenge of targeting specific CNS pathways while minimizing effects on other neurological functions. The blood-brain barrier significantly influences CNS pharmacokinetics, with lipophilicity, molecular size, and transporter interactions determining drug penetration into the central compartment.

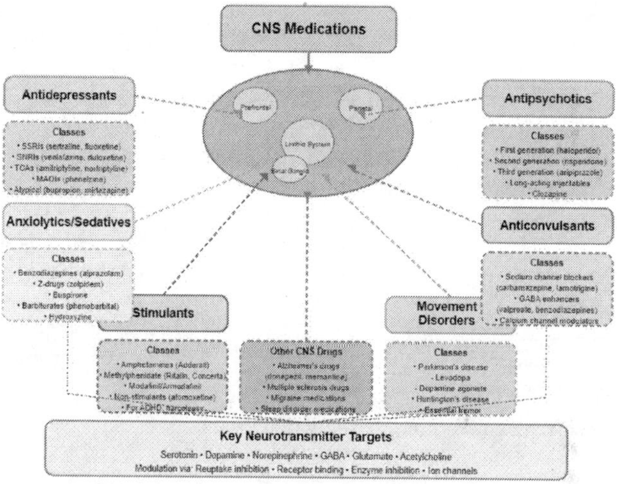

Figure 9.2: Drugs Acting on Central Nervous System

Antidepressants and Mood Stabilizers

Antidepressant medications address major depressive disorder and related conditions through enhancing monoaminergic neurotransmission. Selective serotonin reuptake inhibitors (SSRIs) including fluoxetine, sertraline, and escitalopram selectively block serotonin transporter proteins, increasing synaptic serotonin concentrations. These agents represent first-line therapy due to their favorable safety profile, though sexual dysfunction, gastrointestinal effects, and potential for discontinuation syndrome require consideration. Serotonin-norepinephrine reuptake inhibitors (SNRIs) including venlafaxine, duloxetine, and levomilnacipran inhibit reuptake of both serotonin and norepinephrine, potentially offering advantages in pain syndromes and treatment-resistant depression. Atypical antidepressants provide alternatives through diverse mechanisms: bupropion inhibits norepinephrine and dopamine reuptake with minimal serotonergic effects; mirtazapine enhances noradrenergic and serotonergic transmission through alpha-2 adrenergic antagonism and 5-HT2/3 receptor blockade; and vortioxetine combines serotonin reuptake inhibition with modulation of multiple serotonin receptor subtypes. Tricyclic antidepressants (amitriptyline, nortriptyline) nonselectively inhibit monoamine reuptake while blocking multiple receptor types, resulting in significant anticholinergic, antihistaminic, and alpha-adrenergic effects limiting their first-line use despite established efficacy. Monoamine oxidase inhibitors (phenelzine, tranylcypromine) prevent monoamine degradation, necessitating dietary tyramine restrictions and careful medication reconciliation to prevent hypertensive crisis and serotonin syndrome. Mood stabilizers address bipolar disorder through diverse mechanisms. Lithium modulates multiple neurotransmitter systems and signaling pathways, demonstrating proven antimanic, antidepressant, and antisuicidal properties despite a narrow therapeutic index requiring regular monitoring of serum levels, renal function, and thyroid parameters. Anticonvulsants including valproate, carbamazepine, and lamotrigine provide mood-stabilizing effects through modulation of sodium channels, GABA transmission, and glutamatergic function. Second-generation antipsychotics increasingly serve as primary or adjunctive mood stabilizers based on demonstrated efficacy in acute mania and maintenance treatment.

Antipsychotic Medications

Antipsychotic medications address schizophrenia and other psychotic disorders through dopamine receptor antagonism and modulation of additional neurotransmitter systems. First-generation (typical) antipsychotics including haloperidol and fluphenazine primarily block dopamine D2 receptors, effectively treating positive symptoms (hallucinations, delusions) but with limited efficacy for negative symptoms (apathy, social withdrawal) and cognitive deficits. These agents produce dose-dependent extrapyramidal symptoms through nigrostriatal dopamine blockade, including acute dystonia, akathisia, parkinsonism, and tardive dyskinesia with long-term use. Second-generation (atypical) antipsychotics including risperidone, olanzapine, quetiapine, and aripiprazole demonstrate 5-HT2A/D2 receptor binding ratios favoring serotonergic antagonism, potentially explaining their reduced extrapyramidal liability. These agents show variable efficacy for negative symptoms and cognitive impairment, with individual compounds demonstrating distinct receptor binding profiles influencing their therapeutic and adverse effect patterns. Metabolic effects including weight gain, hyperglycemia, and dyslipidemia represent significant concerns with many atypical antipsychotics, necessitating baseline assessment and ongoing monitoring of metabolic parameters.

Table 9.2: Drugs Acting on Central Nervous System

Drug Class	Generic Examples	Mechanism of Action	Indications
SSRIs	Sertraline Fluoxetine Escitalopram	Inhibit serotonin reuptake	Depression Anxiety disorders OCD PTSD
SNRIs	Venlafaxine Duloxetine Desvenlafaxine	Inhibit serotonin and norepinephrine reuptake	Depression Anxiety Neuropathic pain Fibromyalgia
TCAs	Amitriptyline Nortriptyline Imipramine	Multiple neurotransmitter effects	Depression Neuropathic pain Migraine prevention
MAOIs	Phenelzine Selegiline Tranylcypromine	Inhibit monoamine oxidase	Treatment-resistant depression Atypical depression
Atypical Antidepressants	Bupropion Mirtazapine Trazodone	Various mechanisms	Depression Smoking cessation

Drug Class	Generic Examples	Mechanism of Action	Indications
			Insomnia
First-Generation Antipsychotics	Haloperidol Chlorpromazine Fluphenazine	Block dopamine D2 receptors	Schizophrenia Bipolar disorder Acute agitation
Second-Generation Antipsychotics	Risperidone Olanzapine Quetiapine Aripiprazole	Block multiple receptors	Schizophrenia Bipolar disorder Depression (adjunct) Autism
Benzodiazepines	Diazepam Lorazepam Alprazolam Clonazepam	Enhance GABA effects	Anxiety Insomnia Seizures Muscle spasm
Non-benzodiazepine Hypnotics	Zolpidem Eszopiclone Zaleplon	Selective GABA modulation	Insomnia
Mood Stabilizers	Lithium Valproic acid Lamotrigine	Multiple mechanisms	Bipolar disorder Mania Maintenance therapy
Stimulants	Methylphenidate Amphetamine Lisdexamfetamine	Increase dopamine/norepinephrine	ADHD Narcolepsy
Non-stimulants for ADHD	Atomoxetine Guanfacine	Various mechanisms	ADHD

Drug Class	Generic Examples	Mechanism of Action	Indications
	Clonidine		
Anti-Parkinson's Agents	Levodopa/carbidopa Pramipexole Ropinirole	Replace/mimic dopamine	Parkinson's disease
Anti-Alzheimer's Agents	Donepezil Memantine Rivastigmine	Cholinesterase inhibition or NMDA antagonism	Alzheimer's disease Dementia
Anti-epileptics	Carbamazepine Lamotrigine Levetiracetam Valproic acid	Various mechanisms	Epilepsy Neuropathic pain Mood disorders

Clozapine remains the gold standard for treatment-resistant schizophrenia despite requiring intensive monitoring for agranulocytosis, seizures, myocarditis, and other adverse effects. Long-acting injectable antipsychotic formulations address nonadherence through extended-release preparations administered at intervals ranging from two weeks to three months, improving treatment consistency while necessitating careful dose titration and monitoring for sustained adverse effects.

Anxiolytics and Hypnotics

Anxiety disorders and insomnia represent common conditions requiring thoughtful pharmacological management balancing efficacy against dependence potential. Benzodiazepines enhance gamma-aminobutyric acid (GABA) activity through binding to specific sites on GABA-A receptors, increasing chloride conductance and neuronal inhibition. Individual agents differ primarily in pharmacokinetic parameters, with alprazolam, lorazepam, and clonazepam commonly employed for anxiety disorders, and temazepam, triazolam, and estazolam utilized for insomnia. Despite rapid efficacy, concerns regarding tolerance, dependence, cognitive impairment, and withdrawal limit their long-term utility, with particular caution warranted in elderly patients due to increased fall and fracture risk. Nonbenzodiazepine hypnotics (zolpidem, zaleplon, eszopiclone) selectively bind to the benzodiazepine omega-1 receptor subtype, theoretically providing hypnotic effects with reduced anxiety and muscle relaxation properties, though dependence and complex sleep behaviors remain concerns. Buspirone offers anxiolytic effects through partial 5-HT1A receptor agonism without sedation, cognitive impairment, or dependence liability, though its delayed onset limits utility for acute anxiety. Antidepressants, particularly SSRIs and SNRIs, represent first-line pharmacotherapy for most anxiety disorders based on sustainable efficacy without dependence concerns, despite requiring weeks for full therapeutic effect. Hydroxyzine provides anxiolytic effects through histamine H1 receptor antagonism, offering an alternative for intermittent anxiety symptoms. Orexin receptor antagonists (suvorexant, lemborexant) represent a novel hypnotic class inhibiting wakefulness-promoting orexin signaling, providing potential advantages in maintaining normal sleep architecture.

Anticonvulsants and Medications for Neurological Disorders

Neurological disorders require specialized pharmacotherapy addressing diverse pathophysiological mechanisms. Epilepsy treatment employs anticonvulsants targeting various aspects of neuronal excitability. Sodium channel blockers (phenytoin, carbamazepine, lamotrigine, lacosamide) reduce repetitive neuronal firing through modulation of voltage-gated sodium channels. Calcium channel modulators (ethosuximide, gabapentin, pregabalin) reduce neurotransmitter release through effects on presynaptic calcium influx. GABA enhancers (benzodiazepines, barbiturates, tiagabine, vigabatrin) potentiate inhibitory neurotransmission through various mechanisms affecting GABA availability or receptor function. Synaptic vesicle protein 2A (SV2A) modulators (levetiracetam, brivaracetam) affect neurotransmitter release through binding to this presynaptic protein. Multiple-mechanism anticonvulsants (valproate, topiramate, zonisamide, perampanel) affect various targets simultaneously. Selection considerations include seizure type, comorbidities, potential adverse effects, and drug interaction profiles. Parkinson's disease pharmacotherapy addresses dopaminergic deficiency through several approaches. Levodopa, administered with peripheral decarboxylase inhibitors (carbidopa, benserazide), provides the dopamine precursor crossing the blood-brain barrier for conversion to dopamine within remaining nigrostriatal neurons. Dopamine agonists (pramipexole, ropinirole, rotigotine) directly stimulate dopamine receptors without requiring enzymatic conversion. Monoamine oxidase-B inhibitors (selegiline, rasagiline) prevent dopamine degradation, while catechol-O-methyltransferase inhibitors (entacapone, tolcapone) extend levodopa's duration of action by preventing its peripheral metabolism. Multiple sclerosis treatments include immunomodulatory therapies (interferon beta, glatiramer acetate), cell trafficking inhibitors (fingolimod, natalizumab), B-cell depleting agents (ocrelizumab), and small-molecule immune modulators (dimethyl fumarate, teriflunomide). Alzheimer's disease management employs cholinesterase inhibitors (donepezil, rivastigmine, galantamine) enhancing cholinergic transmission, and N-methyl-D-aspartate (NMDA) receptor antagonists (memantine) modulating glutamatergic activity, though these provide symptomatic benefit without modifying disease progression.

PAIN MANAGEMENT MEDICATIONS

Pain management employs multiple medication classes targeting various mechanisms in nociceptive processing pathways. Optimal therapy addresses the specific pain type (nociceptive, neuropathic, mixed) while minimizing adverse effects through appropriate agent selection, dose optimization, and multimodal approaches. Chronic pain management requires balanced consideration of analgesic efficacy, functional improvement, and long-term safety.

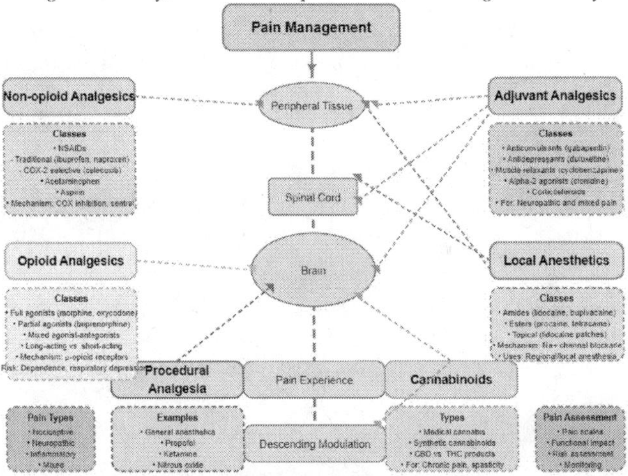

Figure 9.3: Pain Management Medications

Non-opioid Analgesics

Non-opioid analgesics provide the foundation for stepwise pain management through diverse mechanisms. Acetaminophen (paracetamol) exerts analgesic and antipyretic effects through central cyclooxygenase inhibition and potential modulation of endocannabinoid and serotonergic systems, offering efficacy for mild-to-moderate pain without peripheral anti-inflammatory properties. Its favorable gastrointestinal and platelet safety profile supports utility across diverse populations, though hepatotoxicity risk necessitates careful dosing, particularly with chronic use, liver disease, and alcohol consumption. Nonsteroidal anti-inflammatory drugs (NSAIDs) including ibuprofen, naproxen, and diclofenac inhibit cyclooxygenase enzymes, reducing prostaglandin synthesis responsible for inflammation, pain, and fever. These agents demonstrate particular efficacy for inflammatory conditions while carrying risks of gastrointestinal ulceration, renal dysfunction, and cardiovascular events. Selective cyclooxygenase-2 inhibitors (celecoxib) provide similar analgesic efficacy with reduced gastrointestinal toxicity but without eliminating cardiovascular concerns. Topical analgesics including NSAID preparations, capsaicin, and lidocaine patches offer localized pain relief with minimal systemic absorption, providing valuable options for focal pain syndromes and patients with contraindications to systemic therapy.

Table 9.3: Pain Management Medications

Drug Class	Generic Examples	Mechanism of Action	Indications
Non-opioid Analgesics	Acetaminophen	Inhibit central prostaglandins	Mild pain Fever
NSAIDs	Ibuprofen Naproxen Diclofenac	Inhibit cyclooxygenase	Inflammatory pain Fever Dysmenorrhea
COX-2 Selective NSAIDs	Celecoxib	Selectively inhibit COX-2	Inflammatory pain Arthritis
Mild Opioids	Codeine Tramadol	Bind mu-opioid receptors	Moderate pain
Strong Opioids	Morphine Oxycodone Hydromorphone Fentanyl	Bind mu-opioid receptors	Severe pain Cancer pain Post-op pain
Atypical Opioids	Buprenorphine Tapentadol	Partial agonist or mixed	Moderate-severe pain Opioid use

		mechanism	disorder
Topical Analgesics	Lidocaine Diclofenac Capsaicin	Local effects	Localized pain Neuropathic pain Musculoskeletal pain
Anticonvulsants for Pain	Gabapentin Pregabalin Carbamazepine	Decrease neuronal excitability	Neuropathic pain Fibromyalgia Trigeminal neuralgia
Antidepressants for Pain	Duloxetine Amitriptyline Nortriptyline	Enhance descending inhibition	Neuropathic pain Fibromyalgia Chronic pain
Muscle Relaxants	Cyclobenzaprine Baclofen Tizanidine	Various mechanisms	Muscle spasm Spasticity
Migraine Abortives - Triptans	Sumatriptan Rizatriptan Zolmitriptan	5-HT1B/1D agonists	Acute migraine
Migraine Preventives	Propranolol Topiramate Amitriptyline	Various mechanisms	Frequent migraines
CGRP Antagonists	Erenumab Galcanezumab Rimegepant	Block calcitonin gene-related peptide	Migraine prevention and treatment
Corticosteroids	Prednisone Dexamethasone Methylprednisolone	Anti-inflammatory effects	Inflammatory pain Nerve compression Cancer pain

Opioid Analgesics

Opioid analgesics provide effective management for moderate-to-severe pain through activation of mu, kappa, and delta opioid receptors in the central nervous system and peripheral tissues. These agents are classified by their receptor activity (full agonists, partial agonists, mixed agonist-antagonists) and pharmacokinetic properties. Full mu-opioid receptor agonists including morphine, oxycodone, and hydromorphone demonstrate dose-dependent analgesia without ceiling effects, though adverse effects similarly increase with dose escalation. Tramadol combines weak mu-opioid receptor agonism with serotonin and norepinephrine reuptake inhibition, providing multimodal analgesia with reduced respiratory depression risk compared to conventional opioids. Buprenorphine, a partial mu-opioid receptor agonist with kappa receptor antagonism, offers potential safety advantages through its ceiling effect on respiratory depression while maintaining analgesic efficacy. Methadone demonstrates unique pharmacology combining mu-opioid receptor agonism with N-methyl-D-aspartate (NMDA) receptor antagonism and serotonin/norepinephrine reuptake inhibition, providing efficacy for both nociceptive and neuropathic pain. Its complex pharmacokinetics include long and variable half-life, necessitating careful titration and monitoring. Common opioid adverse effects include constipation, nausea, sedation, respiratory depression, and urinary retention, with long-term complications including hormonal disturbances, immunosuppression, hyperalgesia, and dependence. Risk mitigation strategies incorporate prescription drug monitoring programs, opioid agreements, urine drug testing, and naloxone co-prescribing.

Adjuvant Analgesics for Neuropathic and Chronic Pain

Neuropathic pain, resulting from somatosensory nervous system damage or dysfunction, often responds inadequately to conventional analgesics, necessitating specialized approaches. Anticonvulsants demonstrate efficacy through various mechanisms affecting neuronal hyperexcitability. Gabapentinoids (gabapentin, pregabalin) bind to the alpha-2-delta subunit of voltage-gated calcium channels, reducing excitatory neurotransmitter release. These agents show particular benefit in diabetic peripheral neuropathy, postherpetic neuralgia, and fibromyalgia, though dizziness, somnolence, and peripheral edema may limit tolerability. Carbamazepine remains the gold standard for trigeminal neuralgia through sodium channel stabilization. Antidepressants provide analgesia independent of their mood-enhancing effects through modulation of descending pain inhibitory pathways. Tricyclic antidepressants (amitriptyline, nortriptyline) demonstrate established efficacy for various neuropathic conditions, though anticholinergic effects limit utility, particularly in elderly patients. Serotonin-norepinephrine reuptake inhibitors (duloxetine, venlafaxine) offer improved tolerability while maintaining efficacy for diabetic neuropathy, fibromyalgia, and chronic musculoskeletal pain. Local anesthetics including lidocaine infusions and topical formulations provide sodium channel blockade, interrupting aberrant pain signaling with minimal systemic effects. N-methyl-D-aspartate (NMDA) receptor antagonists (ketamine, memantine) address central sensitization contributing to chronic pain states, though side effect profiles often limit their utility outside specialized pain management settings. Emerging approaches include cannabinoids modulating endocannabinoid systems involved in pain processing.

Medications for Specific Pain Syndromes

Specialized pain syndromes often require targeted pharmacological strategies addressing their distinct pathophysiologies. Migraine management encompasses both abortive and preventive approaches. Acute treatment utilizes triptans (sumatriptan, rizatriptan) as serotonin 5-HT1B/1D receptor agonists causing cranial vasoconstriction and inhibition of inflammatory neuropeptide release; ergot alkaloids with similar but less selective mechanisms; nonsteroidal anti-inflammatory drugs for mild-to-moderate attacks; and newer calcitonin gene-related peptide (CGRP) receptor antagonists (ubrogepant, rimegepant) offering novel mechanisms without vasoconstrictor effects. Preventive therapy employs beta-blockers (propranolol, metoprolol), anticonvulsants (topiramate, valproate), antidepressants (amitriptyline), calcium channel blockers (verapamil), and monoclonal antibodies targeting CGRP or its receptor (erenumab, galcanezumab, fremanezumab, eptinezumab). Trigeminal neuralgia responds specifically to carbamazepine and oxcarbazepine through their sodium channel-stabilizing properties, with lamotrigine and baclofen serving as alternatives. Fibromyalgia management employs central-acting agents addressing neurotransmitter imbalances, including serotonin-norepinephrine reuptake inhibitors (duloxetine, milnacipran), gabapentinoids (pregabalin), and low-dose amitriptyline. Complex regional pain syndrome requires multimodal approaches potentially including bisphosphonates to address bone resorption, calcium channel blockers for vasomotor symptoms, and ketamine infusions for refractory cases. Cancer pain management follows World Health Organization guidelines incorporating opioids, non-opioid analgesics, and adjuvants while addressing specific mechanisms including neuropathic components from chemotherapy or direct tumor involvement, bone pain from metastases, and visceral pain from organ infiltration.

ANTICANCER DRUGS

Anticancer drugs have evolved dramatically with enhanced understanding of cancer biology, enabling targeted approaches addressing specific molecular pathways and immune interactions. Contemporary cancer treatment typically employs multimodal strategies combining systemic therapy with surgery, radiation, and supportive care. Pharmacists contribute significantly to oncology care through chemotherapy preparation, dosing calculations, supportive care management, drug interaction evaluation, and patient education regarding complex regimens.

Traditional Cytotoxic Chemotherapeutic Agents

Cytotoxic chemotherapy remains foundational in cancer treatment through targeting rapidly dividing cells via multiple mechanisms. Alkylating agents (cyclophosphamide, ifosfamide, cisplatin, carboplatin, oxaliplatin) form covalent bonds with DNA, creating cross-links that inhibit replication and transcription. These broadly active agents find application across multiple malignancies but carry risks including myelosuppression, nausea, nephrotoxicity, and secondary malignancies. Antimetabolites interfere with nucleic acid synthesis through structural similarity to endogenous metabolites: methotrexate inhibits dihydrofolate reductase; fluoropyrimidines (5-fluorouracil, capecitabine) inhibit thymidylate synthase; and nucleoside analogs (gemcitabine, cytarabine) incorporate into DNA, causing chain termination. Antimicrotubule agents disrupt mitotic spindle formation through either stabilization (taxanes including paclitaxel and docetaxel) or destabilization (vinca alkaloids including vincristine and vinblastine) of microtubules, preventing cell division. Topoisomerase inhibitors interfere with enzymes controlling DNA topology: topoisomerase I inhibitors (irinotecan, topotecan) stabilize the cleavage complex, preventing religation; topoisomerase II inhibitors (etoposide, doxorubicin) induce DNA strand breaks. Anthracyclines (doxorubicin, epirubicin) combine topoisomerase II inhibition with free radical generation and DNA intercalation, demonstrating broad antitumor activity but with cumulative dose-dependent cardiotoxicity limiting lifetime exposure. Platinum compounds (cisplatin, carboplatin, oxaliplatin) form intra- and inter-strand DNA crosslinks while generating reactive oxygen species, with individual agents showing distinct toxicity profiles despite similar mechanisms.

Targeted Therapy

Targeted therapy represents a paradigm shift from traditional cytotoxic approaches by addressing specific molecular alterations driving malignant growth. Tyrosine kinase inhibitors (TKIs) block intracellular signaling pathways essential for cancer cell proliferation and survival. Epidermal growth factor receptor (EGFR) inhibitors (erlotinib, gefitinib, osimertinib) target specific mutations in non-small cell lung cancer; BCR-ABL inhibitors (imatinib, dasatinib, nilotinib) address the pathognomonic translocation in chronic myeloid leukemia; and vascular endothelial growth factor receptor (VEGFR) inhibitors (sorafenib, sunitinib, pazopanib) disrupt angiogenesis essential for tumor growth. Monoclonal antibodies offer targeted approaches through various mechanisms: trastuzumab targets HER2 amplification in breast and gastric cancers; rituximab binds CD20 on B-cell malignancies; bevacizumab inhibits VEGF-mediated angiogenesis; and cetuximab targets EGFR in colorectal and head/neck cancers. Antibody-drug conjugates combine monoclonal antibody specificity with potent cytotoxic payloads, enabling targeted delivery to cancer cells expressing specific antigens. Proteasome inhibitors (bortezomib, carfilzomib) disrupt protein homeostasis critical for multiple myeloma cell survival. Mammalian target of rapamycin (mTOR) inhibitors (everolimus, temsirolimus) interrupt signaling pathways regulating cell growth and metabolism. PARP inhibitors (olaparib, niraparib) exploit synthetic lethality in tumors with defective DNA repair mechanisms, particularly those with BRCA mutations. CDK4/6 inhibitors (palbociclib, ribociclib, abemaciclib) disrupt cell cycle progression in hormone receptor-positive breast cancer. These targeted approaches often enable more selective cancer cell killing with reduced effects on normal tissues, though unique toxicity profiles and resistance mechanisms present ongoing challenges.

Table 9.4: Oncology Drugs and Supportive Care Medications

Drug Class	Generic Examples	Mechanism of Action	Indications
Alkylating Agents	Cyclophosphamide Cisplatin Temozolomide	Damage DNA	Various solid tumors Lymphomas Leukemias
Antimetabolites	5-Fluorouracil Methotrexate Gemcitabine	Interfere with DNA/RNA synthesis	Breast cancer Colorectal cancer Leukemias
Antitumor Antibiotics	Doxorubicin Bleomycin Mitomycin	DNA intercalation/damage	Breast cancer Lymphomas Sarcomas
Plant Alkaloids	Paclitaxel Vincristine Etoposide	Disrupt microtubules or topoisomerase	Breast cancer Lung cancer Leukemias

Kinase Inhibitors	Imatinib Erlotinib Sorafenib	Block specific enzymes in cancer cells	CML GIST Lung cancer Renal cell carcinoma
Monoclonal Antibodies	Rituximab Trastuzumab Bevacizumab	Target specific proteins on cancer cells	Lymphoma Breast cancer Colorectal cancer
Hormonal Agents - Anti-estrogens	Tamoxifen Fulvestrant	Block estrogen effects	Breast cancer
Hormonal Agents - Aromatase Inhibitors	Letrozole Anastrozole Exemestane	Block estrogen production	Breast cancer
Antiandrogens	Bicalutamide Enzalutamide Apalutamide	Block androgen effects	Prostate cancer
Immunotherapy - Checkpoint Inhibitors	Pembrolizumab Nivolumab Ipilimumab	Enhance T-cell activity against cancer	Melanoma Lung cancer Many others
CAR-T Cell Therapy	Tisagenlecleucel Axicabtagene ciloleucel	Genetically modified T cells	Leukemia Lymphoma
Proteasome Inhibitors	Bortezomib Carfilzomib	Inhibit protein degradation	Multiple myeloma
Antiemetics - 5-HT3 Antagonists	Ondansetron Palonosetron	Block serotonin receptors	Chemotherapy-induced nausea
Antiemetics - NK1 Antagonists	Aprepitant Fosaprepitant	Block substance P	Chemotherapy-induced nausea
Colony Stimulating Factors	Filgrastim Pegfilgrastim	Stimulate neutrophil production	Neutropenia prevention

Immunotherapy and Biological Response Modifiers

Cancer immunotherapy harnesses the immune system's potential to recognize and eliminate malignant cells. Immune checkpoint inhibitors remove inhibitory signals that normally prevent excessive immune activation. Programmed death-1 (PD-1) inhibitors (pembrolizumab, nivolumab) and PD-L1 inhibitors (atezolizumab, durvalumab) block the interaction between PD-1 on T cells and PD-L1 on tumor cells, reversing T-cell exhaustion and restoring antitumor immunity. Cytotoxic T-lymphocyte-associated protein 4 (CTLA-4) inhibitors (ipilimumab) block an early checkpoint in T-cell activation, promoting expansion of effector T cells. These agents have revolutionized treatment across multiple malignancies, though immune-related adverse events affecting virtually any organ system require prompt recognition and management. Chimeric antigen receptor (CAR) T-cell therapy represents a personalized approach where patient T cells are genetically engineered to express receptors targeting specific tumor antigens before reinfusion, demonstrating remarkable efficacy in certain hematologic malignancies but with significant toxicities including cytokine release syndrome and neurotoxicity. Cytokines including interferons and interleukins modulate immune responses through complex signaling networks, with established roles in specific malignancies despite substantial toxicity. Bispecific T-cell engagers simultaneously bind T cells and tumor cells, bringing them into proximity to facilitate immune-mediated killing. Cancer vaccines attempt to enhance recognition of tumor-associated antigens, with sipuleucel-T for prostate cancer representing the first FDA-approved therapeutic cancer vaccine. These immune-based approaches often demonstrate unique response patterns including delayed effects, pseudoprogression, and potential for durable responses in subset populations.

Hormonal Therapies and Supportive Care Medications

Hormone-dependent malignancies, particularly breast and prostate cancers, benefit from endocrine manipulation disrupting growth signals. Breast cancer hormonal therapy includes selective estrogen receptor modulators (tamoxifen) that competitively bind estrogen receptors with tissue-specific agonist/antagonist effects; aromatase inhibitors (letrozole, anastrozole, exemestane) that prevent peripheral estrogen synthesis in postmenopausal women; selective estrogen receptor degraders (fulvestrant) that downregulate estrogen receptor expression; and luteinizing hormone-releasing hormone (LHRH) agonists (goserelin) that suppress ovarian function in premenopausal women. Prostate cancer hormonal approaches include androgen deprivation therapy through LHRH agonists (leuprolide) or antagonists (degarelix); androgen synthesis inhibitors (abiraterone); and androgen receptor antagonists (enzalutamide, apalutamide) blocking androgen binding, nuclear translocation, and DNA binding. Supportive care medications address treatment-related toxicities and enhance quality of life. Antiemetics prevent chemotherapy-induced nausea and vomiting through targeting specific neurotransmitter pathways: 5-HT3 receptor antagonists (ondansetron, palonosetron); neurokinin-1 receptor antagonists (aprepitant); dopamine antagonists (metoclopramide); and corticosteroids (dexamethasone). Colony-stimulating factors including granulocyte colony-stimulating factors (filgrastim, pegfilgrastim) reduce neutropenia risk and enable dose-dense chemotherapy regimens, while erythropoiesis-stimulating agents (epoetin alfa, darbepoetin alfa) address chemotherapy-induced anemia in selected patients. Bone-modifying agents including bisphosphonates (zoledronic acid) and RANK ligand inhibitors (denosumab) prevent skeletal-related events in patients with bone metastases while reducing cancer treatment-induced bone loss. Pain management follows oncology-specific protocols addressing various pain mechanisms including tumor infiltration, procedural pain, and treatment-related neuropathy.

Summary

Antimicrobial agents combat infectious diseases through targeted mechanisms disrupting pathogen structures and functions while minimizing host toxicity. Antibacterial classifications include beta-lactams inhibiting cell wall synthesis, protein synthesis inhibitors like macrolides and aminoglycosides, DNA/RNA synthesis disruptors including fluoroquinolones, and cell membrane destabilizers such as polymyxins—each selected based on suspected pathogens, infection site, antimicrobial spectrum, and resistance patterns. Antiviral medications target specific viral replication steps including attachment, uncoating, genome replication, and assembly, while antifungals disrupt ergosterol synthesis or fungal cell membranes. Antimicrobial stewardship principles guide appropriate agent selection, dosing optimization, and treatment duration minimization to combat increasing resistance threats. Central nervous system drugs modulate neurotransmitter systems including serotonin, norepinephrine, dopamine, and gamma-aminobutyric acid to treat psychiatric and neurological conditions. Antidepressants including SSRIs, SNRIs, and atypical agents address mood disorders through various neurotransmitter effects, while antipsychotics target dopaminergic and serotonergic pathways in schizophrenia and bipolar disorder. Anxiolytics provide symptomatic relief through GABA potentiation, and anticonvulsants stabilize neuronal membranes through diverse mechanisms. Pain management approaches employ multimodal strategies targeting different pain pathways. Non-opioid analgesics including acetaminophen and NSAIDs inhibit prostaglandin synthesis peripherally or centrally, while opioids activate mu-receptors producing potent analgesia alongside risk for respiratory depression and dependence. Adjuvant agents including anticonvulsants and antidepressants specifically address neuropathic pain mechanisms. Oncology medications encompass traditional cytotoxic chemotherapies disrupting cell division, targeted therapies addressing specific molecular pathways, immunotherapies enhancing immune recognition of cancer cells, and hormonal therapies modulating hormone-dependent tumor growth. Treatment regimens typically combine multiple agents with complementary mechanisms while requiring intensive supportive care to manage associated toxicities.

Multiple Choice Questions

1. A patient is diagnosed with community-acquired pneumonia and has a penicillin allergy (rash). Which of the following would be the most appropriate antibiotic selection?
   a) Amoxicillin-clavulanate
   b) Azithromycin
   c) Ceftriaxone
   d) Doxycycline
2. Which of the following antibiotics requires therapeutic drug monitoring to minimize nephrotoxicity?
   a) Azithromycin
   b) Gentamicin
   c) Doxycycline
   d) Ciprofloxacin
3. A patient with HIV is taking efavirenz, tenofovir disoproxil fumarate, and emtricitabine. The patient reports significant insomnia and vivid dreams. Which medication is most likely causing these side effects?
   a) Efavirenz
   b) Tenofovir disoproxil fumarate
   c) Emtricitabine
   d) The combination of all three medications
4. Which of the following antidepressants would be most appropriate for a patient with major depressive disorder and insomnia?
   a) Fluoxetine
   b) Bupropion
   c) Mirtazapine
   d) Venlafaxine
5. A patient with schizophrenia has been taking risperidone for 6 months and reports significant weight gain and elevated

blood glucose. Which of the following would be the most appropriate alternative antipsychotic with a lower risk of metabolic side effects?

a) Olanzapine
b) Quetiapine
c) Aripiprazole
d) Clozapine

6. Which of the following would be the most appropriate first-line prophylactic medication for migraine prevention in a young woman with no other medical conditions?

a) Propranolol
b) Topiramate
c) Amitriptyline
d) Valproic acid

7. A patient with chronic neuropathic pain has failed trials of gabapentin and duloxetine. Which of the following would be the most appropriate next step in therapy?

a) Acetaminophen
b) Ibuprofen
c) Pregabalin
d) Tramadol

8. Which of the following is a true statement regarding naloxone?

a) It is a partial opioid agonist used for treatment of opioid use disorder
b) It is an opioid antagonist used for reversal of opioid overdose
c) It is a synthetic opioid used for severe pain
d) It is a mixed opioid agonist-antagonist used for moderate pain

9. A patient receiving cisplatin-based chemotherapy would most likely benefit from prophylactic antiemetic therapy with:

a) Prochlorperazine alone
b) Ondansetron alone
c) Dexamethasone and ondansetron
d) Aprepitant, dexamethasone, and ondansetron

10. A patient with breast cancer is receiving a chemotherapy regimen associated with febrile neutropenia risk of 20%. Which of the following would be most appropriate?

a) No prophylaxis; treat neutropenia if it occurs
b) Prophylactic antibiotics

c) Prophylactic granulocyte colony-stimulating factor (G-CSF)
d) Reduction in chemotherapy dose

Self-Assessment Questions

1. Explain how factors including likely pathogens, local resistance patterns, patient risk factors, and pharmacokinetic/pharmacodynamic principles guide appropriate therapy choices.
2. Compare and contrast the mechanisms of action, spectrum of activity, pharmacokinetic properties, and toxicity profiles of major antibiotic classes explaining how these properties influence clinical application.
3. Evaluate the pharmacological management of HIV infection, explaining the roles of different antiretroviral drug classes in combination regimens, potential resistance concerns, monitoring parameters, and strategies for managing adverse effects and drug interactions.
4. Describe the antimicrobial stewardship interventions that could optimize therapy for a patient receiving broad-spectrum antibiotics, explaining the evidence-based approaches to de-escalation, duration optimization, dose adjustment, and route conversion.
5. Explain how receptor selectivity relates to efficacy and adverse effect profiles.
6. Analyze the pharmacological management of schizophrenia, comparing first-generation versus second-generation antipsychotics in terms of receptor binding profiles, efficacy for positive and negative symptoms, metabolic risk, and movement disorders.
7. Explain the mechanisms, applications, limitations, and monitoring requirements for both abortive therapies
8. Explain the rationale for combining agents with different mechanisms and strategies for evaluating treatment response.
9. Compare and contrast the risk assessment, monitoring requirements, and harm reduction strategies for patients receiving chronic opioid therapy, explaining appropriate tools for evaluating misuse risk, documenting functional improvement, and addressing aberrant behaviors.
10. Analyze the supportive care medications used alongside chemotherapy regimens, explaining how antiemetics, colony-stimulating factors, and antimicrobials should be selected and scheduled based on specific chemotherapy protocols and individual risk factors.

Bibliography

1. Tamma PD, Aitken SL, Bonomo RA, Mathers AJ, van Duin D, Clancy CJ. Infectious Diseases Society of America guidance on the treatment of antimicrobial resistant gram-negative infections. Clin Infect Dis. 2022;74(12):2089-2114.
2. Workowski KA, Bachmann LH, Chan PA, Johnston CM, Muzny CA, Park I, et al. Sexually transmitted infections treatment guidelines, 2021. MMWR Recomm Rep. 2021;70(4):1-187.
3. American Psychiatric Association. The American Psychiatric Association practice guideline for the treatment of patients with schizophrenia. 3rd ed. Washington, DC: American Psychiatric Association Publishing; 2021.
4. Gelenberg AJ, Freeman MP, Markowitz JC, Rosenbaum JF, Thase ME, Trivedi MH, et al. Practice guideline for the treatment of patients with major depressive disorder. 3rd ed. Am J Psychiatry. 2010;167(10):1-152.
5. Chou R, Hartung D, Turner J, Blazina I, Chan B, Levander X, et al. Opioid treatments for chronic pain. Comparative effectiveness review No. 229. Rockville, MD: Agency for Healthcare Research and Quality; 2020.
6. Dowell D, Haegerich TM, Chou R. CDC guideline for prescribing opioids for chronic pain—United States, 2016. JAMA. 2016;315(15):1624-1645.
7. National Comprehensive Cancer Network. NCCN Clinical Practice Guidelines in Oncology: Antiemesis. Version 1.2021. Plymouth Meeting, PA: National Comprehensive Cancer Network; 2021.
8. Hesketh PJ, Kris MG, Basch E, Bohlke K, Barbour SY, Clark-Snow RA, et al. Antiemetics: American Society of Clinical Oncology clinical practice guideline update. J Clin Oncol. 2017;35(28):3240-3261.
9. Goodman LS, Brunton LL, Chabner B, Knollmann BC. Goodman & Gilman's the pharmacological basis of therapeutics. 13th ed. New York: McGraw-Hill; 2018.
10. Smith HS, Raffa RB, Pergolizzi JV Jr, Taylor R Jr, Tallarida RJ. Combining opioid and adrenergic mechanisms for chronic pain. Postgrad Med. 2014;126(4):98-114

CHAPTER 10

SPECIAL POPULATIONS

Author

Mr. Gourab Saha, Associate Professor,
Department of Pharmaceutics, College of Pharmaceutical Sciences, Berhampur, Mohada, Odisha, India

Abstract

Special populations require modified pharmaceutical care approaches due to physiological differences affecting drug response, disposition, and safety profiles. Pediatric pharmacy addresses age-dependent variations across neonatal, infant, child, and adolescent groups, with developmental pharmacokinetic changes affecting absorption, distribution, metabolism, and excretion requiring weight-based or body surface area calculations, specialized formulations addressing swallowing difficulties, and particular vigilance for medications lacking pediatric labeling or safety data. Geriatric pharmacy focuses on multimorbidity, polypharmacy, and age-related physiological changes including reduced renal function, altered body composition, and diminished homeostatic mechanisms, necessitating deprescribing approaches, fall risk assessment, anticholinergic burden evaluation, and medication regimen simplification to enhance adherence and minimize adverse effects. Pregnancy and lactation considerations balance maternal benefit against fetal or infant risk using classification systems that evaluate reproductive toxicity and transplacental or breast milk transfer, with recommendations varying by trimester, condition severity, and alternative therapy availability. Renal and hepatic impairment significantly alter drug clearance pathways, requiring systematic dosage adjustments based on quantitative organ function assessment, with kidney dysfunction necessitating modifications for renally eliminated medications based on creatinine clearance calculations, and liver impairment affecting highly extracted drugs through altered metabolism and protein binding, requiring Child-Pugh classification-guided interventions. Therapeutic approaches across these populations emphasize individualized therapy, heightened monitoring, and interdisciplinary collaboration to optimize medication effectiveness while minimizing iatrogenic harm.

Keywords: *Pharmacokinetics; Physiological alterations; Dose individualization; Organ dysfunction; Vulnerability*

Learning Objectives

After completion of the chapter, the learners should be able to:

- Calculate pediatric medication doses using weight-based, body surface area, and age-based methods with appropriate safety checks.
- Apply geriatric-specific prescribing principles including Beers Criteria and STOPP/START criteria to optimize medication therapy in older adults.
- Evaluate medication risks during pregnancy and lactation using FDA pregnancy categories and lactation safety data.
- Recommend appropriate dosage adjustments for patients with varying degrees of renal impairment based on drug properties and kidney function.
- Modify medication regimens for patients with hepatic impairment based on Child-Pugh classification and drug metabolism pathways.
- Develop monitoring plans addressing population-specific medication risks including growth effects in pediatrics, fall risk in geriatrics, fetal effects in pregnancy, and organ function in impaired patients.

PEDIATRIC PHARMACY

Pediatric pharmacy encompasses the art and science of providing pharmaceutical care to infants, children, and adolescents. This specialized practice recognizes that children are not simply "small adults" but rather individuals with distinct physiological, pharmacokinetic, and pharmacodynamic characteristics that evolve throughout development. Medication therapy in pediatric patients requires careful consideration of age-appropriate dosing, suitable formulations, developmental pharmacology, and unique monitoring parameters to ensure both safety and efficacy.

Developmental Pharmacokinetics

Developmental changes in absorption, distribution, metabolism, and excretion significantly influence drug disposition throughout childhood. Gastric pH progresses from relative neutrality in neonates toward adult acidity by approximately two years of age, affecting ionization and subsequent absorption of pH-dependent medications. Gastric emptying time and intestinal transit demonstrate reduced efficiency and predictability in neonates and young infants, introducing variability in oral drug absorption rates. Skin permeability remains increased in premature and term neonates, potentially enhancing absorption of topically applied substances with systemic toxicity risk. Body composition varies markedly with age, with neonates demonstrating higher total body water percentage and lower adipose tissue proportion compared to older children and adults. These differences alter the volume of distribution for water-soluble and lipophilic medications, necessitating weight-based dosing adjustments. Plasma protein binding capacity is reduced in neonates due to lower albumin concentrations and reduced protein binding affinity, potentially increasing the free fraction of highly protein-bound drugs with subsequent enhanced pharmacological effects or toxicity. Hepatic drug metabolism undergoes significant maturation throughout development, with phase I oxidative pathways mediated by cytochrome P450 enzymes displaying variable ontogeny patterns. CYP3A7 predominates in fetal life but diminishes postnatally, while CYP3A4, CYP2D6, and CYP1A2 demonstrate delayed maturation, reaching adult capacity at different developmental stages. Phase II conjugation pathways, particularly glucuronidation, show significant immaturity in neonates, affecting medications requiring this metabolic pathway. Renal function matures progressively, with glomerular filtration rate approaching adult values by 6-12 months of age when normalized to body surface area, though absolute capacity remains lower throughout childhood.

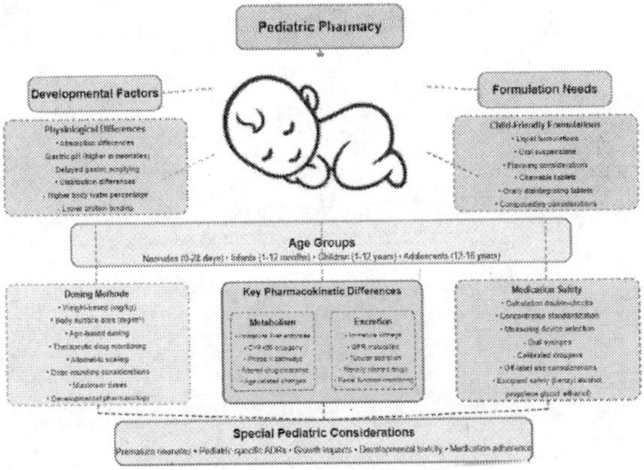

Figure 10.1: Pediatric Pharmacy

Medication Formulations and Administration Techniques

Age-appropriate formulation selection remains fundamental to pediatric medication safety and adherence. Liquid formulations including solutions and suspensions accommodate flexible dosing requirements while eliminating swallowing difficulties common in younger patients. However, these preparations often contain potentially problematic excipients including preservatives, sweeteners, and alcohol that require careful evaluation, particularly in neonates and infants. Measuring devices including oral syringes and calibrated cups should accompany liquid medications to prevent dosing errors associated with household spoons. Solid dosage forms present swallowing challenges for younger children, with tablets generally considered appropriate after age 6-7 years, though individual development determines actual capability. Dispersible tablets and orally disintegrating formulations offer alternatives for children transitioning from liquids to conventional solid forms. Extemporaneous compounding addresses the frequent absence of commercially available pediatric formulations, though stability, bioavailability, and excipient safety require thorough consideration. Beyond formulation selection, administration techniques significantly influence therapeutic outcomes.

Table 10.1: Pediatric Pharmacokinetic Considerations

Parameter	Neonates (0-28 days)	Infants (1-12 months)	Children (1-12 years)	Adolescents (12-18 years)
Gastric pH	Increased (>4)	Gradually decreases	Adult values by age 2	Adult values
Gastric Emptying	Delayed, irregular	Approaches adult values	Similar to adults	Adult values
GI Transit Time	Prolonged	Variable	Similar to adults	Adult values
Gastric Enzymes	Reduced activity	Developing	Near adult levels	Adult values
Body Water %	75-80%	60-65%	60-65%	55-60%
Body Fat %	10-15%	20-25%	20-30%	10-25%
Plasma Proteins	Decreased albumin, binding affinity	Gradually increasing	Near adult levels	Adult values
Blood-Brain Barrier	More permeable	Developing	Near adult function	Adult function
Phase I Metabolism	Reduced (30-50% of adult)	Developing (50-70% of adult)	May exceed adult values	Adult values or higher

Parameter	Neonates (0-28 days)	Infants (1-12 months)	Children (1-12 years)	Adolescents (12-18 years)
Phase II Metabolism	Significantly reduced	Gradually developing	Variable by pathway	Adult values
CYP Enzyme Development	CYP3A7 predominant Limited CYP3A4, 2D6, 1A2	CYP3A4 developing Limited 2D6, 1A2	Variable enzyme maturation	Adult values
Glomerular Filtration	30-40% of adult values	50-80% of adult values	Reaches adult values by 1 year (per BSA)	Adult values
Tubular Secretion	Reduced	Gradually developing	Near adult function	Adult function
Renal Blood Flow	Reduced	Increasing	Proportional to kidney size	Adult values
Half-life	Often prolonged	Variable, approaching adult values	May be shorter than adults	Adult values

Nasogastric and gastrostomy tube administration necessitates assessment of medication compatibility with enteral feeding formulas, adequate tube flushing protocols, and consideration of potential adsorption to tubing materials. Intravenous administration in pediatric patients requires precise calculation of appropriate concentrations and infusion rates based on fluid restrictions and vascular access limitations. Small-volume parenteral medications often necessitate dilution for accurate administration, introducing potential for calculation and preparation errors. Inhalation delivery techniques must accommodate developmental capabilities, with transition from nebulizers to metered-dose inhalers with valved holding chambers and eventually dry powder inhalers as coordination and inspiratory capacity develop.

Medication Safety Considerations

Pediatric patients face disproportionate medication safety challenges due to weight-based dosing requirements, developmental variability, and communication limitations. Dosing errors represent the most common medication error type in pediatric settings, with ten-fold miscalculations particularly problematic due to decimal point placement errors and confusion between milligram and microgram units. Standardized medication ordering processes, including mandatory weight documentation, dose calculation verification, and maximum dose alerts, provide essential safeguards.

Table 10.2: Pediatric Medication Administration Considerations

Age Group	Preferred Dosage Forms	Administration Challenges
Premature Neonates	IV solutions Oral liquids	Limited IV access Small fluid volumes Immature organs
Full-term Neonates	IV solutions Oral liquids	Bitter taste rejection Need for precision Limited blood volume
Infants (1-12 months)	Oral liquids Oral drops Rectal formulations	Spitting out medication Taste preferences Positioning challenges
Toddlers (1-3 years)	Oral liquids Chewable tablets ODTs	Refusal behavior Limited cooperation Taste sensitivity
Preschool (3-5 years)	Oral liquids Chewable tablets ODTs Oral sprays	Fear of medication Autonomy issues Swallowing difficulties
School-age (6-11 years)	Chewable tablets Tablets Liquids Inhalers	Pill swallowing School administration Independence vs. supervision
Adolescents (12-18 years)	Adult formulations Tablets/capsules Inhalers Transdermal	Adherence issues Privacy concerns Risk-taking behavior

Age Group	Preferred Dosage Forms	Administration Challenges
Special Needs	Formulation based on capabilities	Cognitive limitations Physical disabilities Sensory issues
NICU Patients	IV infusions Micro-drop oral	Limited access sites Fluid restrictions Drug compatibility
PICU Patients	IV infusions Specialized formulations	Multiple medications Sedation issues Organ dysfunction
Oncology Patients	Various routes	Immunocompromised status Taste changes Multiple medications

Dose range checking incorporating both minimum and maximum parameters helps identify potential underdosing and overdosing situations before administration. Therapeutic duplication monitoring holds particular importance in pediatric practice where multiple formulations or concentrations of the same medication may be prescribed simultaneously. Electronic health record systems with pediatric-specific functionality, including weight-based dose calculators and pediatric-specific clinical decision support, significantly enhance medication safety. Medication reconciliation processes must incorporate age-appropriate interview techniques and multiple information sources, recognizing that children often receive medications across various settings including school, childcare facilities, and multiple caregivers' homes. Adverse drug reaction identification presents unique challenges in non-verbal or pre-verbal children who cannot report subjective symptoms, necessitating careful observation for behavioral changes, feeding pattern alterations, or developmental regression that might indicate medication-related problems. Pharmacists must consider developmental stages when providing medication education, adapting communication strategies to the cognitive capabilities of both pediatric patients and their caregivers while emphasizing proper administration techniques, expected effects, and concerning symptoms requiring healthcare provider notification.

Common Pediatric Therapeutic Challenges

Certain therapeutic areas present recurring challenges in pediatric pharmacy practice, requiring specialized knowledge and approaches.

Antimicrobial therapy demands careful consideration of age-specific pathogens, developmental pharmacokinetics affecting dosing intervals, and appropriate formulation selection balancing palatability against therapeutic needs. Weight-based dosing calculations, particularly for medications requiring frequent adjustment with growth, necessitate systematic approaches to prevent errors. Asthma management requires age-appropriate device selection transitioning from nebulizers to spacers with metered-dose inhalers and eventually dry powder inhalers as coordination develops. Controlled substance management, particularly for attention-deficit/hyperactivity disorder, requires navigating complex regulatory requirements while addressing medication security, school administration policies, and appropriate monitoring parameters. Pain management incorporates developmental considerations in pain assessment tools, analgesic selection, and route of administration based on developmental capabilities. Seizure disorders necessitate careful balance between therapeutic efficacy and potential cognitive or behavioral adverse effects particularly concerning in developing brains. Psychiatric medication utilization requires thoughtful consideration of off-label prescribing realities, long-term neurodevelopmental impact, and monitoring parameters adapted to developmental stage. Neonatal pharmacy represents a subspecialized area addressing extremely low birth weight infants with profoundly immature organ systems, requiring microinfusion techniques, extensive medication compatibility knowledge, and specialized formulation considerations to address unique physiological challenges including limited fluid tolerance, immature renal and hepatic function, and unique disease states including respiratory distress syndrome and patent ductus arteriosus.

GERIATRIC PHARMACY

Geriatric pharmacy addresses the unique medication management needs of older adults, recognizing the physiological changes, multiple comorbidities, and complex medication regimens characteristic of this population. The pharmacist's role extends beyond traditional dispensing to include comprehensive medication therapy management, deprescribing initiatives, and interdisciplinary collaboration addressing both medication appropriateness and functional outcomes. Geriatric pharmacy practice balances evidence-based disease management against quality-of-life considerations and patient-specific goals.

Age-Related Pharmacokinetic and Pharmacodynamic Changes

Physiological aging significantly influences medication disposition and response, necessitating therapeutic modifications. Absorption undergoes relatively minor alterations with aging, including reduced gastric acid secretion, delayed gastric emptying, and decreased gastrointestinal blood flow, though these changes rarely necessitate specific dosage adjustments. Distribution changes substantially due to body composition alterations including decreased total body water (reducing distribution volume for water-soluble drugs), increased adipose proportion (expanding distribution volume for lipophilic compounds), and reduced serum albumin concentration (increasing free fraction of highly protein-bound medications).

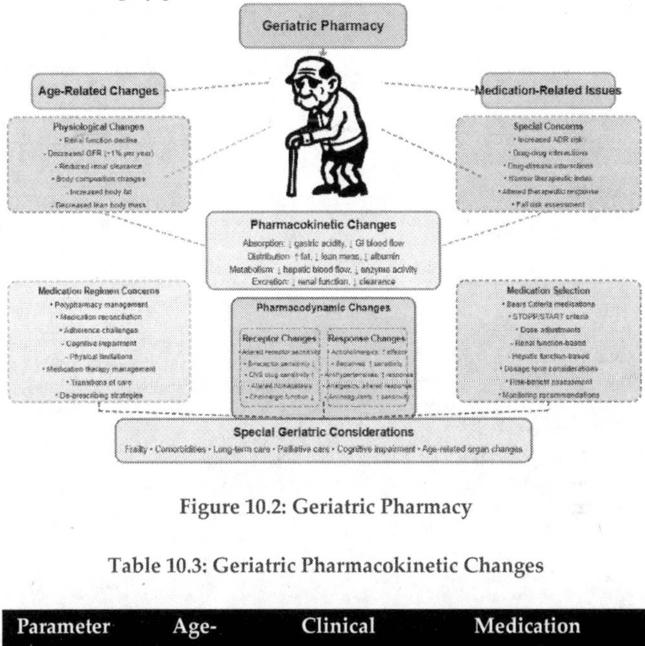

Figure 10.2: Geriatric Pharmacy

Table 10.3: Geriatric Pharmacokinetic Changes

Parameter	Age-Related Change	Clinical Significance	Medication Examples
Gastric Acid Production	Decreased	Reduced dissolution of basic drugs Increased dissolution of acidic drugs	Iron salts (↓ absorption) Ketoconazole (↓ absorption) Aspirin (↑ absorption)
Gastric Emptying	Delayed	Delayed absorption Prolonged exposure to	Acetaminophen (delayed effect) NSAIDs (increased

Parameter	Age-Related Change	Clinical Significance	Medication Examples
		irritants	irritation)
GI Blood Flow	Decreased	Reduced absorption rate	Most orally administered drugs
First-Pass Metabolism	Decreased	Increased bioavailability of some drugs	Propranolol Lidocaine Morphine
Body Fat %	Increased	Increased Vd of lipophilic drugs Prolonged elimination	Benzodiazepines Amiodarone Phenothiazines
Body Water %	Decreased	Decreased Vd of hydrophilic drugs Higher plasma concentrations	Digoxin Lithium Aminoglycosides
Serum Albumin	Decreased	Increased free fraction of highly protein-bound drugs	Warfarin Phenytoin Valproic acid
Alpha-1-Acid Glycoprotein	Increased	Decreased free fraction of basic drugs	Lidocaine Propranolol TCAs
Hepatic Blood Flow	Decreased (30-40%)	Reduced first-pass metabolism Decreased clearance	Beta-blockers Calcium channel blockers Opioids
Hepatic Mass	Decreased (25-30%)	Reduced metabolism capacity	Most hepatically cleared drugs
Phase I Metabolism	Decreased	Reduced clearance of many drugs	Benzodiazepines Warfarin Phenytoin
Phase II Metabolism	Relatively preserved	Less affected than Phase I	Lorazepam Oxazepam Temazepam

Parameter	Age-Related Change	Clinical Significance	Medication Examples
Renal Blood Flow	Decreased (1% per year after 40)	Reduced drug clearance	Aminoglycosides Digoxin Lithium
Glomerular Filtration	Decreased	Reduced clearance of renally eliminated drugs	Most antibiotics Gabapentin Metformin
Tubular Secretion	Decreased	Reduced elimination of actively secreted drugs	Penicillins Cephalosporins Methotrexate

These distribution changes potentially alter initial dosing requirements and influence duration of action. Hepatic metabolism demonstrates variable age-related changes with modest reduction in liver mass and hepatic blood flow potentially reducing first-pass metabolism and clearance of flow-dependent drugs. Phase I oxidative reactions show greater age-related decline compared to phase II conjugation pathways, though considerable interindividual variability exists. Renal excretion undergoes predictable age-related decline with glomerular filtration rate typically decreasing approximately 1% annually after age 40, though significant interindividual variation necessitates individualized assessment rather than age-based assumptions. Creatinine clearance estimation in older adults requires careful interpretation since reduced muscle mass may maintain normal serum creatinine despite significant functional decline. Pharmacodynamic sensitivity increases for many medication classes, particularly those affecting central nervous system function, including benzodiazepines, opioids, and antipsychotics. This enhanced sensitivity reflects changes in receptor density, affinity, and signal transduction efficiency, alongside reduced homeostatic reserve capacity. Consequently, older adults often require lower initial doses with more gradual titration despite potentially requiring similar maintenance doses as younger adults once steady state is achieved.

Polypharmacy and Medication Appropriateness

Polypharmacy, commonly defined as concurrent use of five or more medications, affects approximately two-thirds of older adults and presents multifaceted challenges. While often reflecting appropriate management of multiple comorbidities, polypharmacy increases risk for adverse drug events, drug-drug interactions, medication nonadherence, geriatric syndromes, and healthcare utilization. Medication appropriateness assessment employs both explicit criteria and implicit judgment. Explicit criteria including the Beers Criteria, STOPP/START criteria, and various country-specific frameworks identify potentially inappropriate medications based on unfavorable risk-benefit profiles in older adults. These systematic approaches highlight medications associated with increased fall risk (benzodiazepines, sedative-hypnotics, anticholinergics), cognitive impairment (strongly anticholinergic agents, benzodiazepines), and other geriatric-specific concerns. However, these criteria serve as screening tools rather than absolute contraindications, requiring clinical judgment regarding individual appropriateness. Implicit approaches including the Medication Appropriateness Index evaluate medication use considering indication, effectiveness, dosage, practicality, drug-drug interactions, drug-disease interactions, duplication, duration, and cost. This patient-centered approach requires comprehensive knowledge of the individual's clinical status, preferences, and goals of care. Deprescribing represents the systematic process of identifying and discontinuing medications where existing or potential harms outweigh benefits within the context of individual patient care goals, current level of functioning, life expectancy, and preferences. This process involves prioritizing medications for discontinuation, implementing gradual dose reduction when appropriate to minimize withdrawal or rebound effects, and monitoring for improvement or recurrence of symptoms. Therapeutic classes frequently targeted for deprescribing include proton pump inhibitors beyond short-term indications, benzodiazepines, antipsychotics prescribed for behavioral symptoms, hypoglycemic agents targeting aggressive glycemic control, and statins in very elderly patients without established cardiovascular disease.

Geriatric Syndromes and Medication-Related Problems

Geriatric syndromes—clinical conditions common in older adults with multifactorial etiology and substantial impact on quality of life and functional status—frequently involve medication contributions requiring pharmacist identification and intervention. Cognitive impairment may result from medications with anticholinergic properties (antihistamines, tricyclic antidepressants, bladder antimuscarinics), benzodiazepines, nonbenzodiazepine hypnotics, and certain antiepileptics.

Table 10.4: Potentially Inappropriate Medications in Older Adults (Based on Beers Criteria)

Drug Class	Concern	Alternative Approaches
First-generation Antihistamines	Anticholinergic effects Sedation Confusion Urinary retention	Second-generation antihistamines Intranasal corticosteroids Topical treatments
Antispasmodics	Strong anticholinergic effects Uncertain effectiveness	Dietary modifications Pelvic floor therapy Alternative antispasmodics
Antipsychotics	Increased stroke risk Cognitive decline Mortality in dementia	Non-pharmacological approaches Address underlying causes Lowest effective dose for shortest time
Benzodiazepines	Cognitive impairment Delirium Falls Fractures	Non-pharmacological anxiety management SSRIs Buspirone
Non-Benzodiazepine Hypnotics	Similar adverse effects as benzodiazepines Minimal efficacy	Sleep hygiene Cognitive behavioral therapy Low-dose trazodone
Barbiturates	High risk of physical dependence Overdose at low doses Tolerance	Alternative anticonvulsants Avoid entirely unless for seizures
Antidepressants (TCAs)	Strong anticholinergic effects Sedation Orthostatic hypotension	SSRIs SNRIs Alternative agents

Sulfonylureas (long-acting)	Prolonged hypoglycemia	Shorter-acting sulfonylureas DPP-4 inhibitors Other antidiabetics
NSAIDs (chronic use)	GI bleeding Renal injury Heart failure exacerbation Hypertension	Acetaminophen Topical NSAIDs Physical therapy
Skeletal Muscle Relaxants	Anticholinergic effects Sedation Increased fall risk	Physical therapy Topical analgesics Non-pharmacological approaches
Proton Pump Inhibitors	C. difficile infection Bone loss Hypomagnesemia	Short-term use H2 blockers Lowest effective dose
Peripheral Alpha-1 Blockers	Orthostatic hypotension Syncope Falls	Alternative antihypertensives Alternative BPH treatments
Antiarrhythmics	Toxicity risk QT prolongation Limited efficacy in atrial fibrillation	Rate control strategies Alternative rhythm control Lower doses
Estrogens	Carcinogenic potential Cardiac risk Limited effectiveness for prevention	Non-hormonal approaches for symptoms Localized vaginal therapy for atrophy

Comprehensive medication review using validated anticholinergic burden scales helps identify cumulative exposure across multiple medications. Falls represent multifactorial events with significant medication contributions including psychotropics (benzodiazepines, antipsychotics, antidepressants), cardiovascular agents causing orthostatic hypotension, hypoglycemic agents, and opioid analgesics. Fall risk assessment must evaluate both medication properties and patient-specific vulnerabilities, with interventions potentially including medication discontinuation, dose reduction, regimen simplification, or administration timing modifications. Urinary incontinence may be precipitated or exacerbated by diuretics, medications with anticholinergic properties paradoxically causing overflow incontinence, alpha-blockers reducing urethral resistance, and sedatives limiting mobility for toileting. Functional decline frequently involves sedating medications limiting mobility and participation in activities of daily living. Medication adherence challenges affect approximately 50% of older adults, resulting from complex regimens, cognitive impairment, sensory limitations affecting medication identification, physical dexterity issues with packaging, financial constraints, and health beliefs. Adherence assessment employs multiple methods including refill pattern analysis, pill counts, medication event monitoring systems, and validated screening tools. Interventions include regimen simplification, medication synchronization, adherence packaging, administration aids, caregiver engagement, and motivational interviewing addressing underlying beliefs and concerns.

Tailoring Medication Regimens for Older Adults

Optimizing medication regimens for older adults requires systematic approaches addressing individual needs, preferences, and limitations. Initial regimen design employs the principles of "start low, go slow, but get to goal when appropriate," recognizing increased pharmacodynamic sensitivity while avoiding therapeutic nihilism that might deny beneficial treatments. Medication selection considerations include simplified dosing schedules preferring once-daily regimens; formulation appropriateness addressing swallowing difficulties through liquid options, orally disintegrating tablets, or transdermal systems; and medication burden evaluation balancing therapeutic benefit against regimen complexity. Disease-drug and drug-drug interaction management holds particular importance given multiple comorbidities and polypharmacy prevalence. Specific consideration should address renal dosing adjustments using accurate estimation methods such as the Cockcroft-Gault equation with actual body weight unless extremes of body composition suggest alternative approaches. Therapeutic drug monitoring provides valuable safeguards for medications with narrow therapeutic indices, altered pharmacokinetics in older adults, or variable absorption and metabolism patterns. Medication therapy management services offer comprehensive approaches including thorough medication reconciliation across transitions of care, therapeutic duplication identification, regimen simplification, cost-effectiveness evaluation, and adherence support. Collaborative care models incorporating pharmacist expertise demonstrate improved outcomes including reduced adverse drug events, improved medication appropriateness, decreased healthcare utilization, and enhanced quality of life. Prescribing cascades—where medications prescribed to treat adverse effects of other medications lead to further prescribing—require particular vigilance for identification and intervention. End-of-life medication management involves reevaluation of preventive medications with delayed benefit against palliative medications providing immediate symptom relief, all within the context of the patient's stated goals and values.

PREGNANCY AND LACTATION

Medication management during pregnancy and lactation navigates the tension between maternal therapeutic needs and potential fetal or infant exposure risks. The physiological changes of pregnancy significantly alter drug disposition, while both pregnancy and lactation involve complex risk-benefit considerations requiring evidence-based approaches to minimize unnecessary medication avoidance while preventing adverse outcomes. Pharmaceutical care during these life stages requires extensive knowledge of pregnancy-induced physiological changes, potential teratogenic effects, and medication transfer into breast milk.

Physiological Changes in Pregnancy Affecting Pharmacokinetics

Pregnancy induces profound physiological alterations affecting all pharmacokinetic parameters, with changes evolving throughout gestation. Absorption undergoes various modifications including decreased gastric motility and increased intestinal transit time, potentially delaying absorption of orally administered medications. Increased gastric pH resulting from reduced acid secretion and esophageal reflux may alter ionization and subsequent absorption of pH-dependent drugs. Nausea and vomiting, particularly during the first trimester, may compromise medication absorption and necessitate alternative routes. Distribution changes significantly due to expanded plasma volume (approximately 50% increase), reduced albumin concentration (decreasing from approximately 4.3 g/dL to 3.8 g/dL), increased α_1-acid glycoprotein, and expanded extracellular fluid. These alterations increase the apparent volume of distribution for many drugs, potentially necessitating loading dose adjustments, while reduced plasma protein binding increases free fraction of highly protein-bound medications.

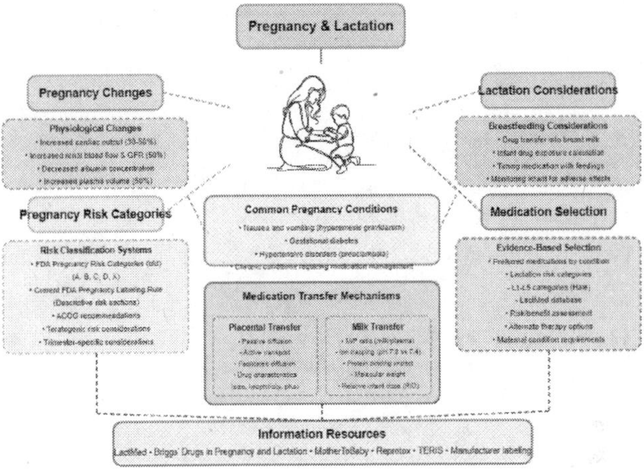

Figure 10.3: Pregnancy and Lactation

The developing fetoplacental unit establishes an additional pharmacokinetic compartment with placental transfer determined by molecular weight, protein binding, lipid solubility, ionization state, and placental transporter activity. Metabolism undergoes complex changes with pregnancy hormones including estrogen and progesterone influencing hepatic enzyme activity. Cytochrome P450 enzymes demonstrate variable alterations: CYP1A2 activity decreases (reducing caffeine and theophylline metabolism), while CYP2D6, CYP3A4, and CYP2C9 activities increase, potentially necessitating dose adjustments for substrates. Excretion capacity increases with renal plasma flow rising approximately 50% and glomerular filtration rate increasing 40-65% from prepregnancy baseline. This enhanced elimination may require dosage increases for predominantly renally cleared medications to maintain therapeutic concentrations. These complex and evolving pharmacokinetic changes necessitate thoughtful monitoring and potential dose adjustments throughout pregnancy, with particular attention during the postpartum period as these parameters return to pre-pregnancy states over variable timeframes.

Table 10.5: Pregnancy Risk Categories and Medication Considerations

Pregnancy Trimester	Physiological Changes	High-Risk Medications	Safer Alternatives
First Trimester (0-13 weeks)	Organogenesis Nausea/vomiting Early plasma volume expansion	Isotretinoin Warfarin ACE inhibitors/ARBs Thalidomide Live vaccines Tetracyclines	Acetaminophen Penicillins Cetirizine Insulin Low molecular weight heparins Levothyroxine
Second Trimester (14-26 weeks)	Increased plasma volume Increased cardiac output Increased GFR Decreased gastric motility	Same as first trimester Fluoroquinolones NSAIDs (prolonged use) Benzodiazepines	Same as first trimester Histamine-2 blockers Topical corticosteroids Most asthma medications Metformin (case-by-case)
Third Trimester (27-40 weeks)	Maximal plasma volume expansion Decreased albumin concentration Compressed gastric emptying Maximal cardiac output	Same as second trimester NSAIDs (risk of premature closure of ductus arteriosus) Tocolytics (long-term) Oral hypoglycemics	Same as second trimester Low-dose aspirin (if indicated) Calcium channel blockers Magnesium sulfate (preeclampsia)
Labor and Delivery	Rapid fluid shifts Altered blood flow Variable gastric emptying	Ergot alkaloids NSAIDs Long-acting opioids	Regional anesthetics Short-acting opioids Oxytocin Magnesium sulfate

Pregnancy Trimester	Physiological Changes	High-Risk Medications	Safer Alternatives
Postpartum	Rapid fluid redistribution Hormonal changes Breast milk production	Consideration of breastfeeding effects	Many medications compatible with breastfeeding
Lactation Safety Considerations			
Infant Age	<2 months: limited drug metabolism 2-6 months: developing metabolism >6 months: more mature systems	High molecular weight drugs Drugs with long half-lives Drugs with active metabolites	Short-acting medications Low milk transfer drugs Low oral bioavailability drugs
Milk Characteristics	Colostrum: protein-rich Mature milk: higher fat content Hindmilk: highest fat content	Lithium Amiodarone Antineoplastics Radioactive compounds	Many antibiotics Most antihypertensives Insulin Thyroid hormones
Timing Considerations	Peak milk concentration typically 1-3 hours after maternal dose	Long-acting medications with narrow therapeutic indices	Short-acting medications timed after breastfeeding
Special Situations	Premature infants Multiple infants Maternal conditions requiring high-risk medications	Cytotoxic agents Drugs of abuse Radioactive compounds	Case-by-case evaluation Temporary pumping and discarding Alternative infant feeding

Teratogenicity and Pregnancy Risk Categories

Teratogenicity—the capacity of a substance to cause developmental abnormalities—requires careful assessment when evaluating medication use during pregnancy. Teratogenic potential depends on multiple factors including the specific agent, dose, duration of exposure, gestational timing, maternal metabolism, placental transfer, and fetal susceptibility. Critical periods of organogenesis occur primarily during weeks 3-8 post-conception (weeks 5-10 of pregnancy), representing the window of greatest vulnerability for structural malformations, though central nervous system development remains sensitive throughout pregnancy. Historically, the FDA pregnancy risk category system (Categories A, B, C, D, X) provided a framework for risk assessment, though its limitations included oversimplification of complex risk data and failure to distinguish between risks at different gestational stages. This system was replaced in 2015 with the Pregnancy and Lactation Labeling Rule (PLLR) requiring descriptive risk summaries incorporating available human and animal data, clinical considerations regarding timing and duration of exposure, and dose-dependent effects. Well-established teratogens include thalidomide causing phocomelia and other limb reductions; isotretinoin associated with craniofacial, cardiac, and central nervous system malformations; valproic acid linked to neural tube defects and neurodevelopmental impacts; warfarin causing nasal hypoplasia and stippled epiphyses during first-trimester exposure with different risks in later pregnancy; and angiotensin-converting enzyme inhibitors and angiotensin receptor blockers associated with renal tubular dysgenesis, oligohydramnios, and resultant fetal complications primarily during second and third trimesters. Pregnancy exposure registries collect observational data on medication effects when used during pregnancy, providing valuable information beyond premarketing animal studies. Preconception planning represents an ideal opportunity for medication regimen optimization, including transitioning from teratogenic medications to safer alternatives, stabilizing chronic conditions, and establishing baseline parameters for monitoring during pregnancy.

Medication Use During Lactation

Breastfeeding offers substantial health benefits for both infant and mother, with medication concerns representing a leading cause of premature breastfeeding discontinuation. Thoughtful evaluation of medication safety during lactation balances these benefits against potential risks from drug exposure through breast milk. Medication transfer into breast milk depends on multiple factors including maternal plasma concentration, molecular weight, protein binding, lipid solubility, ionization state, and half-life. The milk-to-plasma ratio provides an estimation of relative drug concentration in breast milk compared to maternal plasma, though this measure alone inadequately characterizes infant exposure. Relative infant dose (RID), calculated as the infant's daily dose via breast milk divided by the maternal daily dose on a weight-adjusted basis, offers more clinically relevant assessment, with values below 10% generally considered acceptable for most medications. Infant characteristics significantly influence risk, with premature neonates demonstrating reduced drug elimination capacity, while older infants with established hepatic and renal function metabolize and excrete medications more efficiently. Strategic timing of maternal medication administration relative to breastfeeding sessions can minimize infant exposure, with administration immediately after breastfeeding or before the infant's longest sleep period maximizing clearance before the next feeding. Medications generally considered compatible with breastfeeding include most antibiotics (with cephalosporins and penicillins preferred over fluoroquinolones and tetracyclines), anticonvulsants (with levetiracetam and lamotrigine preferred over phenobarbital and primidone), many antihypertensives (particularly beta-blockers such as labetalol, metoprolol, and propranolol), thyroid replacement, and most asthma medications. Medications of concern include cytotoxic antineoplastics, radioactive compounds, drugs of abuse, and selected psychotropics with sedation potential or long half-lives. Resources including LactMed database and the Medications and Mother's Milk reference provide evidence-based recommendations incorporating available data on milk concentrations, reported adverse effects, and pharmacokinetic principles.

Chronic Disease Management During Pregnancy and Lactation

Chronic disease management during pregnancy and lactation requires balancing maternal health needs against potential fetal or infant medication exposure. Asthma management employs a stepwise approach similar to non-pregnant patients, with inhaled corticosteroids (particularly budesonide) representing the preferred controller medication based on extensive safety data. Uncontrolled asthma poses greater risk to fetal development through maternal hypoxemia than medication therapy. Diabetes management targets tight glycemic control with insulin representing the gold standard therapy during pregnancy. Oral agents demonstrate varying safety profiles with metformin increasingly utilized, particularly in gestational diabetes, while sulfonylureas show inconsistent safety data and thiazolidinediones remain contraindicated. Continuous glucose monitoring and insulin pump therapy offer advantages for selected patients. Hypertension treatment employs methyldopa, labetalol, and nifedipine as preferred agents based on established safety, while angiotensin-converting enzyme inhibitors and angiotensin receptor blockers remain contraindicated throughout pregnancy. Blood pressure targets balance preeclampsia prevention against uteroplacental perfusion maintenance. Epilepsy management requires careful preconception planning to transition from valproic acid when possible and establish monotherapy with the lowest effective dose of preferred agents including lamotrigine or levetiracetam. Uncontrolled seizures present greater risk than medication exposure, necessitating continued therapy despite potential risks. Depression treatment considers both untreated depression risks including poor self-care, substance use, and preterm birth, against selective serotonin reuptake inhibitor (SSRI) exposure associated with transient neonatal symptoms and potential small increased risk of persistent pulmonary hypertension. Sertraline and citalopram demonstrate favorable profiles when treatment is necessary. Thyroid disorders require careful monitoring and dose adjustment throughout pregnancy with levothyroxine requirements typically increasing 30-50% during pregnancy due to increased thyroxine-binding globulin and placental deiodinase activity. Overt hypothyroidism requires immediate treatment to prevent neurodevelopmental consequences, while subclinical hypothyroidism management varies based on thyroid antibody status and degree of thyroid-stimulating hormone elevation.

RENAL AND HEPATIC IMPAIRMENT

Renal and hepatic impairment significantly influence pharmacokinetics and pharmacodynamics, necessitating systematic approaches to medication dosage adjustment and therapy selection. These organ systems represent primary pathways for drug elimination, with dysfunction potentially leading to accumulation, toxicity, or reduced therapeutic effect for prodrugs requiring activation. Pharmaceutical care for patients with renal or hepatic impairment requires thorough understanding of altered drug disposition, appropriate assessment methods, and practical adjustment strategies.

Assessing Renal Function and Its Impact on Drug Therapy

Renal function assessment provides the foundation for appropriate medication dosing in kidney disease. Glomerular filtration rate (GFR) estimation employs various equations with distinct advantages and limitations. The Cockcroft-Gault equation, developed in 1976 using creatinine clearance rather than GFR as its endpoint, remains widely utilized in pharmaceutical applications despite known limitations including overestimation in obesity and underestimation in elderly patients with reduced muscle mass. The Modification of Diet in Renal Disease (MDRD) equation and more recent Chronic Kidney Disease Epidemiology Collaboration (CKD-EPI) equation provide more accurate GFR estimation normalized to body surface area (mL/min/1.73m^2) but require conversion to absolute GFR for medication dosing applications. Cystatin C-based equations offer advantages in patients with altered muscle mass but remain less widely available. Acute kidney injury assessment requires serial monitoring with recognition that serum creatinine lags behind actual GFR changes, potentially delaying appropriate intervention. Pharmacokinetic alterations in renal impairment extend beyond reduced glomerular filtration to include changes in absorption from edema and altered gastric pH; distribution changes from altered protein binding, volume status, and tissue perfusion; and potential impacts on non-renal elimination pathways. Medications eliminated primarily through renal excretion (defined as >60-70% unchanged renal elimination) typically require significant dosage adjustment proportional to GFR reduction.

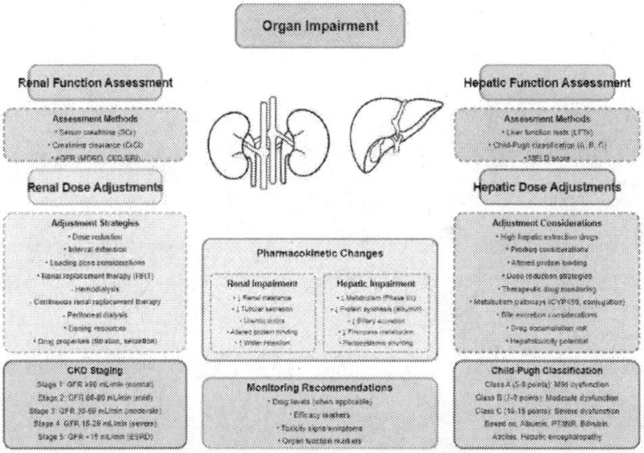

Figure 10.4: Renal and Hepatic Impairment Medication Adjustments

Adjustment strategies include dose reduction, interval extension, or combined approaches based on the medication's time-dependent versus concentration-dependent efficacy profile and toxicity characteristics. Narrow therapeutic index medications including aminoglycosides, vancomycin, and digoxin require particularly careful monitoring with potential therapeutic drug monitoring. Nephrotoxic medication management employs preventive strategies including adequate hydration, dose adjustment, avoidance of concurrent nephrotoxins, and duration limitation. High-risk medications requiring particular attention include nonsteroidal anti-inflammatory drugs, aminoglycosides, amphotericin B formulations, calcineurin inhibitors, and iodinated contrast media.

Table 10.6: Medication Adjustments in Renal Impairment

Drug Class	Examples	Monitoring Parameters
Antibiotics - Aminoglycosides	Gentamicin Tobramycin Amikacin	Drug levels (peak and trough) Creatinine Audiometry Vestibular function
Antibiotics - Beta-lactams	Penicillins Cephalosporins Carbapenems	Clinical response Creatinine Neurological status
Antibiotics - Fluoroquinolones	Ciprofloxacin Levofloxacin Moxifloxacin	QT interval Seizure activity Glucose Tendon integrity
Cardiovascular - ACEIs/ARBs	Lisinopril Enalapril Valsartan	Potassium Creatinine Blood pressure Symptoms of hypotension
Cardiovascular - Digoxin	Digoxin	Digoxin levels Potassium ECG Signs of toxicity
Antidiabetics - Metformin	Metformin	Renal function Lactic acid (if symptoms) Vitamin B12
Antidiabetics - SGLT2 inhibitors	Empagliflozin Dapagliflozin Canagliflozin	Renal function Genital infections Volume status
Antidiabetics - DPP-4 inhibitors	Sitagliptin Saxagliptin	Renal function Glycemic control

Drug Class	Examples	Monitoring Parameters
Anticoagulants - DOACs	Apixaban Rivaroxaban Dabigatran	Renal function Bleeding signs CBC
Opioid Analgesics	Morphine Hydromorphone Codeine	Respiratory rate Sedation Mental status
Gabapentinoids	Gabapentin Pregabalin	Sedation Dizziness Myoclonus Mental status
Bisphosphonates	Alendronate Risedronate Zoledronic acid	Renal function Calcium Symptoms of renal deterioration
Diuretics	Furosemide Hydrochlorothiazide Spironolactone	Electrolytes Renal function Volume status Blood pressure

Medication Management in Renal Replacement Therapy

Renal replacement therapies including hemodialysis, peritoneal dialysis, and continuous renal replacement therapy (CRRT) introduce additional complexity to medication management. Drug removal during hemodialysis depends on multiple factors including molecular weight (with enhanced removal below 500-1000 daltons), protein binding (with free fraction available for dialytic clearance), volume of distribution (with extensive tissue distribution reducing dialytic removal), and dialysis parameters including membrane type, blood and dialysate flow rates, and treatment duration. Highly dialyzable medications demonstrating significant removal (>30%) include many water-soluble antibiotics, lithium, and certain antiseizure medications, potentially requiring supplemental post-dialysis dosing. Dosing strategies in intermittent hemodialysis include administration after dialysis sessions for significantly dialyzable medications, scheduled administration during the final dialysis hour, or supplemental doses following dialysis completion. Peritoneal dialysis provides continuous but less efficient solute clearance compared to hemodialysis, with drug removal primarily determined by molecular weight, protein binding, and peritoneal membrane characteristics. Medication dosing in peritoneal dialysis typically follows guidelines for advanced chronic kidney disease (GFR 10-15 mL/min) with specific adjustments for selected agents. Continuous renal replacement therapies, including continuous venovenous hemofiltration (CVVH), continuous venovenous hemodialysis (CVVHD), and continuous venovenous hemodiafiltration (CVVHDF), provide ongoing solute clearance in critically ill patients. Drug clearance in these modalities depends on the specific technique employed, flow rates, membrane characteristics, and physicochemical drug properties. Dosing typically requires individualization based on residual renal function, specific CRRT parameters, and the clinical context, with therapeutic drug monitoring providing valuable guidance when available. Medications requiring particular attention in dialysis patients include phosphate binders, vitamin D analogs, erythropoiesis-stimulating agents, iron preparations, and antihypertensives requiring careful timing relative to dialysis sessions to manage fluid shifts and resultant blood pressure fluctuations.

Hepatic Function Assessment and Pharmacokinetic Implications

Hepatic impairment affects medication disposition through multiple mechanisms with less predictable patterns compared to renal dysfunction. Assessment of hepatic function for medication dosing purposes presents substantial challenges given the liver's diverse functions and limited correlation between standard laboratory parameters and actual metabolic capacity. Traditional liver function tests including aminotransferases (ALT, AST) primarily indicate hepatocellular injury rather than functional capacity, while synthetic function markers including albumin and prothrombin time better reflect hepatic functional reserve but respond slowly to acute changes. Child-Pugh classification, though developed for prognostic purposes in cirrhosis, represents the most widely utilized system for medication dosing guidance, incorporating serum albumin, prothrombin time, bilirubin, and the clinical parameters of ascites and encephalopathy to categorize impairment as class A (mild), B (moderate), or C (severe). The Model for End-Stage Liver Disease (MELD) score offers an alternative assessment incorporating serum creatinine, bilirubin, and international normalized ratio without subjective clinical parameters, though medication dosing guidance using this system remains limited. Pharmacokinetic alterations in hepatic impairment vary by specific liver pathology and disease severity. Absorption may be affected by portosystemic shunting, altered first-pass metabolism, delayed gastric emptying, and intestinal edema. Distribution changes result from hypoalbuminemia increasing free fraction of highly protein-bound drugs, ascites and edema expanding apparent volume of distribution for water-soluble compounds, and altered body composition in advanced disease. Metabolism demonstrates complex changes with potentially reduced phase I oxidative capacity, particularly in advanced cirrhosis, while phase II conjugation pathways generally maintain activity until late-stage disease. Specific cytochrome P450 enzyme activities demonstrate variable alteration patterns based on the underlying liver pathology. Biliary excretion may be impaired in cholestatic conditions, affecting medications eliminated through this pathway. These diverse and unpredictable changes necessitate individualized approaches to medication selection and dosing.

Table 10.7: Medication Adjustments in Hepatic Impairment

Drug Class	Examples	Monitoring Parameters
Benzodiazepines	Diazepam (avoid) Midazolam (reduce) Lorazepam (safer)	Sedation Mental status Respiratory rate Hepatic encephalopathy
Opioid Analgesics	Morphine (reduce) Oxycodone (reduce) Fentanyl (monitor)	Sedation Respiratory rate Mental status
NSAIDs	All NSAIDs	GI bleeding Renal function Fluid retention Platelet function
Statins	Atorvastatin (reduce) Simvastatin (avoid) Pravastatin (safer)	Liver enzymes Muscle symptoms CK if symptomatic
Anticoagulants	Warfarin (careful monitoring) Apixaban (preferred DOAC) Rivaroxaban (avoid in severe)	INR (potentially unreliable) Bleeding signs Hepatic function
Antiepileptics	Phenytoin (monitor free levels) Carbamazepine (reduce) Levetiracetam (safer)	Free drug levels Therapeutic effect Toxicity signs Liver function
Beta-blockers	Propranolol (significant reduction) Metoprolol (reduce) Atenolol (safer)	Heart rate Blood pressure Signs of beta-blockade

Antidepressants	TCAs (reduce) SSRIs (mild reduction) Mirtazapine (reduce)	Mental status Therapeutic effect Side effects Serotonin syndrome
Antipsychotics	Haloperidol (reduce) Risperidone (reduce) Quetiapine (reduce)	Mental status Extrapyramidal symptoms QT interval Sedation
Proton Pump Inhibitors	Omeprazole (mild reduction) Pantoprazole (preferred) Esomeprazole (mild reduction)	Therapeutic effect Liver function
Diuretics	Furosemide Spironolactone (portal HTN) Hydrochlorothiazide	Electrolytes Renal function Hepatic encephalopathy Fluid status
Antidiabetics	Metformin (caution) Sulfonylureas (reduce/avoid) DPP-4 inhibitors (safer)	Glucose Lactic acidosis signs Liver function
Antibiotics	Macrolides (reduce) Fluoroquinolones (variable) Penicillins (minimal changes)	Therapeutic effect Signs of toxicity Liver function

Medication Selection and Monitoring in Hepatic Dysfunction

Medication therapy in hepatic dysfunction requires thoughtful consideration of both altered pharmacokinetics and the vulnerable functional status of the compromised liver. High hepatic extraction ratio drugs, which undergo substantial first-pass metabolism, demonstrate disproportionately increased bioavailability in liver disease due to portosystemic shunting and reduced enzymatic capacity. These medications, including propranolol, lidocaine, and morphine, typically require significant initial dose reduction with careful titration based on clinical response. Conversely, low extraction ratio drugs show less dramatic alterations in hepatic clearance until advanced disease stages. Medications undergoing predominant phase I metabolism through cytochrome P450 enzymes generally require more substantial adjustment compared to those eliminated through phase II conjugation or renal excretion. Dosing strategy selection incorporates the medication's therapeutic index, availability of therapeutic drug monitoring, and clinical context. Conservative initial dosing with careful upward titration represents the standard approach, though this must balance against providing inadequate therapy for the underlying condition. Potentially hepatotoxic medications require thorough risk-benefit assessment with enhanced monitoring when benefits outweigh risks. Baseline liver function documentation, regular monitoring intervals based on known hepatotoxicity patterns, and patient education regarding concerning symptoms provide essential safeguards. Different hepatotoxicity mechanisms require specific monitoring approaches: predictable, dose-dependent toxicity (acetaminophen) benefits from therapeutic drug monitoring and dose limitation; hypersensitivity reactions (phenytoin) necessitate symptom monitoring including rash, fever, and eosinophilia; and idiosyncratic reactions (isoniazid) require regular transaminase monitoring despite their unpredictable nature. Specific therapeutic classes requiring particular attention include sedatives and opioids with potential to precipitate or worsen hepatic encephalopathy; antihypertensives with altered metabolism and potential for exacerbating portal hypertension; and diuretics requiring careful electrolyte monitoring in the context of secondary hyperaldosteronism. Patients with advanced liver disease receiving multiple medications benefit from comprehensive medication therapy management to assess for drug-drug interactions, optimize therapeutic regimens, monitor for adverse effects, and ensure appropriate laboratory monitoring.

Summary

Special populations require modified approaches to medication therapy addressing unique physiological, pharmacokinetic, and pharmacodynamic considerations. Pediatric pharmacy accommodates developmental changes across multiple age categories from neonates through adolescents, with weight-based dosing requirements, age-specific pharmacokinetic parameters, limited available dosage forms, and vulnerability to calculation errors. Pediatric medication selection addresses growth and developmental impacts, excipient toxicity concerns including benzyl alcohol and propylene glycol, and distinct adverse effect profiles. Appropriate administration often requires compounded formulations and specialized delivery devices with caregiver education. Geriatric pharmacy addresses physiological changes of aging including reduced renal function, hepatic metabolism alterations, decreased muscle mass affecting distribution volume, and increased adipose tissue prolonging lipophilic drug elimination. Polypharmacy management becomes paramount given average medication counts exceeding five in older adults, creating complex interaction potentials and adherence challenges. Medication appropriateness tools including Beers Criteria and STOPP/START criteria identify potentially inappropriate medications while deprescribing frameworks guide systematic medication reduction. Pregnancy and lactation present dynamic physiological states requiring trimester-specific risk-benefit assessments. FDA pregnancy categories (A,B,C,D,X) are being replaced with narrative pregnancy and lactation labeling providing more nuanced guidance, while lactation risk considers milk concentration, oral bioavailability, and infant developmental stage. Renal impairment necessitates medication adjustments based on elimination pathways, with creatinine clearance estimates guiding dosage modifications for renally cleared drugs, while hepatic impairment classified through Child-Pugh scoring affects metabolism of drugs undergoing significant hepatic biotransformation. Across all special populations, individualized therapy approaches balance condition management with population-specific vulnerabilities through careful medication selection, appropriate monitoring, and ongoing reassessment.

Multiple Choice Questions

1. A 3-year-old child weighing 15 kg requires amoxicillin for otitis media. The recommended dose is 40 mg/kg/day divided every 8 hours. Which of the following would be the appropriate dose per administration?
   a) 200 mg
   b) 400 mg
   c) 600 mg
   d) 40 mg
2. Which of the following liquid medications contains an excipient that should be avoided in neonates and young infants?
   a) Amoxicillin suspension with artificial sweetener
   b) Acetaminophen liquid with sorbitol
   c) Prednisolone solution with propylene glycol
   d) Diphenhydramine syrup with corn syrup solids
3. According to the Beers Criteria, which of the following medications should generally be avoided in older adults due to increased risk of adverse effects?
   a) Lisinopril
   b) Metoprolol
   c) Diphenhydramine
   d) Metformin
4. A 75-year-old patient with insomnia is currently taking zolpidem 10 mg at bedtime. Based on geriatric prescribing principles, which of the following would be most appropriate?
   a) Continue current therapy as prescribed
   b) Increase to zolpidem 10 mg plus melatonin
   c) Reduce to zolpidem 5 mg at bedtime
   d) Switch to a benzodiazepine with longer half-life
5. Which of the following medications is classified as FDA Pregnancy Category X under the old categorization system and is contraindicated in pregnancy?
   a) Labetalol
   b) Methyldopa
   c) Warfarin
   d) Amoxicillin
6. A woman in her first trimester of pregnancy presents with severe nausea and vomiting. Which of the following would be the most appropriate initial recommendation?

a) Ondansetron
b) Doxylamine/pyridoxine combination
c) Metoclopramide
d) Prochlorperazine

7. Which of the following antibiotics would be contraindicated for a breastfeeding mother due to potential adverse effects in the infant?
a) Amoxicillin
b) Azithromycin
c) Ciprofloxacin
d) Tetracycline

8. A patient with a creatinine clearance of 15 mL/min is prescribed enoxaparin for deep vein thrombosis. Which of the following would be the most appropriate adjustment?
a) No adjustment needed
b) Reduce dose by 25%
c) Reduce dose by 50%
d) Switch to an alternative anticoagulant

9. For a patient with Child-Pugh Class C liver disease, which of the following medications would require the most significant dosage adjustment?
a) Lisinopril
b) Morphine
c) Levothyroxine
d) Cephalexin

10. A pediatric patient requires acetaminophen for fever. The correct weight-based approach for dosing would be:
a) 5-10 mg/kg every 4-6 hours
b) 10-15 mg/kg every 4-6 hours
c) 25-50 mg/kg every 4-6 hours
d) 50-100 mg/kg every 4-6 hours

Self-Assessment Questions

1. Explain how developmental changes in absorption, distribution, metabolism, and excretion affect medication dosing, selection, and monitoring.
2. Evaluate the appropriate selection, preparation, and administration of liquid medications for young children, explaining techniques for ensuring dosing accuracy, addressing palatability concerns, and avoiding potentially harmful excipients.
3. Design a medication reconciliation process for an elderly patient transitioning from hospital to long-term care, explaining strategies to identify discrepancies, resolve inappropriate prescribing, and ensure communication across care settings.
4. Analyze the application of the Beers Criteria and STOPP/START criteria in medication therapy management for older adults, explaining how these tools should be integrated with clinical judgment when reviewing geriatric medication regimens.
5. Explain the process for identifying inappropriate medications, prioritizing discontinuation targets, implementing gradual dose reductions, and monitoring for withdrawal or disease recurrence.
6. Explaining how the FDA pregnancy labeling system provides information about teratogenic risk, reproductive toxicity, and clinical considerations across different trimesters.
7. Explain how properties including molecular weight, protein binding, lipophilicity, and ionization state affect infant exposure and how this information guides clinical recommendations for lactating women.
8. Explain how treatment goals, medication selection, and monitoring requirements change during pregnancy.
9. Evaluate the dosage adjustment strategies for patients with varying degrees of renal impairment, explaining how different approaches should be selected based on drug properties and patient-specific factors.
10. Analyze the medication management considerations for patients with hepatic impairment, explaining how Child-Pugh classification guides dosing decisions and how pharmacokinetic alterations affect different drug classes.

Bibliography

1. American Academy of Pediatrics Committee on Drugs. Drugs for pediatric emergencies. Pediatrics. 1998;101(1):e13.
2. Kearns GL, Abdel-Rahman SM, Alander SW, Blowey DL, Leeder JS, Kauffman RE. Developmental pharmacology—drug disposition, action, and therapy in infants and children. N Engl J Med. 2003;349(12):1157-1167.
3. Batchelor HK, Marriott JF. Formulations for children: Problems and solutions. Br J Clin Pharmacol. 2015;79(3):405-418.
4. By the American Geriatrics Society Beers Criteria® Update Expert Panel. American Geriatrics Society 2019 Updated AGS Beers Criteria® for potentially inappropriate medication use in older adults. J Am Geriatr Soc. 2019;67(4):674-694.
5. Mangoni AA, Jackson SHD. Age-related changes in pharmacokinetics and pharmacodynamics: Basic principles and practical applications. Br J Clin Pharmacol. 2004;57(1):6-14.
6. Bowie MW, Slattum PW. Pharmacodynamics in older adults: A review. Am J Geriatr Pharmacother. 2007;5(3):263-303.
7. Bookstaver PB, Bland CM, Griffin B, Stover KR, Eiland LS, McLaughlin M. A review of antibiotic use in pregnancy. Pharmacotherapy. 2015;35(11):1052-1062.
8. Anderson GD. Pregnancy-induced changes in pharmacokinetics: A mechanistic-based approach. Clin Pharmacokinet. 2005;44(10):989-1008.
9. Verbeeck RK, Musuamba FT. Pharmacokinetics and dosage adjustment in patients with renal dysfunction. Eur J Clin Pharmacol. 2009;65(8):757-773.
10. Huang E, MacArthur RB, Louie S, Sielaff TD, Zamek-Gliszczynski MJ, Smith DE, et al. Pharmacokinetic considerations in the management of drugs in patients with liver disease. Adv Drug Deliv Rev. 2022;188:114379.

CHAPTER 11

NON-STERILE AND STERILE MANUFACTURING

Author

Mr. Wilberforce Kasangaki, PG Scholar,
Department of Regulatory Affairs, Ramanbhai Patel College of Pharmacy, CHARUSAT, Changa, Gujarat, India

Abstract

Pharmaceutical manufacturing encompasses both sterile and non-sterile preparation techniques required for specialized medication production beyond commercial availability. Non-sterile compounding transforms raw ingredients into patient-specific formulations including capsules, suspensions, ointments, and suppositories using pharmaceutical calculations ensuring accurate concentration, beyond-use dating based on stability data, and proper documentation meeting regulatory requirements including USP <795> standards and DQSA provisions. Sterile compounding applies aseptic techniques to prepare injections, ophthalmics, and other contamination-sensitive products, following USP <797> classifications of risk levels, environmental monitoring requirements, personnel qualification procedures, and beyond-use dating limitations that prevent microbiological or particulate contamination. Equipment and techniques for pharmaceutical preparation include electronic balances, ointment mills, powder blenders, laminar airflow workbenches, biological safety cabinets, and automated compounding devices, each requiring specific operation protocols, maintenance procedures, and performance verification to ensure accurate, consistent product generation. Quality assurance programs integrate environmental monitoring, personnel training, process validation, finished product testing, and comprehensive documentation systems that verify preparation integrity through particulate analysis, sterility testing, endotoxin evaluation, and potency assessment when applicable. These manufacturing principles enable pharmacies to face unmet medication needs through standardized processes that maintain product integrity, ensure patient safety, and fulfill regulatory obligations while providing therapy options unavailable through commercial channels.

Keywords: *Aseptic technique; Beyond-use dating; Environmental controls; Preparation validation; Regulatory compliance*

Learning Objectives

After completion of the chapter, the learners should be able to:

- Implement USP <795> standards for non-sterile compounding including appropriate garbing, documentation, and beyond-use dating determination.
- Apply aseptic technique principles following USP <797> guidelines for preparing sterile compounds across different risk levels.
- Operate specialized compounding equipment including electronic balances, laminar flow hoods, biological safety cabinets, and automated compounding devices.
- Design facility-appropriate environmental monitoring programs including viable and non-viable particle testing, surface sampling, and pressure differential verification.
- Develop comprehensive quality assurance protocols for both sterile and non-sterile preparations including process validation, personnel training, and end-product testing.
- Perform calculations necessary for preparing accurate compounded formulations including aliquoting, dilution, and concentration conversions.

NON-STERILE COMPOUNDING

Non-sterile compounding represents the art and science of creating customized medication preparations that are not required to be sterile. This practice addresses therapeutic needs unmet by commercially available products, including unique dosage forms, strengths, combinations, or formulations free from specific allergens or excipients. Non-sterile compounding requires thorough understanding of pharmaceutical principles including physical and chemical compatibility, stability considerations, and appropriate beyond-use dating to ensure both safety and efficacy of the final preparation.

Regulatory Guidelines and Standards

Non-sterile compounding operates within a comprehensive regulatory framework designed to ensure preparation quality and patient safety. The United States Pharmacopeia Chapter <795> establishes the foundational standards for non-sterile preparations, outlining requirements for facilities, equipment, personnel training, documentation, and quality control procedures. These standards classify compounded preparations based on complexity levels, with simple, moderate, and complex preparations requiring progressively more rigorous controls. Regulatory oversight varies by jurisdiction, with state boards of pharmacy typically providing direct supervision of compounding pharmacies, while the Food and Drug Administration maintains federal authority, particularly regarding bulk drug substances and interstate distribution. The Drug Quality and Security Act of 2013 clarified the regulatory boundaries between traditional pharmacy compounding and larger-scale compounding operations functioning as outsourcing facilities. Documentation requirements include master formulation records detailing specific components, quantities, procedures, equipment, and quality control checks for each preparation. Compounding records document the actual preparation process for each batch, including component lot numbers, quantities used, preparation date, assigned beyond-use date, and personnel involved. Proper documentation supports quality assurance, regulatory compliance, and appropriate clinical use while enabling investigation of any quality or safety concerns that might arise. Training and competency assessment for compounding personnel must address not only technical skills but also understanding of underlying pharmaceutical principles, potential stability issues, and contamination prevention strategies appropriate to non-sterile operations.

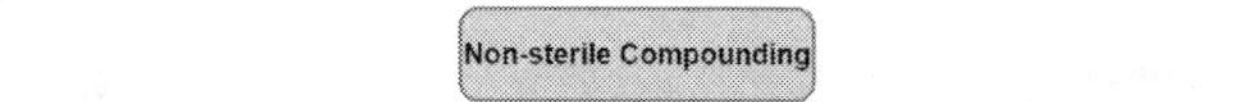

Figure 11.1: Non-sterile Compounding Process Flow

Table 11.1: Non-sterile Compounding Equipment and Uses

Equipment	Purpose	Cleaning/Maintenance
Electronic Balance	Accurate weighing of ingredients	Clean after each use Calibrate regularly Protect from dust Annual certification
Mortar and Pestle	Reducing particle size Mixing ingredients	Clean immediately after use Dedicate for specific uses Store dry
Spatulas	Transferring materials Mixing on ointment slabs	Clean after each use Inspect for damage Store properly
Graduated Cylinders	Measuring liquid volumes	Rinse immediately Dry inverted Inspect for chips/cracks
Ointment Mill	Reducing particle size in semisolids Creating homogeneous mixtures	Clean immediately Disassemble completely Lubricate moving parts
Ointment Slab	Mixing ointments and creams	Clean immediately Store protected Inspect for scratches
Pill Tiles	Mixing small quantities Capsule filling	Clean immediately Inspect for damage Store protected
Hot Plate/Magnetic Stirrer	Heating and mixing solutions	Clean after cooling Check electrical safety Calibrate temperature
Capsule Machines	Filling capsules uniformly	Clean thoroughly Store disassembled Check for damage
Suppository Molds	Forming suppositories	Clean immediately Store properly Check for damage

Equipment	Purpose	Cleaning/Maintenance
Electronic Homogenizer	Creating uniform suspensions/emulsions	Clean immediately Check electrical safety Inspect blades
Water Bath	Controlled heating	Regular water changes Check heating element Descale as needed
Unguator/Electronic Mortar and Pestle	Automated mixing of semisolids	Clean thoroughly Check electrical safety Maintain as directed

Formulation Development and Stability Considerations

Formulation development for compounded preparations requires systematic consideration of multiple pharmaceutical factors to ensure preparation stability, accuracy, and therapeutic efficacy. Vehicle selection significantly influences both physical and chemical stability while affecting palatability, administration ease, and potential excipient-related concerns. Aqueous vehicles provide appropriate matrices for water-soluble drugs but may promote hydrolysis of susceptible compounds. Non-aqueous vehicles including glycerin, propylene glycol, and fixed oils offer alternatives for water-sensitive medications but introduce different stability considerations. Chemical stability assessment considers potential degradation pathways including hydrolysis, oxidation, photolysis, and racemization. pH optimization represents a critical stability factor for many preparations, particularly those containing ionizable compounds with pH-dependent solubility and stability profiles. Buffer systems maintain pH within optimal ranges, preventing significant fluctuations that might compromise stability or therapeutic effect. Antioxidants including sodium metabisulfite, ascorbic acid, and butylated hydroxytoluene protect susceptible compounds from oxidative degradation, while chelating agents such as ethylenediaminetetraacetic acid (EDTA) bind trace metals that might otherwise catalyze oxidation reactions. Preservative selection addresses microbial contamination risk in multi-dose preparations, with systems including parabens, benzalkonium chloride, and potassium sorbate providing broad-spectrum activity when compatible with other formulation components. Beyond-use dating assignment follows systematic approaches outlined in USP <795>, considering water activity, pharmaceutical literature, stability-indicating analytical studies when available, and appropriate safety factors. Conservative dating applies when limited stability data exists, while extended dating requires more substantial supporting evidence through published literature or formal stability studies.

Table 11.2: Non-sterile Compounding Bases and Vehicles

Base/Vehicle Type	Examples	Properties	Incompatibilities
Hydrophilic Ointment Bases	Polyethylene glycol ointment Aquaphor	Water-soluble/washable Absorbs water Minimal occlusion	Strong oxidizers Certain preservatives Incompatible with some ions
Hydrocarbon Bases	White petrolatum Yellow petrolatum Mineral oil	Occlusive Water-repellent Greasy feel	Water-soluble drugs High drug concentrations Hydrophilic substances
Absorption Bases	Hydrophilic petrolatum Lanolin Aquabase	W/O emulsion Some water absorption Occlusive properties	Some preservatives Highly charged molecules Extremes of pH
Water-Washable Bases	Hydrocream Vanishing cream Cetaphil	O/W emulsion Easy spreading Non-greasy	Oil-soluble drugs with poor solubility Substances affecting emulsion stability
Water-Soluble Bases	Polyethylene glycol Carbomer gels	Water-soluble Greaseless Washes off easily	Strong electrolytes Quaternary compounds Some preservatives

Base/Vehicle Type	Examples	Properties	Incompatibilities
Oral Solution Vehicles	Simple syrup Ora-Sweet Ora-Plus	Sweet taste Viscosity for suspension Preservative systems	Substances affecting pH Compounds incompatible with preservatives Oxidation-sensitive drugs
Suspending Agents	Methylcellulose Carboxymethylcellulose Xanthan gum	Increase viscosity Prevent settling Controlled flocculation	Strong electrolytes Extreme pH Certain preservatives
Suppository Bases	Cocoa butter Polyethylene glycol Witepsol	Melting/dissolving properties Drug release characteristics Physical stability	Water content >5% Substances affecting melting point Certain preservatives
Capsule Diluents	Lactose Microcrystalline cellulose Starch	Flow properties Compactibility Compatibility	Drugs that degrade lactose Moisture-sensitive drugs (with hygroscopic diluents) Incompatible drug-excipient combinations
Flavoring Agents	Fruit flavors Mint flavors Vanilla	Taste masking Patient acceptance Compatibility	Incompatible flavors pH-sensitive flavors Drug-flavor interactions
Sweetening Agents	Sucrose Saccharin	Improve palatability	Drug-sweetener

Base/Vehicle Type	Examples	Properties	Incompatibilities
	Stevia	Viscosity (sugar) Diabetic considerations	interactions Incompatible preservatives Formulations for diabetics (sucrose)
Preservative Systems	Parabens Benzalkonium chloride Sorbic acid	Prevent microbial growth Extend shelf life System-specific activity	Incompatible surfactants Absorption by certain containers Inactivation by certain ingredients

Common Dosage Forms and Preparation Techniques

Non-sterile compounding encompasses diverse dosage forms addressing specific therapeutic needs through appropriate preparation techniques. Oral liquid preparations including solutions, suspensions, and emulsions accommodate patients with swallowing difficulties, allow flexible dosing, and enhance palatability through flavoring agents. Solution preparation requires attention to solubility parameters, with cosolvents, pH adjustment, or solubilizing agents employed when needed for poorly soluble compounds. Suspensions incorporate insoluble medications requiring particle size reduction through levigation with appropriate wetting agents before incorporation into the suspending vehicle. Uniform dispersion maintenance requires suspending agents such as methylcellulose or xanthan gum, with thorough patient education regarding proper shaking before use. Topical preparations address dermatological conditions through various forms including ointments, creams, gels, and lotions, each with distinct characteristics affecting drug release, absorption, and patient acceptance. Ointments provide occlusive bases appropriate for chronic, dry skin conditions, with incorporation of active ingredients through either dissolution or levigation techniques. Creams offer more cosmetically acceptable water-in-oil or oil-in-water emulsions suitable for less severe conditions, requiring careful emulsification techniques to ensure stability. Gels provide transparent, non-greasy matrices particularly suitable for hairy areas, with proper dispersion techniques preventing aggregation of gelling agents. Solid oral dosage forms including capsules and troches require precise powder mixing, often employing geometric dilution techniques to ensure uniform drug distribution. Capsule preparation demands attention to powder flow properties, density considerations affecting capsule size selection, and appropriate punching techniques to ensure complete filling. Suppositories offer alternative delivery routes for patients unable to take oral medications, with molding techniques requiring temperature control appropriate to the selected base, typically cocoa butter or polyethylene glycol.

Special Considerations in Non-sterile Compounding

Special considerations in non-sterile compounding address unique challenges associated with specific patient populations and medication classes. Pediatric compounding requires careful dose calculation, appropriate concentration selection to enable accurate measurement, palatability enhancement without introducing problematic excipients, and consideration of age-appropriate dosage forms. Excipient selection for pediatric preparations demands particular scrutiny, avoiding alcohol, propylene glycol, benzyl alcohol, and certain preservatives in concentrations inappropriate for neonates and infants. Veterinary compounding addresses species-specific physiological differences affecting drug disposition, administration challenges, and palatability preferences varying widely across animal species and individuals. Flavor selection for companion animals must consider species-specific preferences, with cats generally favoring fish or meat flavors and dogs accepting sweeter options. Transdermal veterinary preparations offer alternatives for difficult-to-medicate animals, though absorption variability necessitates careful monitoring of therapeutic response. Hormone compounding for bioidentical hormone replacement therapy requires precise weighing of potent substances, thorough mixing to ensure dose uniformity, and appropriate vehicle selection affecting drug release and absorption. Hormones present occupational exposure concerns requiring containment strategies including dedicated equipment, appropriate personal protective equipment, and proper cleaning protocols to prevent cross-contamination. Hazardous drug compounding follows USP <800> standards with designated compounding areas, appropriate engineering controls, personal protective equipment requirements, and specific decontamination and waste management protocols. Appropriate beyond-use dating assignment requires consideration of stability data limitations, with conservative approaches when formulation-specific stability studies are unavailable. Quality control strategies incorporate physical inspection, pH measurement, weight variation assessment for solid dosage forms, and when appropriate, analytical testing to verify active ingredient content and uniformity.

STERILE MANUFACTURING

Sterile compounding involves the preparation of medications requiring sterility for safe administration, including injections, ophthalmic preparations, and other products intended for introduction into normally sterile body spaces. This specialized practice area demands rigorous adherence to aseptic technique, environmental controls, and validation procedures to prevent potentially serious harm from microbial contamination, pyrogens, or particulate matter. The exacting standards for sterile compounding reflect the significant risks associated with introducing contaminants directly into the bloodstream or other sterile tissues.

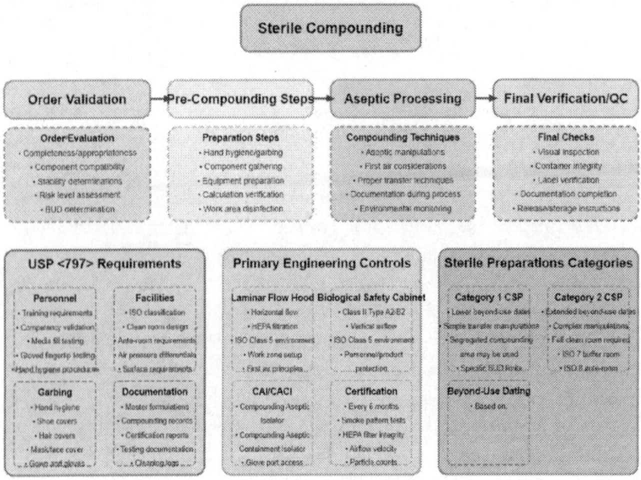

Figure 11.2: Sterile Compounding Requirements

Regulatory Standards and Facility Requirements

Sterile compounding operates under comprehensive regulatory oversight designed to ensure preparation sterility and safety. United States Pharmacopeia Chapter <797> establishes the minimum standards for sterile compounding across all practice settings, with requirements for facilities, environmental monitoring, personnel qualifications, cleaning procedures, and quality assurance programs. These standards classify compounded sterile preparations (CSPs) based on risk levels determined by preparation complexity, starting components, and manipulation extent. Category 1 CSPs have shorter beyond-use dates (BUDs) based on storage conditions and may be prepared in environments with less stringent requirements, while Category 2 CSPs with extended BUDs require more rigorous environmental conditions and testing.

Table 11.3: Sterile Compounding Requirements and Standards

Category	USP <797> Requirements	Implementation Methods
Facility Design	Primary and secondary engineering controls Buffer and ante-rooms Pressure differentials HEPA filtration	Proper room classification Regular certification Airflow visualization Appropriate surfaces
Environmental Monitoring	Viable air sampling Surface sampling Fingertip testing Media fill tests	Established sampling plans Regular testing schedule Trending of results Immediate action for excursions
Personnel Qualifications	Training requirements Competency assessment Aseptic technique validation Continuing education	Structured training program Regular competency assessments Media fill testing Hand hygiene monitoring
Garbing Requirements	Hand hygiene Shoe covers Hair covers Face masks Sterile gloves Sterile gowns	Proper garbing sequence Quality of materials Regular garbing assessment Dedicated garbing area
Cleaning and Disinfection	Defined frequencies Approved agents Surface compatibility Sporicidal agents	Cleaning schedules Rotation of agents Staff training Material compatibility testing
Beyond-Use Dating	Risk level-based dating Stability data requirements Storage condition	Stability literature review Testing when required Conservative dating

Category	USP <797> Requirements	Implementation Methods
	specifications Extended dating requirements	policies Proper storage conditions
Quality Assurance	Process validation End-product testing Quality control Error reporting	QA program development Regular process audits Trending of data CAPA implementation
Hazardous Drug Handling	USP <800> requirements Containment strategies PPE specifications Waste management	C-PECs for hazardous drugs Dedicated equipment Enhanced PPE Closed-system transfer devices
Documentation Systems	Master formulation records Compounding records Testing records Quality control	Standardized forms Electronic systems Regular reviews Record retention
Verification and Release	Visual inspection Weight/volume checks Label verification Final pharmacist check	Standardized checking process Independent verification Technology assistance Documentation of checks
Training Requirements	Initial training Ongoing education Competency assessment Remedial training	Structured curriculum Regular refreshers Documented assessment Feedback mechanisms

Facility design requirements include segregated compounding areas with appropriate air quality specifications, requiring HEPA filtration, defined airflow patterns, and pressure differentials creating cascading positive pressure from cleanest to less clean areas. Primary engineering controls (PECs) including laminar airflow workbenches (LAFW) and biological safety cabinets (BSC) provide ISO Class 5 environments for direct compounding activities. Secondary engineering controls encompass the clean room suite with anterooms serving as transition spaces for hand hygiene, garbing, and materials transfer. Airflow design prevents intrusion of less clean air into cleaner spaces through positive pressure relationships, with hazardous drug compounding requiring negative pressure to contain potential contaminants. Surface characteristics throughout compounding areas must resist particle shedding, facilitate effective cleaning, and withstand regular disinfection with appropriate agents. Material selection for walls, floors, ceilings, and fixtures excludes porous surfaces, exposed wood, or other elements that might harbor contamination or resist cleaning. Personnel flow and material transfer pathways minimize contamination risk through defined procedures, appropriate pass-throughs, and unidirectional movement from cleaner to less clean areas.

Aseptic Technique and Personnel Requirements

Aseptic technique represents the cornerstone of sterile compounding, encompassing specialized procedures preventing contamination introduction during preparation. Personnel requirements begin with comprehensive training covering theoretical foundations of microbiology, contamination sources, and practical aspects of aseptic manipulation. Initial qualification includes aseptic technique verification through media-fill tests simulating most challenging compounding activities routinely performed, with periodic requalification maintaining demonstrated competency. Hand hygiene serves as the foundation of aseptic technique, employing antimicrobial soap with specific scrubbing procedures followed by alcohol-based hand sanitizers before donning sterile gloves. Garbing sequence follows specified procedures with non-shedding coveralls, shoe covers, hair covers, facial hair covers, masks, and sterile gloves creating protective barriers between personnel and the sterile compounding environment. Garb quality must meet standards for particle generation and permeability, with sterile components required for direct contact with critical sites. First air principles guide proper manipulation within primary engineering controls, maintaining critical sites (vial stoppers, syringe tips, ampule necks) within the HEPA-filtered airflow path without obstruction from hands, arms, or objects that might disrupt the protective air curtain. Touch contamination prevention requires conscious technique development, maintaining awareness of sterile versus non-sterile surfaces and employing non-touch transfer methods when possible. Material preparation before introduction into primary engineering controls includes removal of outer packaging and thorough disinfection with sterile 70% isopropyl alcohol or other appropriate agents, allowing sufficient contact time for effective microbial reduction. Workflow organization minimizes unnecessary movement, material transfer, and interruptions that might compromise aseptic conditions or introduce contamination opportunities.

Sterile Compounding Processes and Techniques

Sterile compounding encompasses multiple preparation types requiring specific techniques ensuring final product sterility and accuracy.

Table 11.4: Sterile Compounding Equipment and Techniques

Equipment	Purpose	Maintenance/Certification
Laminar Flow Hood	Primary engineering control HEPA-filtered air ISO Class 5 environment	6-month certification Daily cleaning Monthly deep clean Prefilter maintenance
Biological Safety Cabinet	Hazardous drug compounding Personnel protection Product protection	6-month certification Daily cleaning HEPA filter integrity Airflow verification
Compounding Aseptic Isolator	Isolator technology Microbial protection Negative/positive pressure	6-month certification Glove integrity testing Transfer system checks Pressure differential monitoring
HEPA Filters	Remove particulates Maintain air quality ISO classification	Integrity testing Leak testing Pressure monitoring Replacement as needed
Automated Compounding Devices	IV admixture preparation TPN compounding Multi-ingredient preparations	Daily calibration Tubing changes Software updates Preventive maintenance
Syringes	Measuring and transferring Drug administration Compounding component	Single-use only Visual inspection Proper disposal Sterility maintenance

Equipment	Purpose	Maintenance/Certification
Needles	Transfer between containers Filter sterilization Reconstitution	Single-use only Proper disposal Safety mechanism verification Integrity check
Filter Needles/Devices	Remove particulates Sterilization Ampule filtration	Single-use only Integrity verification Proper disposal Pressure limitations
Peristaltic Pumps	Controlled filling Automated transfers Repetitive operations	Regular calibration Tubing replacement Motor maintenance Accuracy checks
Sterilization Equipment	Terminal sterilization Component preparation Equipment sterilization	Regular validation Preventive maintenance Calibration Performance qualification
Media Fill Test Kits	Process validation Personnel qualification Aseptic technique verification	Appropriate media Proper storage Sterility verification Expiration monitoring
Environmental Monitoring Tools	Viable/non-viable monitoring Pressure differential Temperature/humidity	Instrument calibration Media quality checks Software validation Sensor maintenance
Incubators	Media growth Test incubation Microbial identification	Temperature mapping Calibration Cleaning protocols Performance qualification
IV Workflow Management Systems	Barcode verification Gravimetric checks Process documentation Error prevention	Software updates Camera/scale calibration Database maintenance Performance verification

Intravenous admixture preparation represents the most common sterile compounding activity, involving addition of medications to fluid containers for parenteral administration. This process employs syringes with appropriate needle sizes for medication withdrawal and transfer, with careful attention to maintain needle sterility throughout the procedure. Vial manipulation requires specific techniques for both liquid and powder formulations, with multiple-dose vials receiving particular attention to maintain sterility during repeated access. Ampule opening employs alcohol-soaked gauze supporting clean breaks while preventing glass particle contamination, with filtration needles recommended for solution withdrawal. Total parenteral nutrition compounding represents complex preparation involving precise additions of dextrose, amino acids, electrolytes, vitamins, trace elements, and sometimes lipid emulsions, typically utilizing automated compounding devices for large-volume preparations requiring multiple additives. Compatibility assessment remains critical with careful consideration of component concentrations, order of mixing, and potential precipitation or degradation reactions. Patient-controlled analgesia preparation requires precise concentration verification, appropriate reservoir selection, and meticulous labeling ensuring safe administration rates. Ophthalmic preparation demands heightened attention to sterility, with specialized filtration frequently employed and particulate matter inspection critical for products contacting delicate ocular tissues. Repackaging of commercially available sterile products requires maintenance of sterility throughout the transfer process, with beyond-use dating reflecting both stability limitations and sterility maintenance considerations. Batch preparation involves production of multiple identical units within a single compounding sequence, requiring careful planning, component staging, and systematic procedures maintaining aseptic conditions throughout extended compounding activities.

Sterility Testing and Quality Control

Quality control for sterile preparations encompasses multiple strategies verifying both preparation accuracy and sterility assurance. Visual inspection represents the most fundamental quality check, examining preparations against light/dark backgrounds for particulate matter, container integrity, appropriate solution clarity, and absence of visible contamination. More sophisticated methods include filter integrity testing for sterilizing filtration processes, automated compounding device verification, and gravimetric analysis confirming appropriate solution densities. Environmental monitoring programs assess air quality, surface contamination, and personnel aseptic technique through systematic sampling. Viable air sampling quantifies microorganisms present in compounding environments, typically employing impaction samplers collecting microorganisms on growth media for subsequent incubation and colony counting. Surface sampling utilizes contact plates or swabs to evaluate cleaning effectiveness and identify potential bioburden reservoirs requiring intervention. Fingertip sampling assesses garbing effectiveness and aseptic technique by testing gloved fingertips for microbial contamination following compounding activities. Action levels established for each monitoring type trigger appropriate responses when exceeded, including investigation, cleaning, retraining, or facility modification. Sterility testing follows USP <71> methodology for selected preparations, particularly those intended for storage beyond immediate use or prepared in larger batches. Direct inoculation or membrane filtration techniques transfer samples to appropriate growth media supporting both aerobic and anaerobic organisms, with extended incubation periods allowing detection of slow-growing contaminants. Endotoxin testing employs Limulus Amebocyte Lysate (LAL) assays detecting bacterial endotoxins that might cause pyrogenic reactions despite preparation sterility, particularly important for intrathecal, intraocular, or large-volume parenteral preparations. Potency testing verifies active ingredient concentration through appropriate analytical methods, with particular importance for narrow therapeutic index medications, pediatric preparations, or products with extended beyond-use dating.

EQUIPMENT AND TECHNIQUES

Pharmaceutical compounding requires specialized equipment and refined techniques to ensure preparation accuracy, consistency, and quality. Equipment selection, maintenance, calibration, and proper utilization significantly influence final preparation characteristics and therapeutic outcomes. Mastery of fundamental techniques across various dosage forms enables pharmacists to address diverse patient needs through appropriate compounded medications.

Basic Compounding Equipment

Basic compounding equipment provides the foundation for preparation manipulation across various dosage forms. Balances and scales represent perhaps the most critical equipment, with selection based on required accuracy and precision for intended applications. Analytical balances capable of measuring to 0.1 mg support work with potent substances requiring precise quantities, while prescription balances measuring to 1-5 mg suffice for less critical applications. Regular calibration using certified weights ensures ongoing accuracy, with daily functionality verification before use. Calibrated graduated cylinders, conical graduates, and pipettes provide volumetric measurement with selection based on required volume and accuracy needs. Class A glassware offers superior accuracy for critical measurements, while plastic graduates suffice for less exacting applications. Mortar and pestle sets in various materials serve different functions: glass for liquid incorporation and wet grinds; porcelain for general powder processing; and Wedgwood for harder materials requiring greater force. Proper technique employs circular grinding motions from outer edge toward center, ensuring uniform particle size reduction. Spatulas in various configurations address different material handling needs, with stainless steel offering chemical resistance for most applications and non-metallic options preventing potential interactions with reactive compounds. Electronic homogenizers, ointment mills, and mechanical mixers provide more efficient mixing for larger batches or challenging formulations requiring exceptional uniformity. Heating equipment including water baths, hot plates, and melting apparatus supports processes requiring temperature control, with integrated thermometers ensuring appropriate ranges for thermolabile ingredients. Specialized equipment for specific dosage forms includes capsule filling machines, suppository molds, lozenge trays, and tablet compression devices, each requiring specific techniques for optimal utilization.

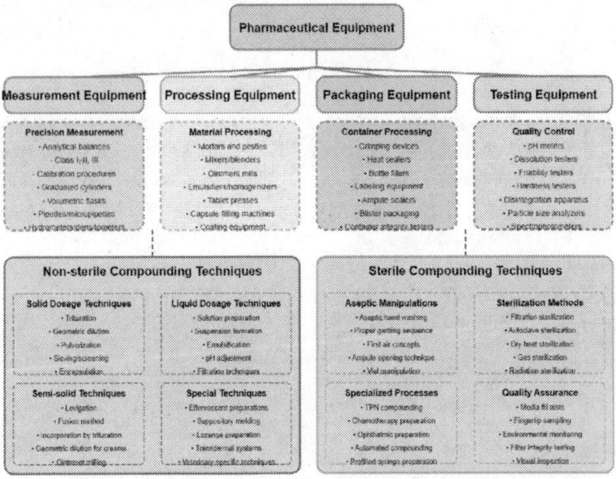

Figure 11.3: Equipment and Techniques for Pharmaceutical Manufacturing

Advanced Compounding Equipment and Technology

Advanced compounding equipment enhances preparation quality, efficiency, and reproducibility for more complex formulations. Automated compounding devices for total parenteral nutrition and other complex fluid admixtures employ computer-controlled pumps delivering precise volumes through a manifold system into final containers. These systems provide gravimetric or volumetric verification, automated calculations, and documentation of all additions while reducing contamination risk and repetitive motion injuries associated with manual compounding. Powder encapsulation equipment ranges from semi-automated devices facilitating consistent filling of moderate batch sizes to fully automated systems for larger-scale production, each requiring appropriate technique for powder distribution, capsule filling, and quality verification. Ointment mills provide superior particle size reduction and dispersion for topical preparations containing insoluble active ingredients, with adjustable roller gaps determining final particle dimensions and resulting texture, absorption characteristics, and therapeutic efficacy. Electronic mortar and pestle systems offer programmable grinding cycles ensuring consistent results for standardized formulations while reducing physical strain during extended processing. Specialized mixing equipment including planetary mixers, high-shear blenders, and magnetic stirring systems provide efficient, thorough mixing for various preparation types, with selection based on viscosity, volume, and required mixing intensity. Filtration equipment ranging from simple filter paper to sophisticated membrane filtration systems removes particulate matter from solutions, with selection based on required particle retention size, chemical compatibility, and flow rate needs. Analytical equipment increasingly appears in compounding pharmacies, including pH meters ensuring appropriate acidity for stability and therapeutic effect, refractometers verifying solution concentration, and in some settings, more sophisticated instrumentation including high-performance liquid chromatography for potency verification of critical preparations.

Specialized Techniques for Various Dosage Forms

Specialized techniques for specific dosage forms ensure optimal preparation characteristics and therapeutic performance. Geometric dilution represents a fundamental technique for uniform incorporation of potent substances into larger powder volumes, beginning with equal volumes of active ingredient and diluent, thoroughly mixing, then progressively adding equal volumes of diluent with thorough mixing between additions. This systematic approach prevents aggregation of active ingredients and ensures dose uniformity in the final preparation.

Trituration employs systematic grinding in a mortar and pestle to reduce particle size, typically proceeding from crystalline materials to fine powder through consistent circular motions applying appropriate pressure. Levigation creates smooth dispersions of insoluble substances in appropriate vehicles, beginning with incorporation of a small quantity of vehicle into the powder to create a concentrated paste before gradual dilution with additional vehicle. Proper levigation prevents particle aggregation and ensures uniform distribution throughout the final preparation. Emulsification techniques create stable dispersions of immiscible liquids through appropriate emulsifying agents and mixing procedures, with oil-in-water or water-in-oil systems selected based on desired characteristics. Primary emulsions formed with concentrated emulsifier solutions provide the foundation for subsequent dilution while maintaining stability. Solubilization strategies for poorly soluble compounds include cosolvency using alcohol, glycerin, or propylene glycol; complexation with cyclodextrins; micellization with surfactants; and pH adjustment exploiting ionization characteristics of weakly acidic or basic compounds. Filtration techniques remove particulate contaminants while potentially providing sterilization for appropriate solutions, with filter selection based on chemical compatibility, required flow rate, and target particle retention size. Encapsulation techniques include punch methods for individual preparations and more efficient plate methods for larger batches, with attention to powder flow properties, density, and compression characteristics ensuring complete, uniform filling.

Equipment Maintenance and Calibration

Equipment maintenance and calibration ensure ongoing accuracy, reliability, and compliance with quality standards. Cleaning protocols for compounding equipment must address both visible residue removal and microbial contamination control, with particular attention to equipment used for potent or hazardous substances requiring specialized decontamination procedures. Material-specific cleaning considerations include avoidance of abrasive cleaners on glass surfaces prone to scratching; thorough drying of metal equipment preventing corrosion; and appropriate disinfectant selection compatible with equipment surfaces without leaving problematic residues. Calibration programs establish regular verification schedules for all measuring devices, with frequency determined by usage patterns, stability of calibration, and criticality of accuracy for specific applications. Balance calibration employs NIST-traceable weights bracketing the typical usage range, with daily calibration verification before use and more comprehensive procedures at established intervals. Volumetric equipment calibration uses gravimetric methods measuring dispensed volumes of purified water under controlled temperature conditions, converting measured weights to volumes using temperature-corrected density values. Temperature monitoring devices require regular verification against certified thermometers ensuring accurate readings for processes where temperature influences stability, sterility, or other critical preparation characteristics. Preventive maintenance schedules address equipment-specific requirements including lubrication of moving parts, seal replacement, filter changes, and software updates for electronic systems. Documentation of all maintenance, calibration, and performance verification activities provides evidence of ongoing compliance with quality standards while establishing equipment history supporting investigation of any preparation issues potentially related to equipment performance. Equipment retirement decisions consider performance history, repair frequency, calibration stability, and availability of replacement parts, with formal decommissioning procedures ensuring discontinued equipment cannot inadvertently return to service.

QUALITY ASSURANCE

Quality assurance in pharmaceutical compounding encompasses systematic processes ensuring consistent preparation of medications meeting appropriate standards for identity, strength, quality, and purity. This multifaceted approach extends beyond final preparation testing to include personnel training, documentation systems, process validation, and continuous quality improvement initiatives. A comprehensive quality assurance program provides the foundation for patient safety while supporting regulatory compliance and preparation reproducibility.

Quality Management Systems

Quality management systems provide the organizational framework supporting consistent preparation quality through defined processes, responsibilities, and continuous improvement mechanisms. Standard operating procedures (SOPs) document all aspects of compounding operations including facility maintenance, equipment operation, compounding processes, testing methods, and documentation requirements. These procedures establish standardized approaches reducing variability while providing training references and ensuring regulatory compliance. Effective SOPs incorporate sufficient detail for consistent execution while remaining accessible to personnel at all experience levels, with regular review and revision maintaining alignment with current practices and regulatory requirements. Personnel qualification programs establish initial training requirements, competency assessment methods, and ongoing education expectations for all staff involved in compounding activities. Structured training progression typically begins with theoretical foundations before advancing to supervised practical experience and culminating in independent competency demonstration. Documentation systems maintain records of all compounding activities, supporting both internal quality verification and external regulatory review. Master formulation records document standardized formulations including complete ingredient lists, preparation procedures, equipment requirements, expected physical characteristics, beyond-use dating justification, and quality control checks. Compounding records document each preparation batch with specific component lot numbers, quantities, preparation date, assigned beyond-use date, and personnel involvement, creating complete preparation traceability. Deviation management systems identify, document, investigate, and resolve departures from established procedures, with appropriate corrective and preventive actions implemented to prevent recurrence. Effective quality management incorporates periodic self-inspection programs systematically reviewing all aspects of compounding operations against internal standards and regulatory requirements, identifying improvement opportunities before they become compliance issues.

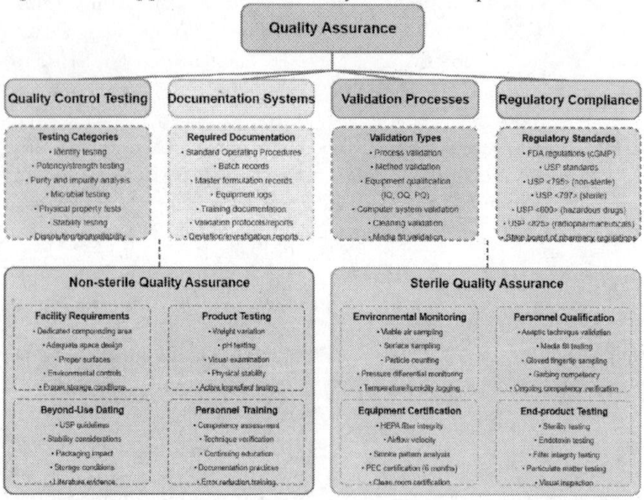

Figure 11.4: Quality Assurance in Pharmaceutical Manufacturing

Beyond-Use Dating and Stability Considerations

Beyond-use dating establishes time limits for safe and effective compounded preparation use based on stability considerations, contamination risk, and supporting evidence. Stability assessment considers multiple degradation pathways including hydrolysis, oxidation, photolysis, thermolysis, and microbial proliferation, with appropriate testing or literature evaluation supporting dating assignments. Chemical stability refers to maintenance of active ingredient potency within acceptable limits, typically 90-110% of labeled strength, while physical stability encompasses appearance, uniformity, pH, and other measurable characteristics affecting preparation usability. USP <795> and <797> provide framework guidance for beyond-use dating based on preparation type, components, storage conditions, and available stability data. Conservative default beyond-use dates apply when preparation-specific stability data remains unavailable, while extended dating requires supporting evidence through published stability studies or direct testing using stability-indicating methods.

Table 11.5: Quality Assurance in Compounding

QA Component	Implementation Methods	Common Challenges
Standard Operating Procedures	Template development Expert review Staff training Accessibility	Keeping current Staff compliance Consistent application Balancing detail with usability
Personnel Training	Structured curriculum Hands-on assessment Knowledge testing Observation	Resource constraints Standardization Measuring effectiveness Staff turnover
Process Validation	Protocol development Risk assessment Statistical analysis Failure investigation	Resource intensity Representative testing Managing failures Determining frequency
Environmental Monitoring	Sampling plans Trend analysis Action limits Excursion management	Interpretation of results Resource constraints Timely testing Action limit establishment
End-product Testing	Risk-based approach	Cost-benefit analysis Method

QA Component	Implementation Methods	Common Challenges
	Sampling plans Test method validation Laboratory controls	development Testing limitations Timely results
Error Reporting	Non-punitive culture Standardized reporting Investigation process Tracking system	Encouraging reporting Thoroughness Timely investigation Effective prevention
Documentation Systems	Standardized forms Electronic systems Record review process Archiving protocols	Completeness Accessibility Consistency Timely review
Equipment Qualification	Protocol development Engineering support Third-party certification Scheduled testing	Resource intensity Technical expertise Scheduling challenges Documentation burden
Raw Material Control	Supplier audit Risk-based testing Quarantine procedures Specification development	Supply chain reliability Testing capabilities Resource constraints Specification development
Change Control	Standardized forms Review committee Risk assessment Communication plan	Resistance to change Thoroughness Timely implementation Unintended consequences
Cleaning Validation	Worst-case approach Analytical methods Acceptance criteria Revalidation schedule	Method development Representative sampling Residue limits Resource intensity

QA Component	Implementation Methods	Common Challenges
Quality Metrics	Data collection systems Statistical analysis Regular review Action planning	Meaningful metrics Data collection burden Analysis capabilities Taking action on results
Recall Procedures	Mock recalls Traceability systems Communication templates Investigation protocols	Traceability challenges Timely execution Effective communication Thoroughness

Stability-indicating analytical methods capable of distinguishing between active ingredients and degradation products provide the gold standard for extended dating justification, though such testing often exceeds capabilities of typical compounding pharmacies. Literature evaluation supporting beyond-use dating requires critical assessment of study relevance, including identical formulation composition, concentration, storage conditions, and container systems. Packaging selection significantly influences preparation stability, with considerations including light protection for photosensitive compounds; moisture permeability for water-sensitive components; oxygen transmission rates for oxidation-prone substances; and compatibility between container materials and formulation components. Storage condition specifications form integral components of beyond-use dating, with refrigeration or freezing often extending permissible storage periods but requiring maintenance of specified temperature ranges throughout the storage period. Patient education regarding proper storage, beyond-use dating significance, and physical indicators of potential degradation complements formal stability assessment in ensuring preparation integrity throughout the intended use period.

Testing and Verification Methods

Testing and verification methods confirm compounded preparation quality through direct assessment of critical attributes. Physical inspection represents the most fundamental verification method, examining preparations for appropriate appearance, consistency, color, clarity, and freedom from visible contamination or physical instability indicators. Weight verification for capsules and other solid dosage forms confirms appropriate fill weight and consistency across a batch, typically measuring a statistically significant sample to verify compliance with established acceptance criteria. pH testing ensures appropriate acidity or alkalinity supporting both stability and therapeutic effect, particularly critical for preparations where pH significantly influences drug solubility, ionization state, or degradation rate. Specific gravity measurement verifies appropriate concentration for solutions where density correlates with composition, providing a simple, non-destructive verification method. More sophisticated analytical testing includes refractometry for concentration verification of solutions with refractive index correlation to strength; spectrophotometric methods quantifying active ingredients based on characteristic light absorption patterns; and chromatographic techniques separating and quantifying active ingredients and potential degradation products. Microbial testing assesses contamination in preserved non-sterile preparations or confirms sterility in preparations requiring absence of viable microorganisms. Dissolution or release testing evaluates drug availability from specific dosage forms, particularly relevant for modified-release preparations where drug liberation patterns significantly influence therapeutic effect. Potency testing verifies active ingredient concentration through appropriate analytical methods, with particular importance for preparations with narrow therapeutic indices, unusual delivery systems, or extended beyond-use dating. Risk-based approaches to testing frequency and methodology balance resource utilization against quality assurance needs, with more comprehensive testing applied to preparations presenting higher patient risk due to administration route, narrow therapeutic index, or complex formulation characteristics.

Documentation and Continuous Quality Improvement

Documentation and continuous quality improvement create the foundation for ongoing quality enhancement while demonstrating regulatory compliance. Comprehensive documentation systems maintain records of personnel qualifications, facility maintenance, equipment calibration, environmental monitoring, compounding activities, and quality control results, supporting both internal quality management and external regulatory review. Electronic documentation systems increasingly supplement or replace paper-based approaches, offering advantages in data accessibility, trend analysis capability, and integration with inventory and dispensing systems. Robust documentation facilitates investigation of any adverse events or quality deviations, providing complete preparation traceability from component receipt through patient dispensing. Continuous quality improvement employs systematic approaches to identifying enhancement opportunities, implementing appropriate changes, and measuring resulting outcomes. Quality metrics including preparation rejection rates, documentation error frequency, environmental monitoring results, and patient outcome measures provide objective data supporting improvement initiatives. Root cause analysis methodologies identify underlying factors contributing to quality issues, moving beyond superficial explanations to address fundamental systemic vulnerabilities. Plan-Do-Study-Act cycles provide structured approaches to improvement implementation, incorporating careful planning, controlled implementation, outcome measurement, and appropriate adjustment based on observed results. Non-punitive error reporting systems encourage personnel to identify potential quality issues without fear of inappropriate consequences, recognizing that system improvement rather than individual blame produces sustainable quality enhancement. Regular quality review meetings examine trending data, significant deviations, and improvement initiatives, maintaining organizational focus on quality advancement while ensuring appropriate resource allocation to highest-priority areas. External quality indicators including professional certification, accreditation program participation, and independent laboratory testing provide objective verification of internal quality systems while demonstrating commitment to excellence extending beyond minimum regulatory compliance.

Summary

Pharmaceutical compounding bridges the gap between commercially available medications and patient-specific therapeutic needs through customized preparation processes. Non-sterile compounding follows USP <795> standards encompassing preparation of oral, topical, and rectal formulations requiring proper documentation, beyond-use dating determination, and stability assessment. This practice addresses unique patient requirements including allergy avoidance, dosage customization, combination therapy, and specialized delivery forms using appropriate equipment including electronic balances, pharmaceutical mills, ointment slabs, and capsule-filling machines. Sterile compounding presents heightened complexity due to infection risk, requiring strict adherence to USP <797> guidelines categorizing preparations by risk level and establishing corresponding beyond-use dating limitations. Aseptic technique forms the foundation of sterile preparation, involving meticulous hand hygiene, appropriate garbing with sterile gloves, gowns, and masks, and strategic material handling to prevent contamination. Primary engineering controls including laminar airflow workbenches and biological safety cabinets provide ISO Class 5 environments for sterile manipulation, while secondary controls maintain appropriate air pressure differentials and particulate reduction in surrounding spaces. Advanced equipment including automated compounding devices, robotic systems, and closed-system transfer devices enhance preparation accuracy and personnel protection particularly when handling hazardous medications. Quality assurance programs incorporate personnel qualification through media-fill testing and aseptic technique evaluation, environmental monitoring using viable and non-viable particulate sampling, and end-product testing including sterility assessment, endotoxin evaluation, and potency determination when appropriate.

Multiple Choice Questions

1. According to USP <795>, which of the following would be classified as a complex non-sterile compounding procedure?
   a) Reconstituting an antibiotic suspension
   b) Mixing two commercial creams together
   c) Preparing capsules from a bulk powder
   d) Making a solution from a commercially available tablet
2. The beyond-use date for a non-preserved aqueous oral solution prepared from ingredients in solid form should not exceed:
   a) 14 days when stored at controlled cold temperature
   b) 30 days when stored at controlled cold temperature
   c) 90 days when stored at controlled cold temperature
   d) 180 days when stored at controlled cold temperature
3. Which of the following represents the proper order of gowning for sterile compounding?
   a) Hand hygiene, shoe covers, hair cover, face mask, gown, sterile gloves
   b) Shoe covers, hand hygiene, hair cover, face mask, gown, sterile gloves
   c) Hair cover, face mask, hand hygiene, gown, shoe covers, sterile gloves
   d) Gown, hand hygiene, hair cover, face mask, shoe covers, sterile gloves
4. According to USP <797>, which of the following would be classified as a high-risk level compounded sterile preparation?
   a) A single transfer of sterile medication from a vial to an IV bag using aseptic technique
   b) Combining multiple sterile products in a single container using closed-system transfers
   c) Preparing a solution from non-sterile components that will be terminally sterilized
   d) Pooling medications from multiple sterile vials to prepare a single patient dose
5. The beyond-use date for a properly prepared high-risk level compounded sterile preparation stored at room temperature should not exceed:
   a) 12 hours
   b) 24 hours
   c) 3 days
   d) 14 days

6. Which of the following is the primary engineering control for sterile compounding of hazardous drugs?
   a) Laminar airflow workbench
   b) Biological safety cabinet
   c) Isolator
   d) Cleanroom
7. Media-fill testing for pharmacy personnel who compound sterile preparations should be performed:
   a) Only upon initial training
   b) Annually
   c) At least every six months
   d) Monthly
8. Which of the following represents the appropriate first step when compounding a cream using the geometric dilution method?
   a) Calculating the quantity of each ingredient
   b) Calibrating the balance
   c) Thoroughly mixing the active ingredient with an approximately equal quantity of the base
   d) Documenting the compounding procedure in the log book
9. In a cleanroom environment, which of the following air quality classifications would be required for the ante-area where personnel hand hygiene and garbing take place?
   a) ISO Class 5
   b) ISO Class 7
   c) ISO Class 8
   d) ISO Class 9
10. Which of the following quality control tests would be most appropriate for evaluating the effectiveness of a pharmacy's cleaning procedures in sterile compounding areas?
   a) Media-fill testing
   b) Fingertip sampling
   c) Surface sampling
   d) Filter integrity testing

Self-Assessment Questions

1. Explain how risk levels are determined, appropriate beyond-use dating is established, and quality control procedures should be implemented for different dosage forms.
2. Explain each required component including calculations, preparation procedure, quality control checks, storage requirements, and stability considerations.
3. Compare and contrast the requirements for compounding hazardous versus non-hazardous medications, explaining the specific containment strategies, personal protective equipment, and environmental controls needed to protect personnel during preparation.
4. Evaluate the critical factors affecting stability in compounded preparations, explaining how physical compatibility, chemical stability, microbial contamination, and packaging interactions should be assessed when establishing beyond-use dates.
5. Explain how the categories of compounded sterile preparations (immediate use, low-risk, medium-risk, high-risk) determine facility requirements, beyond-use dating, and quality assurance processes.
6. Explain the scientific rationale for each step from hand hygiene through final verification and detailing how contamination could occur if procedures are not followed correctly.
7. Compare and contrast the design, function, and appropriate use of different primary engineering controls (laminar airflow workbenches, biological safety cabinets, compounding aseptic isolators), explaining how each provides environmental protection for sterile preparation.
8. Explain the purpose and procedures for media-fill testing, gloved fingertip sampling, and visual observation of technique, including appropriate response to failed competency assessments.
9. Design a comprehensive environmental monitoring program for a sterile compounding facility, explaining the locations, methods, frequencies, and acceptance criteria for viable and non-viable particulate testing in accordance with current standards.
10. Explain the appropriate quality control testing (sterility, endotoxin, potency) based on risk level, intended use, and batch size

Bibliography

1. The United States Pharmacopeial Convention. USP general chapter <797> pharmaceutical compounding—sterile preparations. In: USP 43-NF 38. Rockville, MD: United States Pharmacopeial Convention; 2020.
2. The United States Pharmacopeial Convention. USP general chapter <795> pharmaceutical compounding—nonsterile preparations. In: USP 43-NF 38. Rockville, MD: United States Pharmacopeial Convention; 2020.
3. The United States Pharmacopeial Convention. USP general chapter <800> hazardous drugs—handling in healthcare settings. In: USP 43-NF 38. Rockville, MD: United States Pharmacopeial Convention; 2020.
4. Kastango ES, Bradshaw BD. USP chapter 797: Establishing a practice standard for compounding sterile preparations in pharmacy. Am J Health Syst Pharm. 2004;61(18):1928-1938.
5. Allen LV Jr. The art, science, and technology of pharmaceutical compounding. 5th ed. Washington, DC: American Pharmacists Association; 2016.
6. Trissel LA. Handbook on injectable drugs. 20th ed. Bethesda, MD: American Society of Health-System Pharmacists; 2020.
7. McElhiney LF. Compounding guide for ophthalmic preparations. Washington, DC: American Pharmacists Association; 2013.
8. Pharmaceutical Inspection Co-operation Scheme. PIC/S guide to good practices for the preparation of medicinal products in healthcare establishments. Geneva, Switzerland: Pharmaceutical Inspection Convention, Pharmaceutical Inspection Co-operation Scheme; 2014.
9. The Joint Commission. Medication compounding certification. Oakbrook Terrace, IL: The Joint Commission; 2020.
10. Mixon W, Angelle P, Yoch D. Buyer's guide to compounding equipment: Recommendations from USP compliance experts. Int J Pharm Compd. 2009;13(6):480-490.

CHAPTER 12

EMERGENCY CARE

Author

Dr. Aditi Naidu Patti, Assistant Professor, Department of Pharmacy Practice, Vignan Institute of Pharmaceutical Technology, Duvvada, Visakhapatnam, Andhra Pradesh, India

Abstract

Emergency care in pharmacy settings involves medication management, first response capabilities, toxicology knowledge, and organizational protocols for crisis situations. Emergency medications maintained in pharmacy inventories include life-saving agents addressing anaphylaxis (epinephrine), opioid overdose (naloxone), hypoglycemia (dextrose, glucagon), cardiac arrest (atropine, amiodarone), and status epilepticus (benzodiazepines, levetiracetam), with pharmacist responsibilities including proper storage, expiration monitoring, dosing reference maintenance, and team education regarding appropriate administration. First aid in pharmacy settings requires preparation for common medical emergencies including cardiac events, allergic reactions, hypoglycemia, seizures, bleeding, and respiratory distress, with pharmacist training in basic life support, automated external defibrillator operation, and emergency response protocols coordinated with local emergency medical services. Toxicology basics essential for pharmacist practice include recognition of common poisoning presentations, initial management approaches for substance overdoses, familiarity with antidote mechanisms and indications, poison control center collaboration protocols, and triage decision-making for determining appropriate level of care. Crisis management extends beyond medical emergencies to address disaster response, medication supply chain disruptions, security incidents, and public health emergencies, requiring established communication hierarchies, essential medication stockpiles, alternative dispensing procedures, and coordination with government agencies and healthcare systems. This emergency preparedness helps pharmacists during both individual medical crises and larger-scale emergencies affecting medication access and public health.

Keywords: *Emergency Response; Overdose Management; Antidote; Disaster Preparedness; Life-Threatening Conditions*

Learning Objectives

After completion of the chapter, the learners should be able to:

- Prepare emergency medication kits with appropriate drugs, concentrations, and administration supplies for various practice settings.
- Demonstrate proper response techniques for common pharmacy emergencies including anaphylaxis, cardiac events, hypoglycemia, and seizures.
- Apply toxicology principles to identify and manage common poisoning and overdose scenarios including opioids, acetaminophen, and salicylates.
- Implement triage protocols to determine appropriate levels of care for patients presenting with various emergency conditions.
- Develop pharmacy disaster preparedness plans addressing medication supply maintenance, communication protocols, and coordination with emergency services.
- Recommend appropriate antidotes and supportive treatments for specific toxic exposures based on mechanism of action and patient presentation.

EMERGENCY MEDICATIONS

Emergency medications address acute, potentially life-threatening conditions requiring immediate intervention. These critical agents serve multiple roles in different settings, from community pharmacy response to medical emergencies, to institutional crash cart contents, to emergency medical services deployment. Proper emergency medication management requires thorough understanding of indications, contraindications, dosing, administration techniques, and storage requirements to ensure readiness when seconds matter in patient outcomes.

Cardiac Emergency Medications

Cardiac emergencies represent among the most time-critical situations requiring immediate pharmacological intervention. Epinephrine stands as the cornerstone of cardiac arrest management through its alpha- and beta-adrenergic effects, increasing coronary and cerebral perfusion pressure during cardiopulmonary resuscitation while enhancing myocardial contractility and stimulating spontaneous contractions. Administration in cardiac arrest employs 1 mg (1:10,000 concentration) intravenously or intraosseously every 3-5 minutes, with continuous infusion considerations for post-resuscitation support. Vasopressors including norepinephrine, dopamine, and vasopressin support blood pressure in cardiogenic, distributive, and other shock states through vasoconstriction and variable inotropic effects, with dosing typically weight-based and titrated to target blood pressure or perfusion parameters. Antiarrhythmic agents address various rhythm disturbances with amiodarone used in ventricular fibrillation/pulseless ventricular tachycardia refractory to defibrillation; lidocaine sometimes employed as an alternative; and adenosine serving as both diagnostic and therapeutic agent for supraventricular tachycardias through transient AV node blockade. Antiplatelet and antithrombotic therapy in acute coronary syndromes includes aspirin administration immediately upon suspicion, with additional agents including P2Y12 inhibitors (clopidogrel, ticagrelor) and anticoagulants (unfractionated heparin, enoxaparin) initiated based on specific presentation and planned intervention approach. Rapid administration of these agents significantly influences morbidity and mortality outcomes, making both appropriate stocking and proper administration knowledge essential in emergency settings.

Respiratory Emergency Medications

Respiratory emergencies require prompt pharmacological intervention to maintain oxygenation and ventilation. Bronchodilators represent first-line therapy for bronchospasm, with short-acting beta-2 agonists (albuterol) providing rapid airway smooth muscle relaxation through multiple administration routes including metered-dose inhalers with spacers, nebulization, or in extreme cases, intravenous formulations. Anticholinergic agents (ipratropium) offer complementary bronchodilation through different mechanisms, particularly valuable in COPD exacerbations and when combined with beta-agonists for enhanced effect. Systemic corticosteroids (methylprednisolone, prednisone, dexamethasone) address the inflammatory component of many respiratory emergencies, with early administration reducing symptom duration, hospitalization rates, and relapse frequency despite their delayed onset of action. Magnesium sulfate provides additional bronchodilation in severe asthma exacerbations through smooth muscle relaxation via calcium channel antagonism, typically administered intravenously over 20-30 minutes with careful monitoring for hypotension. Epinephrine serves critical roles in both anaphylaxis and severe asthma unresponsive to conventional therapy, with intramuscular administration (1:1,000 concentration) preferred in anaphylaxis for reliable absorption and rapid effect. Oxygen therapy supports all respiratory emergencies, with delivery systems ranging from simple nasal cannulas to non-rebreather masks and high-flow nasal cannula systems based on patient needs. Naloxone reverses respiratory depression from opioid overdose through competitive mu-receptor antagonism, administered via multiple routes including intranasal, intramuscular, intravenous, and subcutaneous, with dose titration ideally balancing respiratory stimulation against precipitation of withdrawal in opioid-dependent individuals.

Table 12.1: Emergency Medications and Their Uses

Medication Class	Primary Indications	Critical Monitoring Parameters
Vasopressors	Cardiac arrest Hypotension Anaphylaxis Septic shock	Blood pressure Heart rate Peripheral perfusion ECG changes Tissue necrosis (extravasation)
Antiarrhythmics	Ventricular fibrillation Ventricular tachycardia Supraventricular tachycardia Atrial fibrillation	ECG changes Blood pressure QT interval Heart rate Signs of toxicity
Anticonvulsants	Status epilepticus Acute seizures Seizure prophylaxis Alcohol withdrawal	Respiratory status Level of consciousness Seizure control Vital signs Paradoxical reactions
Reversal Agents	Opioid overdose Benzodiazepine overdose Heparin reversal DOAC reversal	Respiratory rate Level of consciousness Withdrawal symptoms
Inotropes	Cardiogenic shock Heart failure Cardiac output augmentation Bradycardia	Blood pressure Heart rate Cardiac output Arrhythmias Signs of toxicity
Analgesics	Acute pain Procedural sedation Trauma Myocardial infarction	Respiratory rate Sedation level Pain score Blood pressure
Sedatives	Procedural sedation	Respiratory status

Medication Class	Primary Indications	Critical Monitoring Parameters
	Mechanical ventilation Agitation Status epilepticus	Hemodynamic parameters Sedation depth Recovery time Paradoxical reactions
Neuromuscular Blockers	Rapid sequence intubation Mechanical ventilation Procedure facilitation Status asthmaticus	Ventilation adequacy Train-of-four monitoring Sedation adequacy Anaphylaxis Malignant hyperthermia
Antidotes	Overdose/poisoning Acetaminophen toxicity Digoxin toxicity Cyanide poisoning	Vital signs Mental status Specific toxicity markers Allergic reactions Electrolyte abnormalities
Emergency Cardiovascular	Bradycardia Hyperkalemia Metabolic acidosis Torsades de pointes	Heart rate ECG changes Acid-base status Electrolytes Signs of toxicity
Respiratory Medications	Asthma/COPD exacerbation Croup Airway edema Bronchospasm	Respiratory rate Oxygen saturation Work of breathing Peak flow/spirometry Side effects
Glucose Regulators	Hypoglycemia Hyperkalemia Calcium channel blocker overdose Sulfonylurea overdose	Blood glucose Mental status Potassium levels Fluid status Rebound effects

Neurological Emergency Medications

Neurological emergencies require specific pharmacological interventions addressing seizures, stroke, and other acute neurological conditions. Benzodiazepines represent first-line therapy for status epilepticus, with midazolam increasingly preferred for non-intravenous administration routes (intramuscular, intranasal, buccal) when vascular access is unavailable; lorazepam demonstrating longer seizure control duration when given intravenously; and diazepam offering rectal administration options particularly valuable in home management plans. Second-line anticonvulsants including fosphenytoin, valproate, and levetiracetam address benzodiazepine-refractory seizures, with specific agent selection considering onset time, administration considerations, and side effect profiles. Hyperosmolar therapy with mannitol or hypertonic saline reduces intracranial pressure in traumatic brain injury and other conditions with cerebral edema, requiring careful administration rate control and monitoring for fluid and electrolyte disturbances. Thrombolytic therapy with tissue plasminogen activator (tPA) remains the primary pharmacological intervention for ischemic stroke within appropriate time windows, requiring rapid recognition, careful patient selection through established criteria, and precise weight-based dosing to balance potential benefit against hemorrhagic conversion risk. Glucose management in neurological emergencies addresses both hypoglycemia with concentrated dextrose solutions (D50W, D10W) and hyperglycemia with insulin therapy, recognizing that both extremes adversely affect neurological outcomes. Antidotes for specific toxicological emergencies affecting the nervous system include flumazenil for benzodiazepine overdose and physostigmine for anticholinergic toxicity, though both carry significant cautions regarding seizure precipitation in certain contexts.

Anaphylaxis and Other Emergency Medications

Anaphylaxis represents a systemic, life-threatening hypersensitivity reaction requiring immediate pharmacological intervention. Epinephrine constitutes the definitive first-line treatment through multiple beneficial effects including alpha-1-mediated vasoconstriction reducing mucosal edema and hypotension; beta-1 cardiac stimulation increasing contractility and heart rate; and beta-2-mediated bronchodilation addressing respiratory symptoms. Intramuscular administration into the anterolateral thigh (vastus lateralis) provides optimal absorption, with 0.3-0.5 mg (0.3-0.5 mL of 1:1,000 concentration) for adults and weight-based dosing for pediatric patients, repeated every 5-15 minutes as needed based on response. Delayed epinephrine administration correlates with increased mortality, making immediate access through emergency kits, autoinjectors, or rapid preparation from ampules critically important. Adjunctive therapies include H1-antihistamines (diphenhydramine) primarily addressing urticaria and pruritus without significant impact on core anaphylactic pathophysiology; H2-antagonists (famotidine, ranitidine) sometimes added for potential additive benefit; and corticosteroids (methylprednisolone, prednisone) potentially reducing risk of biphasic or protracted reactions despite delayed onset. Additional emergency medications include activated charcoal for specific ingestions, administered within appropriate timeframes and when airway protection remains assured; dextrose for hypoglycemia confirmation or empiric administration in altered mental status when glucose measurement is unavailable; and calcium channel blocker or beta-blocker antidotes including calcium chloride, glucagon, and high-dose insulin therapy for significant cardiovascular toxicity. Pharmacy-based emergency kits require regular inspection, temperature monitoring, organization supporting rapid medication identification, and clear protocol guidance including proper dosing, administration techniques, and post-administration monitoring parameters.

Table 12.2: Emergency Response Algorithms and Medications

Emergency Condition	Initial Assessment	First-Line Medications	Secondary Interventions
Cardiac Arrest (VF/VT)	CPR Defibrillation Airway management IV/IO access	Epinephrine 1 mg IV/IO q3-5min Amiodarone 300 mg IV/IO Lidocaine 1-1.5 mg/kg IV/IO	Magnesium 1-2 g IV (Torsades) Sodium bicarbonate (specific indications) Calcium (hyperkalemia) Reversal agents (overdose)
Cardiac Arrest (PEA/Asystole)	CPR Airway management IV/IO access Identify causes	Epinephrine 1 mg IV/IO q3-5min Fluids for hypovolemia Atropine no longer routine	Address reversible causes: - Calcium (hyperkalemia) - Sodium bicarbonate (acidosis, TCA overdose) -Dextrose/Glucagon (hypoglycemia) - Naloxone (opioid overdose)

Emergency Condition	Initial Assessment	First-Line Medications	Secondary Interventions
Anaphylaxis	Airway assessment Vital signs Rash evaluation Auscultation	Epinephrine 0.3-0.5 mg IM (adult) Epinephrine 0.01 mg/kg IM (pediatric) IV fluids	Diphenhydramine 25-50 mg IV/PO Methylprednisolone 125 mg IV Ranitidine 50 mg IV Albuterol for bronchospasm
Status Epilepticus	Airway protection Oxygen IV access Glucose check	Lorazepam 0.1 mg/kg IV/IO Diazepam 0.15-0.2 mg/kg IV/IO Midazolam 0.2 mg/kg IM	Fosphenytoin 20 mg PE/kg IV Valproic acid 40 mg/kg IV Levetiracetam 60 mg/kg IV Phenobarbital 20 mg/kg IV
Acute Coronary Syndrome	Vital signs 12-lead ECG Cardiac markers STEMI vs. NSTEMI	Aspirin 162-325 mg chewed Nitroglycerin 0.4 mg SL Morphine 2-4 mg IV (if needed) P2Y12 inhibitor (per protocol)	Anticoagulant (heparin/enoxaparin) Beta-blocker if appropriate Statin ACE inhibitor Reperfusion strategy meds
Stroke (Ischemic)	NIHSS assessment CT scan Blood glucose Vital signs	Alteplase 0.9 mg/kg IV (if eligible) Aspirin 325 mg (if no tPA) BP management medications	Antiplatelet therapy Statin therapy DVT prophylaxis Swallowing assessment before PO
Acute Heart Failure	Vital signs Oxygen saturation JVD/edema Lung auscultation	Nitroglycerin 0.4 mg SL/spray Furosemide Oxygen therapy	Morphine (selected cases) ACE inhibitor/ARB Nitroprusside (severe HTN) Inotropes

Emergency Condition	Initial Assessment	First-Line Medications	Secondary Interventions
Severe Asthma/COPD	Respiratory assessment Oxygen saturation Work of breathing Peak flow/FEV1	Albuterol nebulizer (continuous or q20min) Ipratropium nebulizer Systemic corticosteroids Oxygen therapy	Magnesium sulfate 2 g IV Terbutaline SC Epinephrine (if severe) BiPAP/intubation considerations
Hyperkalemia	ECG evaluation Vital signs Neurological status Recent medications	Calcium gluconate 1-3 g IV (cardioprotection) Insulin 10 units + Dextrose 25g IV Albuterol nebulizer 10-20 mg	Sodium bicarbonate 50 mEq (acidosis) Kayexalate/Patiromer/SZC (removal) Furosemide (if adequate renal function) Dialysis consideration
Opioid Overdose	Respiratory assessment Level of consciousness Pupil examination Evidence of use	Naloxone 0.4-2 mg IV/IM/IN Titrate to respiratory effect Airway support	Additional naloxone doses Continuous naloxone infusion Supportive care Consider co-ingestants
Diabetic Emergencies (DKA/HHS)	Blood glucose Mental status Vital signs Electrolytes/ABG	IV fluids (0.9% NS) Insulin (0.1 units/kg/hr) Potassium replacement Bicarbonate (severe acidosis only)	Glucose when BG <200-250 Transition to SQ insulin Phosphate replacement Address precipitating cause

Emergency Condition	Initial Assessment	First-Line Medications	Secondary Interventions
Sepsis/Septic Shock	Vital signs Mental status Source identification Lactate level	Broad-spectrum antibiotics IV fluid resuscitation Vasopressors (if hypotensive) Source control	Additional antimicrobials Stress-dose steroids Blood products Glucose control

FIRST AID IN PHARMACY

First aid in pharmacy encompasses the immediate care provided to injured or suddenly ill individuals before complete medical care becomes available. Pharmacists and pharmacy personnel often serve as first responders to medical emergencies occurring within pharmacy settings or surrounding areas due to their healthcare training and accessibility to the public. Effective first aid delivery requires knowledge of assessment techniques, recognition of emergency situations requiring immediate intervention, appropriate response prioritization, and understanding of both pharmacological and non-pharmacological interventions.

Basic Life Support and Emergency Response

Basic life support (BLS) provides the foundation for emergency response within pharmacy settings, focusing on maintaining airway patency, supporting breathing, and ensuring circulation until advanced medical assistance arrives. Current BLS guidelines emphasize high-quality chest compressions as the priority in cardiac arrest, with compression depth of 2-2.4 inches at a rate of 100-120 compressions per minute, allowing complete chest recoil between compressions and minimizing interruptions. The compression-to-ventilation ratio remains 30:2 for single rescuers, with emphasis on compression quality over perfect ventilation in the initial response.

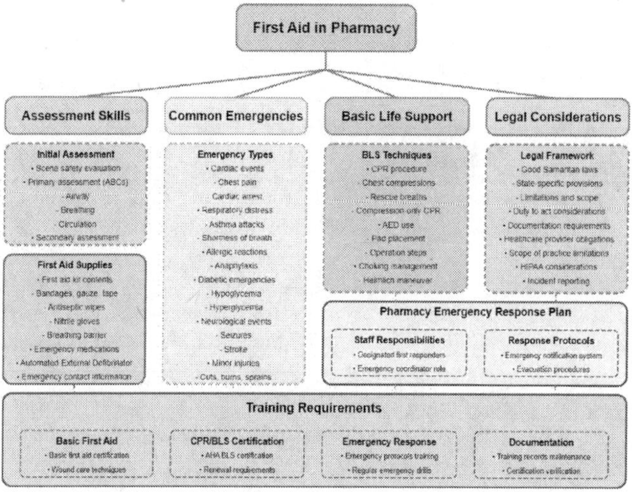

Figure 12.1: First Aid in Pharmacy

Early defibrillation with automated external defibrillators (AEDs) significantly improves survival in witnessed cardiac arrest with shockable rhythms, making pharmacy access to these devices increasingly important, particularly in rural or underserved areas with extended emergency medical services response times. Emergency response organization within pharmacy settings requires clear protocols establishing responsibility chains, communication procedures with emergency services, documentation requirements, and staff role assignments. Regular emergency drills maintain skill proficiency while identifying potential process improvements before actual emergencies occur. Patient assessment follows the primary survey approach (Airway, Breathing, Circulation, Disability, Exposure) identifying immediately life-threatening conditions requiring intervention before more detailed evaluation. Airway assessment determines patency and potential obstruction, with techniques including head tilt-chin lift or jaw thrust maneuvers to establish and maintain airway access. Breathing evaluation assesses respiratory rate, depth, effort, and bilateral chest movement, with rescue breathing or bag-valve-mask ventilation initiated when necessary. Circulation assessment includes pulse presence, rate, quality, and blood pressure when equipment is available, alongside evaluation for external hemorrhage requiring control measures. Disability screening provides rapid neurological assessment using the AVPU scale (Alert, Verbal response, Painful response, Unresponsive) or Glasgow Coma Scale. Exposure involves examining for additional injuries or medical alert identification while maintaining patient dignity and thermal protection.

Table 12.3: First Aid Situations and Pharmacy Interventions

Emergency Situation	Assessment	First Aid Measures	Referral Criteria
Minor Burns	Degree (1st, 2nd, 3rd) Size (% BSA) Location Causative agent	Cool water immersion Remove jewelry/clothing Cover with clean dressing Pain management	Burns >3% BSA 3rd degree burns Face/hands/genitals Circumferential burns Significant pain
Minor Wounds/Cuts	Depth Length Bleeding severity Contamination	Clean with mild soap and water Apply direct pressure Apply appropriate dressing	Deep wounds Heavy bleeding Wounds requiring sutures Signs of infection Animal/human bites
Allergic Reactions	Severity Systems involved Progression rate Previous history	Remove allergen if possible Antihistamine administration Epinephrine if indicated	Difficulty breathing Facial/throat swelling Persistent symptoms History of anaphylaxis
Insect Stings/Bites	Insect type Reaction severity Stinger presence Number of stings	Remove stinger (scrape, don't squeeze) Clean area Cold compress Oral antihistamine	Multiple stings Allergic reaction Signs of infection Tick attachment >24 hours
Sprains/Strains	Mechanism of injury Swelling/bruising Range of	RICE (Rest, Ice, Compression, Elevation) Immobilization if needed	Inability to bear weight Severe pain Obvious deformity

Emergency Situation	Assessment	First Aid Measures	Referral Criteria
	motion Pain severity	Pain management Avoid heat first 48 hours	Popping sound at injury
Headache	Type/location Severity Associated symptoms Triggers/timing	Pain management Hydration Rest in quiet, dark environment Stress reduction	Sudden severe headache "Worst headache ever" Neurological symptoms Persistent/worsening pain
Fever	Temperature Associated symptoms Duration Age of patient	Appropriate antipyretics Hydration Light clothing/covering Lukewarm sponging (children)	Infants <3 months Very high fever (>103°F) Altered mental status Persistent fever >3 days
Gastrointestinal Distress	Symptoms (N/V/D) Duration Associated factors Hydration status	Hydration Diet modification Symptom management Rest	Severe dehydration Blood in stool/vomit Severe abdominal pain Symptoms >3 days
Allergic Skin Reactions	Appearance Distribution Itching severity Potential triggers	Remove allergen Cool compresses Appropriate medications Avoid scratching	Widespread reaction Severe discomfort Involvement of mucous membranes Signs of infection
Eye Injuries/Irritation	Type of injury/irritant Vision	Chemical exposure: flush 15-20 min Foreign body:	Chemical burns Vision changes Embedded objects

Emergency Situation	Assessment	First Aid Measures	Referral Criteria
	changes Pain severity Foreign body presence	don't rub Minor irritation: artificial tears Shield eye if needed	Severe pain/light sensitivity
Heat-Related Illness	Temperature Mental status Sweating presence Associated symptoms	Move to cool area Hydration Cooling methods Position (supine with legs elevated)	Altered mental status Temperature >104°F Persistent symptoms High-risk individuals
Chest Pain	Character Radiation Associated symptoms Risk factors	Rest Position of comfort Aspirin if cardiac suspected Nitroglycerin if prescribed	Any chest pain suspicious for cardiac Difficulty breathing Diaphoresis/nausea Pain >5 minutes
Diabetic Emergencies	Blood glucose Mental status Known diabetic Symptoms	Hypoglycemia: glucose source Hyperglycemia: hydration Position of safety Monitor vital signs	Unconsciousness Inability to swallow Ketoacidosis symptoms No improvement with intervention
Musculoskeletal Pain	Location Severity Duration Aggravating factors	Appropriate analgesics Rest affected area Ice/heat as appropriate Supportive devices	Severe or worsening pain Following trauma Functional limitation Signs of infection

Common Medical Emergencies in Pharmacy Settings

Pharmacy settings encounter various medical emergencies requiring appropriate recognition and response. Syncope (fainting) represents among the most common presentations, resulting from transient cerebral hypoperfusion with potential causes including vasovagal reactions, orthostatic hypotension, cardiac arrhythmias, or hypoglycemia. Initial management involves positioning the patient supine with elevated legs, maintaining airway patency, assessing vital signs when possible, and evaluating for injuries sustained during falls. Distinguishing simple vasovagal syncope from more concerning etiologies requires attention to precipitating factors, associated symptoms, and recovery pattern. Allergic reactions range from localized responses to systemic anaphylaxis, with assessment focusing on respiratory status (stridor, wheezing, respiratory rate), cardiovascular stability (pulse, blood pressure), and cutaneous manifestations (urticaria, angioedema). Management depends on severity, with anaphylaxis requiring immediate epinephrine administration and activation of emergency medical services. Respiratory distress presents through increased work of breathing, accessory muscle use, abnormal respiratory patterns, or cyanosis, with asthma exacerbations, foreign body aspiration, pulmonary embolism, and acute coronary syndrome among potential causes. Initial interventions include positioning for optimal breathing mechanics, supplemental oxygen when available, and appropriate medication administration based on the specific etiology. Diabetic emergencies include hypoglycemia presenting with diaphoresis, tremor, confusion, and potential unconsciousness, managed with oral glucose for conscious patients or injectable glucagon when oral administration is unsafe; and hyperglycemic crises (diabetic ketoacidosis, hyperosmolar hyperglycemic state) typically developing more gradually with polyuria, polydipsia, nausea, and progressive alteration in consciousness, requiring emergency medical service transport for definitive management. Acute coronary syndromes manifest through chest discomfort often described as pressure, tightness, or squeezing, with potential radiation to the jaw, neck, or arms, accompanied by diaphoresis, nausea, dyspnea, or lightheadedness. Immediate response includes positioning for comfort, aspirin administration when not contraindicated, nitroglycerin for those with prescribed medications, and prompt emergency medical service activation with clear communication of suspected cardiac etiology to minimize system delays.

Wound Care and Minor Injuries

Wound care and minor injury management within pharmacy

settings addresses common presentations while identifying conditions requiring advanced medical attention. Wound assessment evaluates several factors determining appropriate management: wound type (abrasion, laceration, puncture, avulsion); contamination level; bleeding severity; depth and involvement of underlying structures; location relative to cosmetically or functionally significant areas; and patient factors including tetanus immunization status, medication use (particularly anticoagulants), and comorbidities affecting healing potential. Bleeding control employs direct pressure as the primary intervention, applied with clean gauze or cloth directly to the bleeding site with continuous pressure for at least 15 minutes without removing initial dressings to check progress. Pressure point use or tourniquet application remains reserved for life-threatening hemorrhage unresponsive to direct pressure. Wound cleansing reduces infection risk through irrigation with normal saline or clean tap water, removing visible contaminants and reducing bacterial burden without cytotoxic antiseptics potentially impairing healing. Appropriate dressing selection considers wound characteristics with occlusive dressings maintaining moist healing environments for partial-thickness wounds; absorbent dressings for exudative wounds; and appropriate securing methods minimizing additional tissue trauma. Minor burn management follows depth assessment with first-degree (superficial) burns involving only the epidermis presenting with erythema and pain without blistering; second-degree (partial-thickness) burns extending into the dermis with blister formation and significant pain; and third-degree (full-thickness) burns destroying all skin layers appearing dry with potentially reduced sensation requiring immediate medical referral. Initial burn treatment includes removing the heat source, cooling the area with room temperature water for 10-15 minutes, avoiding ice application, covering with clean non-adherent dressings, and pain management with appropriate analgesics. Musculoskeletal injuries including sprains, strains, and contusions benefit from the PRICE approach (Protection, Relative rest, Ice, Compression, Elevation) during initial management, with assessment for potential fractures or dislocations requiring medical referral based on deformity, significant swelling, crepitus, or neurovascular compromise.

First Aid Kit Development and Maintenance

First aid kit development for pharmacy settings requires thoughtful consideration of likely emergencies, available space, staff training level, and proximity to advanced medical care. Essential components include personal protective equipment (gloves, face shields, masks) protecting both providers and patients during emergency response; wound care supplies (various bandage sizes, gauze, adhesive tape, antiseptic wipes, non-adherent dressings); basic assessment tools (blood pressure cuff, stethoscope, penlight, thermometer, glucose meter); and emergency medications appropriate to the practice setting and staff training. Emergency medications might include aspirin for suspected cardiac emergencies; oral glucose preparations for hypoglycemia; epinephrine autoinjectors or ampules with appropriate administration supplies for anaphylaxis; albuterol inhalers with spacers for bronchospasm; and naloxone for opioid overdoses in communities with high prevalence. Specialized equipment considerations include automated external defibrillators with appropriate maintenance programs ensuring battery function and current protocol compliance; bag-valve-mask devices for assisted ventilation; and tourniquets or hemostatic agents in settings with higher bleeding risk. Kit organization principles emphasize clear labeling, logical grouping of related items, easily recognizable packaging, inventory lists identifying contents and locations, and tamper-evident seals indicating kit integrity. Maintenance protocols establish regular inspection schedules verifying complete inventory, checking expiration dates, replacing used or outdated supplies, confirming equipment functionality, and documenting all inspections and replacements. Staff training ensures all pharmacy personnel understand kit location, contents, and appropriate utilization based on their training level, with regular review sessions maintaining knowledge currency and addressing questions or concerns. Documentation systems record all emergency responses, interventions provided, supplies used, and outcomes observed, supporting both quality improvement initiatives and risk management requirements while facilitating appropriate supply replacement.

TOXICOLOGY

Toxicology in pharmacy practice encompasses the identification, assessment, and management of poisonings and overdoses from medications, household products, industrial chemicals, plants, and other substances. Pharmacists contribute significantly to toxicology through poison prevention education, toxic exposure recognition, initial management guidance, antidote access, and collaboration with poison control centers. The knowledge of toxicokinetic principles, recognition of toxidromes, knowledge of appropriate interventions, and familiarity with antidote mechanisms provides the foundation for effective toxicological response.

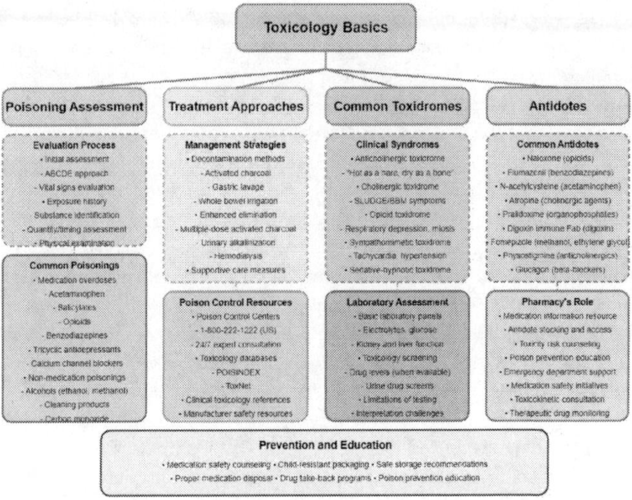

Figure 12.2: Toxicology Basics for Pharmacy Practice

Toxicokinetics and Assessment

Toxicokinetics applies pharmacokinetic principles to toxic substances, examining how absorption, distribution, metabolism, and elimination influence toxicity development, progression, and resolution. Absorption considerations in toxic exposures include route-specific factors: gastrointestinal absorption influenced by formulation characteristics, gastric pH, and presence of food or binding substances; inhalational exposure affected by substance volatility, respiratory rate, and alveolar membrane permeability; dermal absorption determined by lipophilicity, molecular size, and skin integrity; and parenteral exposures bypassing absorption barriers with immediate bioavailability. Modified-release formulations, pharmaceutical excipients, and concretions (particularly with salicylates or iron) can significantly alter absorption profiles and toxicity duration. Distribution patterns influence target organ toxicity, with lipophilic substances crossing the blood-brain barrier causing central nervous system effects; protein binding affecting free fraction available for toxic effects; and volume of distribution influencing elimination strategy selection. Metabolism may either detoxify substances through phase I or II reactions or create more toxic metabolites through bioactivation, exemplified by acetaminophen's hepatotoxic metabolite N-acetyl-p-benzoquinone imine (NAPQI) produced through cytochrome P450 activity. Elimination pathways determine both toxicity duration and potential therapeutic interventions, with renal elimination amenable to enhancement through urine alkalinization for weakly acidic compounds or increased fluid throughput; hepatic clearance potentially augmented through enzyme induction; and specific elimination-enhancing techniques including hemodialysis, hemoperfusion, or multiple-dose activated charcoal for selected toxins. Toxicological assessment begins with thorough history gathering when possible, including substance identity, quantity, time of exposure, intentionality, co-ingestants, and pre-existing medical conditions. Physical examination focuses on vital signs, mental status, pupillary response, skin findings, bowel sounds, and other manifestations suggesting specific toxidromes. Laboratory evaluation may include standard panels (complete blood count, electrolytes, renal and hepatic function, coagulation studies) alongside toxin-specific tests when available and interpretation of arterial or venous blood gases identifying specific acid-base disturbances associated with particular toxins.

Common Toxidromes and Recognition

Toxidromes represent constellations of signs and symptoms characterizing specific poisoning categories, facilitating recognition and appropriate management. The anticholinergic toxidrome results from muscarinic receptor antagonism, classically described as "hot as a hare, blind as a bat, dry as a bone, red as a beet, and mad as a hatter." Clinical manifestations include hyperthermia, tachycardia, mydriasis, dry mucous membranes, flushed skin, urinary retention, decreased bowel sounds, and altered mental status ranging from agitation to delirium. Common causes include antihistamines, tricyclic antidepressants, antipsychotics, and plants containing anticholinergic alkaloids. The cholinergic toxidrome results from excessive cholinergic stimulation through either acetylcholinesterase inhibition or direct receptor agonism. Manifestations follow the "SLUDGE" mnemonic (Salivation, Lacrimation, Urination, Defecation, Gastrointestinal distress, Emesis) alongside miosis, bronchorrhea, bronchospasm, bradycardia, and potential seizures or central nervous system depression.

Table 12.4: Common Toxicological Emergencies and Antidotes

Toxin/Overdose	Clinical Presentation	Initial Management	Specific Antidotes
Acetaminophen	Often asymptomatic initially Later: RUQ pain, nausea/vomiting Delayed hepatotoxicity (24-72h) Coagulopathy, jaundice	Activated charcoal (<1 hour) Obtain levels at ≥4 hours post-ingestion Plot on nomogram Start antidote if indicated	N-acetylcysteine (NAC) - Loading: 150 mg/kg IV or PO - Maintenance: varies by protocol - Continue for 17-21 hours minimum
Opioids	Respiratory depression Miosis (pinpoint pupils) CNS depression Hypotension Hypothermia	Airway management Oxygen supplementation IV access Antidote administration	Naloxone - 0.4-2 mg IV/IM/IN - Titrate to adequate respiration - May need repeat doses - Consider infusion for long-acting opioids
Benzodiazepines	Sedation/somnolence Respiratory depression Ataxia Hyporeflexia Hypothermia	Airway management Supportive care Activated charcoal (if recent ingestion) Consider antidote	Flumazenil (use with caution) - 0.2 mg IV over 30 sec - May repeat up to 1 mg total - Contraindicated in chronic use, seizure history, TCA co-ingestion

Toxin/Overdose	Clinical Presentation	Initial Management	Specific Antidotes
Tricyclic Antidepressants	Anticholinergic effects QRS prolongation QT prolongation Seizures Hypotension	Airway management Activated charcoal Cardiac monitoring Seizure management	Sodium bicarbonate - 1-2 mEq/kg IV bolus - Target arterial pH 7.50-7.55 - For QRS >100 ms or ventricular arrhythmias
Calcium Channel Blockers	Bradycardia Hypotension Heart block Hyperglycemia Mental status changes	Airway management IV access Cardiac monitoring Atropine for bradycardia	Calcium chloride/gluconate High-dose insulin euglycemia therapy Glucagon Lipid emulsion (in refractory cases)
Beta Blockers	Bradycardia Hypotension Bronchospasm Hypoglycemia Seizures (propranolol)	Airway management IV access Cardiac monitoring Atropine for bradycardia	Glucagon - 3-10 mg IV bolus - 1-5 mg/hr infusion High-dose insulin euglycemia therapy Lipid emulsion (in refractory cases)
Organophosphates	SLUDGE syndrome Respiratory weakness Bradycardia Miosis	Decontamination (PPE essential) Airway management Antidote	Atropine - 2-5 mg IV, double q5min until secretions dry Pralidoxime

Toxin/Overdose	Clinical Presentation	Initial Management	Specific Antidotes
	Fasciculations	administration Cardiac monitoring	- 1-2 g IV, then infusion Benzodiazepines for seizures
Cyanide	Altered mental status Metabolic acidosis Elevated lactate Bright red venous blood Bitter almond odor	Airway management 100% oxygen IV access Antidote administration	Hydroxocobalamin - 5 g IV (adult) - 70 mg/kg (pediatric) Sodium thiosulfate - 12.5 g IV (adult)
Carbon Monoxide	Headache Dizziness Nausea Cherry-red skin (late) Normal pulse oximetry	Remove from source 100% oxygen Assess carboxyhemoglobin level Consider hyperbaric oxygen	100% oxygen - Reduces CO half-life from 4-6 hours to 40-80 minutes Hyperbaric oxygen - Consider for severe poisoning
Salicylates	Tachypnea Tinnitus Hyperthermia Mixed acid-base disturbance Altered mental status	Airway management Activated charcoal (multi-dose) IV hydration Correct electrolytes	Sodium bicarbonate - Alkalinize urine (pH >7.5) - Enhance elimination - Prevent CNS penetration Hemodialysis for severe cases
Digoxin	Nausea/vomiting Visual changes Bradyarrhythmias	Activated charcoal Cardiac monitoring Correct	Digoxin Immune Fab - Acute: # vials = amount

Toxin/Overdose	Clinical Presentation	Initial Management	Specific Antidotes
	Hyperkalemia AV blocks	electrolytes Manage arrhythmias	ingested (mg) ÷ 0.5 - Chronic: # vials = (serum level × weight in kg) ÷ 100
Methanol/Ethylene Glycol	Visual disturbances (methanol) High anion gap metabolic acidosis Calcium oxalate crystals (EG) Osmolar gap	Airway management IV access Bicarbonate for acidosis Prevent metabolism	Fomepizole - 15 mg/kg loading, then 10 mg/kg q12h Ethanol (alternative) - Target level 100-150 mg/dL Hemodialysis for severe cases
Iron	Vomiting/diarrhea Abdominal pain Metabolic acidosis Shock Hepatic failure	Abdominal X-ray Whole bowel irrigation IV fluid resuscitation Serum iron level	Deferoxamine - 15 mg/kg/hr IV (max 6-8 g/day) - Blue-gray urine (vin rosé)

Organophosphate insecticides, carbamate insecticides, and certain mushroom species represent common causes. The opioid toxidrome presents with the classic triad of respiratory depression, miosis, and decreased level of consciousness, alongside constipation, hypotension, and hypothermia. Caused by both prescription and illicit opioids, recognition has gained importance with the ongoing opioid epidemic. The sympathomimetic toxidrome results from excessive adrenergic stimulation, presenting with hyperthermia, tachycardia, hypertension, mydriasis, diaphoresis, agitation, and potential seizures. Cocaine, amphetamines, synthetic cathinones, and other stimulants represent typical causes. The sedative-hypnotic toxidrome presents with central nervous system depression, respiratory depression, hypotension, hypothermia, and ataxia, resulting from benzodiazepines, barbiturates, and other sedatives. The serotonin syndrome, resulting from excessive serotonergic activity, presents with the triad of altered mental status, autonomic hyperactivity, and neuromuscular abnormalities, particularly clonus, hyperreflexia, and muscle rigidity pronounced in the lower extremities.

Initial Management

Initial toxicological management follows systematic approaches addressing life-threatening manifestations while limiting ongoing toxin absorption and enhancing elimination when appropriate. Supportive care provides the foundation for all toxicological management, addressing airway protection in patients with depressed consciousness; breathing support for respiratory depression or bronchospasm; circulatory support for hypotension or dysrhythmias; temperature management for hypo- or hyperthermia; and seizure control when present. Specific antidotes, when available, address particular toxins through various mechanisms but never replace fundamental supportive care. Gastrointestinal decontamination aims to reduce toxin absorption, with approaches varying by clinical context. Activated charcoal administration, typically 1 g/kg (50-100 g for adults), adsorbs many toxins when administered within 1-2 hours of ingestion, though contraindications include absent protective airway reflexes, caustic substance ingestion, and substances poorly bound to charcoal (alcohols, metals, lithium). Gastric lavage, once routine, now demonstrates limited efficacy and potential complications, restricting its use to specific scenarios involving potentially lethal ingestions within 60 minutes without safer alternatives. Whole bowel irrigation using polyethylene glycol electrolyte solution mechanically removes unabsorbed substances from the gastrointestinal tract, particularly valuable for sustained-release preparations, substances not adsorbed by activated charcoal, or body packers. Enhanced elimination techniques increase toxin clearance after absorption. Multiple-dose activated charcoal interrupts enterohepatic or enterogastric recirculation of certain toxins including carbamazepine, phenobarbital, and theophylline. Urinary alkalinization enhances elimination of weak acids including salicylates through ion trapping within renal tubules. Extracorporeal removal through hemodialysis or hemoperfusion addresses specific toxins with characteristics amenable to these approaches, including low volume of distribution, low protein binding, water solubility, and molecular weight allowing passage through dialysis membranes. Toxicological consultation through poison control centers (1-800-222-1222 in the United States) provides expert guidance regarding appropriate management strategies, laboratory monitoring, decontamination approaches, antidote indications, and disposition decisions.

Antidotes and Their Mechanisms

Antidotes counteract specific toxins through various mechanisms, providing targeted interventions supplementing supportive care. N-acetylcysteine addresses acetaminophen toxicity through multiple mechanisms: serving as a glutathione precursor replenishing depleted stores; directly binding the toxic metabolite NAPQI; and enhancing sulfate conjugation pathways. Administration follows specific protocols with either 72-hour oral or 21-hour intravenous regimens based on acetaminophen levels plotted on the Rumack-Matthew nomogram. Naloxone reverses opioid toxicity through competitive antagonism at mu, kappa, and delta opioid receptors, rapidly improving respiratory depression and mental status. Dosing begins at 0.4-2 mg intravenously, intramuscularly, or intranasally, with subsequent dose escalation based on response and potential repeated dosing due to naloxone's shorter duration compared to many opioids. Flumazenil antagonizes benzodiazepine effects through competitive binding at the GABA-benzodiazepine receptor complex, but carries significant seizure risk in patients with benzodiazepine dependence or co-ingestants lowering seizure threshold, limiting its routine use. Digoxin-specific antibody fragments (Digibind, DigiFab) bind both circulating and tissue-bound digoxin, rapidly reversing cardiotoxicity, though requiring careful dose calculation based on digoxin level or ingested amount. Fomepizole inhibits alcohol dehydrogenase, preventing toxic metabolite formation in methanol and ethylene glycol poisoning, replacing the traditional ethanol infusion approach with more predictable kinetics and fewer monitoring requirements. Hydroxocobalamin binds cyanide forming cyanocobalamin (vitamin B12), addressing cyanide toxicity from fire smoke inhalation, industrial exposure, or nitroprusside infusions. Physostigmine, a reversible cholinesterase inhibitor, temporarily reverses anticholinergic toxicity through increased acetylcholine availability, though cardiac risk limits its use to severe cases without tricyclic antidepressant involvement. Calcium channel blocker and beta-blocker toxicity antidotes include high-dose insulin-euglycemia therapy, calcium administration, glucagon, vasopressors, and in selected cases, intravenous lipid emulsion, with approaches often combined in severe poisonings. Crotalidae polyvalent immune Fab (CroFab) and other antivenoms neutralize specific venoms through binding toxic components, preventing further tissue damage and systemic effects when administered within appropriate timeframes.

CRISIS MANAGEMENT

Crisis management in pharmacy encompasses the systematic approach to unexpected, potentially harmful situations threatening patient safety, public health, staff welfare, or operational continuity. Effective crisis management integrates preparedness, response coordination, communication strategies, and recovery planning to mitigate negative impacts while maintaining essential services. Pharmacists increasingly recognize crisis management as a core professional responsibility, particularly given their frontline healthcare position during public health emergencies, natural disasters, medication safety events, and workplace emergencies.

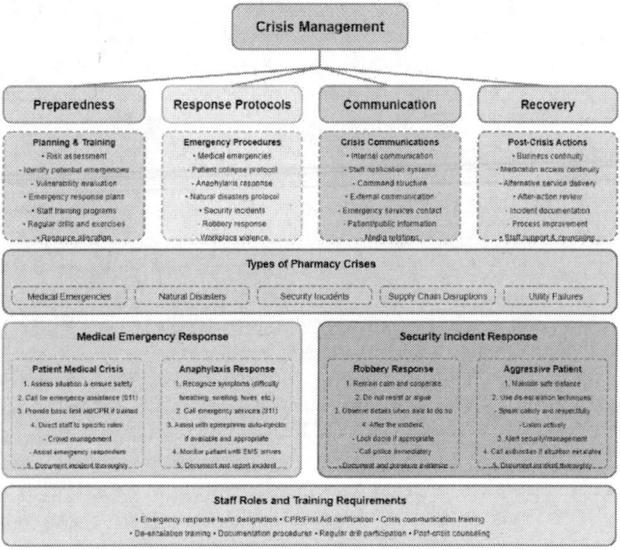

Figure 12.3: Crisis Management in Pharmacy

Crisis Preparedness and Planning

Crisis preparedness establishes the foundation for effective response through systematic assessment, planning, and resource development before emergencies occur. Risk assessment identifies potential crisis scenarios relevant to specific pharmacy settings, considering geographical location (natural disaster vulnerability); patient population characteristics; medication inventory including high-alert or controlled substances; and operational dependencies such as power, water, and supply chain reliability. Prioritization focuses planning efforts on scenarios combining highest likelihood with greatest potential impact on patient care and operational continuity. Emergency operations planning develops detailed response frameworks for identified scenarios, clearly defining activation criteria, command structures, staff roles and responsibilities, communication pathways, resource mobilization procedures, and coordination with external agencies. Continuity of operations planning specifically addresses maintaining essential services during disruptions, identifying minimum functional requirements, alternative operational models, and service prioritization strategies when resources become constrained. Resource planning ensures availability of essential supplies, equipment, and information during crises when normal acquisition channels may be disrupted. Emergency supply caches might include shelf-stable medications addressing common chronic conditions; emergency medications such as insulin, anticonvulsants, and cardiovascular agents; alternative power sources for refrigeration and essential equipment; and communication devices functioning independently from standard infrastructure. Documentation redundancy ensures critical patient information remains accessible during electronic system failures through appropriate backup systems, downtime procedures, and manual alternatives for essential functions. Staff preparation includes regular training on emergency protocols; clear role assignments with identified backups for key positions; skill development supporting role flexibility during crises; and personal preparedness guidance ensuring staff availability during community-wide emergencies. Community integration connects pharmacy emergency planning with broader healthcare system and public health emergency frameworks, establishing relationships with emergency management agencies, hospital systems, and other pharmacies potentially sharing resources or accepting patient transfers during localized emergencies.

Table 12.5: Crisis Management in the Pharmacy Setting

Crisis Type	Warning Signs	Immediate Response	Post-Crisis Actions
Medical Emergency - Customer	Chest pain Difficulty breathing Loss of consciousness Slurred speech Seizure activity	Call 911 Initial assessment Clear immediate area Begin CPR if necessary	Documentation Incident report Staff debriefing Follow-up with patient Equipment check/restock

Crisis Type	Warning Signs	Immediate Response	Post-Crisis Actions
Medical Emergency - Staff	Same as customer Plus: - Unusual behavior - Excessive sweating - Expressed discomfort	Same as customer Plus: - Staff privacy considerations - Coverage for staff duties	Same as customer Plus: - Worker's compensation - Return to work planning - Staff coverage planning
Medication Error - Detected	Wrong patient Wrong drug Wrong dose Wrong directions Wrong formulation	Stop dispensing process Assess potential harm Correct error Document intervention	Root cause analysis Process improvement Staff education Disclosure documentation Follow-up if needed
Medication Error - After Dispensing	Patient report Discovered during review Adverse event report Prescriber notification	Contact patient immediately Assess actual/potential harm Provide correct medication Document event	Same as detected error Plus: - Formal reporting (ISMP, etc.) - Patient follow-up - Prescriber communication
Robbery/Theft	Suspicious behavior Demand for drugs/money Visible	Comply with demands Avoid confrontation Note details for police	Incident report Police report DEA notification (if

Crisis Type	Warning Signs	Immediate Response	Post-Crisis Actions
	weapons Threatening notes/language	Activate silent alarm if safe	controlled) Inventory assessment Security review Staff counseling
Active Shooter	Unusual noises Visible weapons Panic from others Direct threats	Run: Escape if possible Hide: If escape impossible Fight: Last resort Call 911 when safe	Police cooperation Incident documentation Staff counseling Operational assessment Security enhancements
Natural Disaster/Weather Emergency	Weather alerts Power fluctuations Structural concerns Community warnings	Follow emergency protocol Secure medications Evacuate if necessary Protect refrigerated items	Damage assessment Emergency operations plan Inventory verification Patient medication needs Insurance claims
Power Outage	Flickering lights Equipment failures Weather warnings Utility notifications	Secure refrigerated items Backup computer systems Emergency lighting Assess duration	Temperature log review Integrity assessment System recovery Supply replacement Process documentation

Crisis Type	Warning Signs	Immediate Response	Post-Crisis Actions
Computer System Failure	Error messages Slow processing System crashes Network issues	Switch to manual procedures Document all transactions Contact IT support Notify patients of delays	System validation Data reconciliation Backlog processing Process improvement Staff training
Hazardous Material Spill	Visible spill Chemical odor Container damage Exposure symptoms	Evacuate immediate area Contain if trained/equipped Follow SDS guidance Call for assistance if needed	Incident documentation Waste disposal Exposure monitoring Process review Retraining if needed
Disruptive/Aggressive Customer	Raised voice Threatening language Physical agitation Refusal to leave	Maintain safe distance De-escalation techniques Involve management Call security/police if needed	Incident documentation Patient account notes Security review Staff debriefing Customer follow-up if appropriate
Mass Casualty Incident (External)	Emergency notifications Surge of patients Medical supply	Triage pharmacy resources Prepare critical supplies	Supply assessment Documentation review Process evaluation

Crisis Type	Warning Signs	Immediate Response	Post-Crisis Actions
	requests First responder presence	Contact authorities for guidance Prepare staff for surge	Community support Resupply planning
Impaired Healthcare Worker	Medication discrepancies Behavioral changes Performance issues Patient complaints	Private discussion Remove from patient care Document observations Follow reporting requirements	Formal reporting Investigation Treatment referral Return to work planning Monitoring program

Crisis Communication Strategies

Crisis communication facilitates effective information exchange during emergencies, supporting coordinated response while maintaining stakeholder trust. Internal communication systems ensure reliable information flow among staff despite potential infrastructure disruptions. Redundant communication pathways might include standard telecommunications, mobile messaging platforms, radio systems, and designated physical meeting points with established check-in procedures. Clear activation protocols specify triggering criteria, notification sequences, and verification methods confirming message receipt and understanding. External communication addresses multiple stakeholder groups with tailored approaches. Patient communication during crises provides guidance regarding medication access, modified services, alternative resources, and safety information through appropriate channels considering potential technology limitations during emergencies. Healthcare partner communication maintains coordination with physicians, hospitals, other pharmacies, and emergency services through established channels and contact lists regularly updated to reflect personnel changes. Public communication addresses broader community information needs through media relationships, social media platforms, and coordination with public health messaging to ensure consistency. Communication content during crises follows established principles: maintaining transparency while avoiding speculation beyond confirmed facts; acknowledging uncertainty when present while providing clear guidance on known information; balancing comprehensive information against the need for simplicity and actionability; and addressing both immediate concerns and forward-looking guidance supporting informed decision-making. Special communication considerations include addressing language barriers through translated materials or interpreter services; ensuring accessibility for individuals with disabilities through appropriate format alternatives; and recognizing information processing challenges during high-stress situations, necessitating clear, concise messaging with important points repeated through multiple channels. Rumor management strategies proactively monitor information channels for misinformation, establish the pharmacy as a trusted information source through consistent, accurate communication, and develop rapid response capabilities addressing emerging concerns before misinformation becomes entrenched.

Response Coordination and Decision-Making

Response coordination transforms crisis plans into effective action through structured decision-making, resource deployment, and adaptability to evolving situations. Incident command systems provide organizational frameworks scaling from small-scale emergencies to major disasters, establishing clear authority lines, communication channels, and functional responsibilities. Basic incident command components include command (overall direction and public information management); operations (direct response activities); planning (situation assessment and response strategy development); logistics (resource acquisition and deployment); and finance/administration (tracking costs and regulatory compliance). Situation assessment establishes response priorities through systematic information gathering regarding the nature and scope of the emergency; current and projected impacts on pharmacy operations; affected populations and their immediate needs; available resources; and external response activities potentially affecting pharmacy functions. Decision-making frameworks balance urgency against information quality, recognizing that crisis decisions often occur with incomplete information under significant time pressure. Tiered approaches address this tension by making immediate decisions on life-safety issues while gathering additional information for complex operational questions. Resource allocation during crises follows ethical frameworks balancing utilitarian approaches (greatest good for greatest number) against commitments to vulnerable populations with limited alternatives. Medication allocation during shortages might employ crisis standards considering patient acuity, likelihood of benefit, availability of therapeutic alternatives, and conservation strategies extending limited supplies. Collaborative response leverages relationships with other healthcare providers, emergency management agencies, and community organizations to address needs exceeding individual pharmacy capabilities. Mutual aid agreements with other pharmacies establish frameworks for resource sharing, patient redistribution, and staff support during localized emergencies affecting specific facilities. Documentation during crisis response captures key decisions, actions taken, resources deployed, and outcomes observed, supporting both ongoing management and post-event analysis while fulfilling regulatory and legal requirements regarding emergency operations.

Recovery and Post-Crisis Assessment

Recovery transforms crisis response into restored operations while incorporating lessons learned into enhanced future preparedness. Recovery planning ideally begins during the response phase, with dedicated personnel developing strategies for service restoration, resource replenishment, staff support, and transition management. Phased recovery approaches identify immediate priorities for service restoration based on patient needs and operational dependencies, establishing realistic timeframes and resource requirements for each recovery stage. Infrastructure and supply chain restoration addresses physical facilities, technology systems, inventory replacement, and documentation recovery, with temporary alternatives maintaining essential services during extended recovery periods. Pharmaceutical inventory recovery requires systematic approaches addressing medication shortages, storage condition excursions potentially affecting stability, documentation gaps complicating controlled substance reconciliation, and prioritization strategies during gradual supply chain normalization. Staff support recognizes both physical and psychological impacts of crisis events, with programs addressing acute stress reactions, long-term mental health effects, and potential burnout from prolonged emergency operations. Specific interventions might include modified scheduling during recovery phases, access to mental health resources, team debriefing sessions, and recognition of exceptional contributions during the crisis. Post-crisis assessment employs structured approaches including after-action reviews examining all response aspects from initial detection through recovery operations. Effective reviews establish psychologically safe environments encouraging honest evaluation, focus on systems rather than individual blame, examine both successes and failures, and translate findings into concrete improvement actions. Corrective action planning transforms assessment findings into specific improvements with assigned responsibility, resource allocation, implementation timeframes, and verification methods ensuring completion. Plan revision incorporates lessons learned into updated emergency protocols, addressing identified gaps through modified procedures, additional resources, enhanced training, or improved coordination mechanisms. External reporting shares relevant findings with regulatory agencies, professional organizations, and healthcare partners, contributing to collective knowledge advancing broader emergency preparedness while fulfilling reporting obligations for certain emergency types.

Summary

Emergency care within pharmacy practice involves rapid response to acute medical situations through medication expertise, procedural knowledge, and coordination with healthcare teams. Emergency medications require strategic selection, appropriate stocking, and regular verification of frequently used agents including epinephrine for anaphylaxis, naloxone for opioid overdose, dextrose for hypoglycemia, and benzodiazepines for status epilepticus. These medications necessitate specialized packaging ensuring quick identification, rapid administration access, and clear dosing information particularly during high-stress situations. First aid capabilities within pharmacy settings address common scenarios including cardiac events requiring CPR and AED use, allergic reactions requiring epinephrine administration, diabetic emergencies necessitating glucose provision, minor trauma requiring wound assessment and care, and respiratory distress requiring positioning and potential bronchodilator administration. Toxicology principles guide management of poisoning and overdose situations through understanding toxic mechanisms, recognition of toxidromes with characteristic symptom clusters, and implementation of appropriate interventions. Common toxicology scenarios encountered in pharmacy settings include acetaminophen overdose requiring N-acetylcysteine, opioid toxicity necessitating naloxone, and various medication overdoses requiring activated charcoal or specific antidotes. Crisis management extends beyond individual patient emergencies to encompass broader situations including natural disasters, public health emergencies, and mass casualty incidents requiring medication supply coordination, triage systems implementation, and continuity of care planning. Pharmacists contribute significantly during these events through maintaining emergency medication supplies, providing accurate medication information, assisting with alternative therapy recommendations during shortages, and participating in interdisciplinary emergency response teams. Effective emergency response requires regular training, clear communication protocols, appropriate documentation systems, and coordinated follow-up procedures ensuring continuous care transition after initial stabilization.

Multiple Choice Questions

1. Which of the following is the first-line medication for anaphylaxis?
   a) Diphenhydramine
   b) Epinephrine
   c) Methylprednisolone
   d) Albuterol
2. A patient presents to the pharmacy with symptoms of an acute myocardial infarction. After activating emergency services, which of the following medications would be most appropriate to administer if available?
   a) Nitroglycerin
   b) Aspirin
   c) Metoprolol
   d) Morphine
3. A patient experiencing hypoglycemia who is conscious and able to swallow should be given:
   a) Intravenous dextrose 50%
   b) Intramuscular glucagon
   c) 15-20 grams of oral glucose
   d) Subcutaneous regular insulin
4. Which of the following naloxone formulations is designed for administration by laypersons without specific training?
   a) Injectable solution requiring needle assembly
   b) Prefilled syringe for intravenous administration
   c) Nasal spray device
   d) Solution requiring dose calculation based on weight
5. Which of the following toxidromes is characterized by miosis, respiratory depression, bradycardia, and decreased bowel sounds?
   a) Anticholinergic
   b) Cholinergic
   c) Opioid
   d) Sympathomimetic
6. A patient has ingested approximately 30 tablets of acetaminophen 500 mg two hours ago in a suicide attempt. Which of the following is the antidote for acetaminophen toxicity?
   a) Flumazenil

b) Naloxone
c) N-acetylcysteine
d) Activated charcoal

7. Which of the following best describes the role of poison control centers in managing overdose cases?
a) They dispatch emergency medical services to the scene
b) They provide expert toxicology consultation to healthcare providers and the public
c) They stock and distribute antidotes to local hospitals
d) They are responsible for reporting overdoses to law enforcement

8. In a choking adult who becomes unconscious, the appropriate next step is to:
a) Perform a finger sweep to remove the obstruction
b) Position the patient and begin CPR, starting with chest compressions
c) Administer abdominal thrusts while the patient is lying down
d) Place the patient in the recovery position and monitor breathing

9. During a natural disaster, which of the following represents the most appropriate approach to maintaining medication access for chronic disease patients?
a) Limiting all prescription dispensing to 3-day supplies
b) Requiring new prescriptions for all medications regardless of refill status
c) Using professional judgment to provide emergency supplies of maintenance medications
d) Referring all patients to emergency departments for medication needs

10. A patient presents with suspected calcium channel blocker overdose. Which of the following would be the most appropriate antidotal therapy?
a) Calcium gluconate
b) Sodium bicarbonate
c) Flumazenil
d) Protamine sulfate

Self-Assessment Questions

1. Explain how medication selection should be based on likely emergencies, staff training, and community resources.
2. Design an anaphylaxis response protocol for a community pharmacy, including medication selection, dosing guidelines, administration techniques, monitoring parameters, and coordination with emergency medical services.
3. Compare and contrast the presentation and emergency management of hypoglycemia versus hyperglycemic crisis, explaining how pharmacists can recognize each condition
4. Evaluate the appropriate selection and administration of naloxone formulations for opioid overdose reversal in different practice settings, explaining considerations for dose, onset, duration, and patient monitoring.
5. Explain the appropriate use of emergency medications, monitoring procedures, and coordination with emergency medical services.
6. Explain the characteristic signs and symptoms that guide recognition and initial management.
7. Evaluate the appropriate management of acetaminophen overdose, explaining the role of N-acetylcysteine, the significance of the Rumack-Matthew nomogram in treatment decisions, and the clinical monitoring required during therapy.
8. Design a toxicology management protocol for poisoning or overdose presentations in a pharmacy setting, including initial assessment, stabilization measures, coordination with poison control centers, and documentation requirements.
9. Analyze the pharmacy's role in public health emergency response, explaining how medication distribution systems, patient education, and coordination with public health authorities would be implemented during infectious disease outbreaks.
10. Develop a emergency preparedness plan for a pharmacy during natural disasters, explaining procedures for maintaining medication access, ensuring cold chain integrity during power outages, and addressing medication needs of displaced persons.

Bibliography

1. Callaway CW, Donnino MW, Fink EL, Geocadin RG, Golan E, Kern KB, et al. Part 8: Post-cardiac arrest care: 2015 American Heart Association guidelines update for cardiopulmonary resuscitation and emergency cardiovascular care. Circulation. 2015;132(18 Suppl 2):S465-S482.
2. Kleinman ME, Brennan EE, Goldberger ZD, Swor RA, Terry M, Bobrow BJ, et al. Part 5: Adult basic life support and cardiopulmonary resuscitation quality: 2015 American Heart Association guidelines update for cardiopulmonary resuscitation and emergency cardiovascular care. Circulation. 2015;132(18 Suppl 2):S414-S435.
3. Wyckoff MH, Aziz K, Escobedo MB, Kapadia VS, Kattwinkel J, Perlman JM, et al. Part 13: Neonatal resuscitation: 2015 American Heart Association guidelines update for cardiopulmonary resuscitation and emergency cardiovascular care. Circulation. 2015;132(18 Suppl 2):S543-S560.
4. Simons FER, Ebisawa M, Sanchez-Borges M, Thong BY, Worm M, Tanno LK, et al. 2015 update of the evidence base: World Allergy Organization anaphylaxis guidelines. World Allergy Organ J. 2015;8(1):32.
5. Powers WJ, Rabinstein AA, Ackerson T, Adeoye OM, Bambakidis NC, Becker K, et al. Guidelines for the early management of patients with acute ischemic stroke: 2019 update to the 2018 guidelines for the early management of acute ischemic stroke: A guideline for healthcare professionals from the American Heart Association/American Stroke Association. Stroke. 2019;50(12):e344-e418.
6. American College of Emergency Physicians; Clinical policy: Use of intravenous tPA for the management of acute ischemic stroke in the emergency department. Ann Emerg Med. 2015;66(3):322-333.e31.
7. Goldfrank LR, Hoffman RS, Howland MA, Lewin NA, Nelson LS, editors. Goldfrank's toxicologic emergencies. 11th ed. New York: McGraw-Hill Education; 2019.
8. Hoffman RS, Howland MA, Lewin NA, Nelson LS, Goldfrank LR. Goldfrank's toxicologic emergencies. 10th ed. New York: McGraw-Hill Education; 2015.
9. Nelson LS, Lewin NA, Howland MA, Hoffman RS, Goldfrank LR, Flomenbaum NE. Goldfrank's toxicologic emergencies. 9th ed. New York: McGraw-Hill; 2011.
10. Dart RC, Borron SW, Caravati EM, Cobaugh DJ, Curry SC, Falk JL, et al. Expert consensus guidelines for stocking of antidotes in hospitals that provide emergency care. Ann Emerg Med. 2009;54(3):386-394.e1.

CHAPTER 13

PHARMACY MANAGEMENT

Author

Dr. Syed Ansar Ahmed, Associate Professor, Department of Pharmaceutical Chemistry, Indira College of Pharmacy, VishnuPuri, Nanded, Maharashtra, India

Abstract

Pharmacy management combines business operations with clinical services to ensure organizational effectiveness while maintaining patient care quality. Inventory control balances medication availability against financial constraints through systematic approaches including ABC classification prioritizing high-value items, economic order quantity calculations optimizing purchase volumes, perpetual inventory systems tracking real-time stock levels, and vendor management strategies negotiating favorable terms while preventing stockouts of critical medications. Quality management systems establish frameworks for continuous improvement through defined quality metrics, regular performance evaluation, deviation management protocols, and implementation of corrective and preventive actions (CAPA), with structures including Plan-Do-Check-Act cycles and Lean Six Sigma methodologies minimizing error rates while enhancing operational efficiency. Staff training and development builds competent pharmacy teams through structured orientation programs, ongoing competency assessment, performance evaluation systems, career advancement pathways, and succession planning, with educational approaches spanning traditional instruction, simulation exercises, preceptor development, and interprofessional training opportunities that align with organizational goals and regulatory requirements. Financial management ensures pharmacy viability through revenue cycle optimization, third-party contract analysis, expense control measures, budget development processes, and financial performance monitoring using key metrics including prescription volume, gross margin, inventory turnover, labor costs, and various productivity indicators that guide resource allocation decisions

Keywords: *Operational Efficiency; Resource Optimization; Performance Improvement; Workforce Development; Fiscal Responsibility*

Learning Objectives

After completion of the chapter, the learners should be able to:

- Implement inventory management systems that optimize stock levels while minimizing carrying costs and preventing stockouts.
- Develop quality management programs incorporating continuous quality improvement methodologies and regulatory compliance standards.
- Design comprehensive staff training programs addressing technical skills, clinical knowledge, and professional development needs.
- Analyze pharmacy financial performance using key metrics including prescription volume, gross margin, inventory turnover, and labor cost percentages.
- Create strategic plans for pharmacy operations that align with organizational goals, market trends, and evolving healthcare models.
- Apply principles of effective leadership and conflict resolution to manage pharmacy teams in various practice settings.

INVENTORY CONTROL

Inventory management represents a critical function in pharmacy operations, directly influencing financial performance, medication availability, and ultimately patient care. Effective inventory control balances minimizing carrying costs against ensuring medication accessibility, requiring systematic approaches to purchasing, storage, monitoring, and optimization. Well-designed inventory systems support both routine operations and contingency planning while adapting to evolving healthcare delivery models and pharmaceutical market dynamics.

Inventory Management Systems

Inventory management systems provide structured frameworks for medication procurement, tracking, and optimization based on demand patterns and operational requirements. Perpetual inventory systems maintain continuous records of stock levels through real-time transaction recording, offering precise inventory visibility but requiring consistent documentation discipline and technological infrastructure. Periodic inventory systems review stock levels at scheduled intervals through physical counts, requiring less day-to-day maintenance but providing less current information for decision-making. Hybrid approaches combine elements of both systems, typically maintaining perpetual records for high-value, critical, or controlled medications while employing periodic reviews for other inventory categories. Technology integration significantly enhances inventory management capabilities through various implementations. Pharmacy management systems incorporate inventory modules tracking purchases, dispensing transactions, and adjustments while generating replenishment recommendations based on usage patterns and defined parameters. Automated dispensing cabinets in institutional settings provide secured medication storage with integrated tracking, automatically documenting medication removal and generating restocking requests when par levels are approached. Barcode scanning systems reduce manual data entry errors while accelerating transaction processing through automated identification of products during receiving, dispensing, and inventory counting processes.

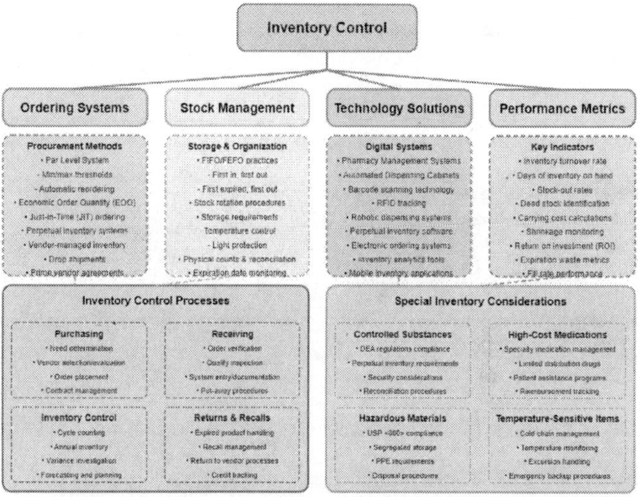

Figure 13.1: Inventory Control Systems and Methods

Radio-frequency identification (RFID) technology offers potential advantages through non-line-of-sight reading capabilities and simultaneous multiple item identification, though implementation costs and standardization challenges have limited widespread adoption. Classification strategies organize inventory into categories supporting tailored management approaches. ABC analysis categorizes items based on value and usage, with "A" items (high value/usage) receiving most intensive management; "B" items (moderate value/usage) warranting regular attention; and "C" items (low value/usage) managed through simplified approaches, optimizing resource allocation across the inventory spectrum.

Table 13.1: Inventory Management Systems and Methods

System/Method	Advantages	Disadvantages
Perpetual Inventory	Accurate stock levels Automated purchasing Reduced stockouts Detailed tracking	Higher implementation cost Requires strict procedures Technology dependent Needs regular auditing
Periodic Inventory	Lower technology requirements Simpler implementation Thorough verification Less daily maintenance	Labor intensive Less accurate between counts Increased stockout risk Delayed problem identification
ABC Analysis	Focused management Optimized control efforts Efficient resource allocation Prioritized attention	Requires regular reassessment May overlook critical low-cost items Complexity in categorization Potential service inconsistency
Just-in-Time (JIT)	Reduced carrying costs Less storage space needed Lower expired product waste Improved cash flow	Vulnerable to supply disruptions Requires reliable suppliers Limited buffer for demand spikes Higher ordering costs
Par Level System	Simple to implement Clear visual indicators Adaptable to seasonality Easy staff training	Manual monitoring required Par level optimization challenges Space allocation issues Less responsive to trends
Economic Order Quantity (EOQ)	Cost optimization Systematic approach	Assumes constant demand Requires accurate cost

System/Method	Advantages	Disadvantages
	Reduced total costs Objective decision-making	data May conflict with vendor minimums Simplifies complex variables
Vendor-Managed Inventory (VMI)	Reduced management burden Supplier expertise leverage Lower emergency orders Improved supplier relationship	Dependence on vendor Less direct control System integration challenges Potential conflicts of interest
Consignment Inventory	Improved cash flow Reduced financial risk Access to expensive items Expanded product offerings	Complex accounting Physical space commitment Supplier relationship dependency Potential contractual complexity
RFID/Barcode Systems	Improved accuracy Reduced manual entry Enhanced tracking Automated data collection	Implementation costs Technical infrastructure needed Staff training requirements System maintenance
Automated Dispensing Cabinets	Controlled access Real-time tracking Reduced diversion risk Improved charge capture	High capital investment Ongoing maintenance costs Space requirements Technical support needs
Min-Max System	Simple implementation Easy to understand Customizable by item Visual management potential	Manual monitoring Level optimization challenges Regular review needed Labor intensive

System/Method	Advantages	Disadvantages
Multi-Echelon Inventory	Reduced total inventory Balanced availability Resource optimization Improved system resilience	Complex coordination Advanced analytics needed Transportation considerations Organizational alignment challenges

Purchasing and Supplier Management

Purchasing functions significantly influence both inventory performance and financial outcomes through strategic approaches to procurement processes. Order point systems initiate purchases when inventory reaches predetermined levels calculated based on usage rates, lead times, safety stock requirements, and economic order quantities. These systems operate independently for each product, triggering replenishment when specific thresholds are crossed without regard to ordering schedules. Periodic ordering systems consolidate purchasing activities into scheduled review cycles, evaluating all inventory categories simultaneously and generating consolidated orders, potentially sacrificing precise timing for operational efficiency and order consolidation benefits. Hybrid models apply different approaches to various product categories based on criticality, value, and usage patterns. Economic order quantity (EOQ) models optimize order sizes by balancing inventory carrying costs against ordering costs, calculating theoretical optimal purchase quantities through formulas incorporating annual usage, ordering costs, and inventory holding cost percentages. While mathematical elegance appeals, practical application requires adjustment for supplier minimum orders, package sizes, quantity discounts, and space constraints. Strategic supplier relationships extend beyond transactional purchasing to collaborative partnerships offering mutual benefits. Primary wholesaler agreements typically provide favorable pricing, extended payment terms, ordering system integration, and inventory management tools in exchange for volume commitments and preferred vendor status. Contract compliance management ensures purchases align with established agreements to maintain negotiated pricing and meet commitment levels while monitoring compliance percentages as key performance indicators. Secondary wholesaler relationships provide alternatives for stock shortages, discontinued items, or advantageous pricing opportunities outside primary contracts. Direct manufacturer purchasing may offer cost advantages for high-volume products, though administrative burden and minimum order requirements must be evaluated against potential savings. Group purchasing organizations (GPOs) aggregate purchasing volume across multiple facilities, leveraging collective bargaining power to negotiate favorable pricing and contract terms while reducing administrative burden through standardized contracting processes.

Medication Storage and Handling

Medication storage and handling practices ensure product integrity, regulatory compliance, and operational efficiency through systematic approaches to physical inventory management. Space allocation balances accessibility against security considerations, with high-use medications positioned for efficient workflow; controlled substances secured according to regulatory requirements; and hazardous drugs segregated with appropriate containment strategies. Organization systems typically employ alphabetical arrangements within therapeutic categories, supporting both efficiency and error reduction through logical grouping. Storage condition requirements vary across pharmaceutical categories, necessitating monitored environments for products with specific temperature, humidity, or light sensitivity parameters. Refrigeration systems for cold chain products require continuous temperature monitoring, emergency power provisions, and alert systems detecting excursions beyond acceptable ranges. Temperature mapping studies verify uniform conditions throughout storage areas, identifying potential problem zones requiring mitigation. Controlled substance security employs multiple safeguards including limited access authorization, perpetual inventory maintenance, regular reconciliation procedures, and documentation of all transactions throughout the medication lifecycle. Physical security measures include secured storage areas with tamper-evident access monitoring, surveillance systems, and segregated storage within primary drug inventory areas. Hazardous drug handling follows USP <800> standards with designated storage areas preventing contamination spread, appropriate engineering controls, personal protective equipment requirements, and specific labeling identifying products requiring special handling. Medication dating management prevents dispensing of expired products through systematic approaches including color-coded labeling identifying expiration quarters; segregated storage for short-dated products; regular expiration reviews; and first-expired-first-out (FEFO) rotation practices ensuring oldest stock receives priority use. Beyond-use dating for repackaged or compounded preparations requires documentation systems tracking both manufacturer expiration dates and preparation-specific stability limitations. Receiving processes verify incoming shipments against purchase orders, inspect for damage or tampering, confirm appropriate storage during transit for temperature-sensitive items, and promptly update inventory records reflecting received quantities.

Inventory Optimization Strategies

Inventory optimization balances service levels against financial considerations through systematic evaluation and refinement of stock levels, purchasing patterns, and usage trends. Key performance indicators provide objective measurement of inventory system effectiveness, including inventory turnover rate (annual cost of goods sold divided by average inventory value); days on hand (average inventory value divided by daily usage cost); service level percentages (proportion of demand fulfilled without delay); and obsolescence rates (expired or unusable inventory as percentage of total stock). Target ranges for these metrics vary based on pharmacy type, accessibility to suppliers, and criticality of medication categories, with critical medications warranting higher service levels despite potential efficiency reductions. Demand forecasting techniques project future medication requirements through various methodologies including historical usage analysis, seasonality pattern identification, therapeutic trend evaluation, and anticipated changes in prescribing patterns or patient populations. Quantitative approaches employ statistical methods analyzing historical dispensing data, while qualitative approaches incorporate clinician input regarding anticipated practice changes, new treatment guidelines, or emerging therapeutic alternatives. Stock level optimization establishes appropriate inventory quantities through systematic parameter setting. Minimum stock levels represent safety thresholds triggering replenishment activities, calculated based on usage variability, supplier reliability, and criticality factors. Maximum stock levels establish upper inventory boundaries preventing overstocking while accommodating usage patterns, physical space constraints, and financial limitations. Lead time management addresses the interval between order placement and receipt, with strategies including supplier performance tracking, advance ordering for predictable demand increases, and alternative sourcing for critical items with extended lead times. Shortage management strategies address both routine stockouts and more significant drug shortage situations through systematic approaches. Alternative sourcing pathways identify secondary suppliers, different package sizes, or therapeutic alternatives when primary products become unavailable. Allocation systems ensure equitable distribution of limited supplies during significant shortages based on patient need, therapeutic alternatives, and conservation opportunities. Therapeutic interchange protocols developed collaboratively with prescribers establish pre-approved substitution pathways when preferred medications become unavailable, streamlining response to shortage situations.

QUALITY MANAGEMENT SYSTEMS

Quality management systems provide structured frameworks ensuring consistent delivery of pharmaceutical services meeting professional standards, regulatory requirements, and patient expectations. These systems integrate quality principles throughout organizational processes rather than treating quality as a separate function, embedding continuous improvement methodologies into routine operations. Effective quality management balances compliance-focused documentation against practical improvement initiatives addressing meaningful outcome measures rather than simply generating paperwork.

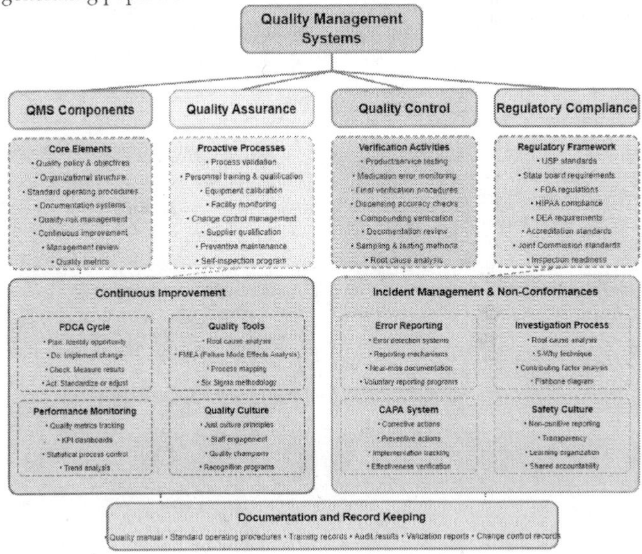

Figure 13.2: Quality Management Systems in Pharmacy

Quality System

Quality system fundamentals establish the philosophical and structural foundation supporting systematic quality management in pharmacy practice. Quality philosophies include several complementary approaches influencing pharmaceutical quality systems. Total Quality Management emphasizes organization-wide commitment to quality with customer focus, continuous improvement, and employee engagement as central tenets. Lean methodology focuses on eliminating waste in all forms—including unnecessary steps, waiting time, excess inventory, and defects requiring rework—while optimizing processes creating value from the customer perspective. Six Sigma employs data-driven approaches to reduce process variation, targeting 3.4 defects per million opportunities through systematic problem-solving methodologies. These philosophies inform practical quality structures with varying emphasis depending on organizational culture and specific quality challenges. Structural components supporting quality management include clearly defined leadership responsibility for quality outcomes; documented policies and procedures establishing standardized processes; training programs ensuring staff competency; monitoring systems identifying deviations from established standards; improvement mechanisms addressing identified gaps; and documentation frameworks demonstrating both compliance and improvement activities. Quality culture development represents perhaps the most challenging yet important aspect of effective quality systems, requiring leadership modeling of quality values; recognition systems rewarding quality contributions; transparent communication regarding quality metrics; and psychological safety allowing open discussion of problems without inappropriate blame. Regulatory frameworks influencing pharmacy quality systems include state board of pharmacy regulations establishing minimum practice standards; accreditation requirements from organizations including The Joint Commission, ACHC, and URAC; federal regulations from agencies including FDA, DEA, and CMS; and professional standards from organizations such as ASHP, APhA, and PCAB. These external requirements establish compliance baselines, while robust internal quality systems typically exceed minimum standards to achieve organizational quality objectives.

Table 13.2: Inventory Control Metrics

Metric	Formula/Calculation	Target Range
Inventory Turnover Ratio	COGS ÷ Average Inventory Value	10-15 for pharmacies Higher for fast-moving items Lower for specialty items
Days of Inventory on Hand	(Average Inventory ÷ COGS) × 365	24-36 days overall 14-21 days for A items 30-45 days for B items 45-60 days for C items
Gross Margin Return on Investment (GMROI)	Gross Profit ÷ Average Inventory Value	>3.0 (excellent) 2.0-3.0 (good) <2.0 (needs improvement)
Stockout Rate	Number of Stockouts ÷ Total Line Items × 100	<1% for critical medications <3% for essential medications <5% overall
Fill Rate	Orders Filled Completely ÷ Total Orders × 100	>98% for prescriptions >95% for other products
Shrinkage Percentage	(Expected Inventory – Actual Inventory) ÷ Expected Inventory × 100	<1% overall <0.5% for controlled substances
Carrying Cost Percentage	Annual Inventory Carrying Costs ÷ Average Inventory Value × 100	15-25% of inventory value
Order Accuracy	Correct Orders ÷ Total Orders × 100	>98% accuracy
Dead Stock Percentage	Value of Non-moving Inventory ÷ Total Inventory Value × 100	<5% of total inventory

Metric	Formula/Calculation	Target Range
Order Cycle Time	Average Days from Order to Receipt	<2 days for routine orders <1 day for critical items
Return on Investment (ROI)	(Net Profit from Inventory ÷ Inventory Investment) × 100	>20% for most pharmacies
Inventory Accuracy	Items with Correct Counts ÷ Total Items Counted × 100	>95% overall >99% for controlled substances

Quality Assurance and Performance Improvement

Quality assurance and performance improvement represent complementary approaches within comprehensive quality management systems. Quality assurance employs preventive strategies ensuring processes consistently meet established standards, while performance improvement focuses on enhancing outcomes beyond current standards through systematic evaluation and refinement. Process standardization creates consistency through detailed procedures specifying critical process steps, acceptable performance parameters, required documentation, and responsibility assignments. Standardized approaches reduce unnecessary variation while accommodating appropriate clinical judgment in patient-specific situations. Standard operating procedures (SOPs) document approved methodologies for routine functions, providing both guidance for current staff and training references for new personnel. Effective SOPs balance sufficient detail for consistent execution against usability concerns, with excessive complexity potentially reducing compliance. Regular review cycles ensure ongoing relevance as practices evolve. Quality metrics provide objective measurement of process performance and outcomes, with selection reflecting organizational priorities, external requirements, and improvement opportunities. Structure metrics assess system capabilities including staffing levels, training completion, and equipment certification. Process metrics evaluate adherence to established procedures such as medication reconciliation completion, required counseling provision, and dispensing accuracy checks. Outcome metrics measure actual results including adverse drug events, hospital readmissions related to medication issues, and patient-reported medication experiences. Balanced scorecard approaches incorporate multiple metric types ensuring comprehensive quality evaluation rather than narrow focus on easily measured parameters. Performance improvement methodologies provide structured approaches to enhancing outcomes through various frameworks. The Plan-Do-Study-Act (PDSA) cycle represents a fundamental improvement model with sequential phases: planning specific interventions with clear objectives; implementing changes on appropriate scale; studying results through data collection and analysis; and acting on findings through standardization of successful interventions or modification of unsuccessful approaches. Root cause analysis investigates significant events or persistent problems through systematic examination of contributing factors, moving beyond superficial explanations to identify fundamental system vulnerabilities. Failure Mode and Effects Analysis (FMEA) proactively evaluates processes for potential failure points before adverse outcomes occur, prioritizing improvement efforts based on severity, probability, and detectability of potential failures.

Table 13.3: Quality Management Systems in Pharmacy

QMS Component	Elements	Implementation Methods
Quality Policy and Objectives	Organizational commitment Specific quality goals Quality metrics Stakeholder focus	Leadership development Staff engagement Clear communication Strategic alignment
Documentation System	SOPs Quality manual Forms and records Policy documents	Document control software Standardized templates Accessibility planning Version control
Risk Management	Risk assessment Mitigation strategies Monitoring systems Contingency planning	FMEA Risk registers Prioritization matrices Regular risk reviews
Personnel Management	Roles and responsibilities Competency requirements Training programs Performance evaluation	Job descriptions Training matrices Competency assessments Performance reviews

QMS Component	Elements	Implementation Methods
Process Management	Process mapping Critical control points Process measures Standardization	Process flow diagrams SIPOC analysis Standard work development Visual management
Customer/Patient Focus	Feedback mechanisms Satisfaction measurement Complaint management Service recovery	Satisfaction surveys Focus groups Comment cards Social media monitoring
Supplier/Vendor Management	Qualification process Performance monitoring Quality agreements Collaborative improvement	Vendor assessment tools Performance scorecards Regular reviews Quality agreements
Corrective and Preventive Action (CAPA)	Issue identification Root cause analysis Action implementation Effectiveness verification	CAPA tracking system Investigation protocols Action planning tools Follow-up procedures
Quality Audits	Internal audit program External audit readiness Audit schedule Findings management	Trained auditors Audit checklists Scheduling system Finding tracking
Management Review	Performance data review Resource allocation Strategic	Regular review meetings Data compilation tools Action tracking

QMS Component	Elements	Implementation Methods
	adjustments Improvement planning	Strategic planning integration
Quality Metrics and KPIs	Safety metrics Efficiency metrics Compliance metrics Financial quality impact	Balanced scorecard approach Dashboard development Automated data collection Regular reporting
Continuous Improvement Systems	Improvement methodology Staff involvement Idea generation Implementation process	PDSA cycles Kaizen events Suggestion systems Improvement teams

Record Management

Record management systems provide evidence of quality system functioning while supporting operational consistency, regulatory compliance, and continuous improvement initiatives. Policy and procedure management establishes governance structures controlling document creation, review, approval, distribution, and revision. Effective systems include standardized formats ensuring consistent structure; approval workflows documenting appropriate review; version control preventing use of outdated documents; accessibility features ensuring staff access to current versions; and regular review cycles maintaining relevance as practices evolve. Electronic document management systems enhance these functions through automated workflows, revision tracking, and integration with training management platforms. Quality event documentation captures deviations from expected processes or outcomes through structured reporting systems. Near-miss documentation records potential errors detected before reaching patients, providing valuable learning opportunities without patient harm. Error reporting systems document actual medication errors reaching patients, capturing event details, contributing factors, and immediate actions taken. Adverse event monitoring tracks unexpected negative outcomes potentially related to medication therapy, distinguishing between preventable and non-preventable events while identifying improvement opportunities. These documentation systems require cultivation of just culture approaches balancing appropriate accountability for individual choices against recognition of system contributions to errors, avoiding blame-focused responses that discourage reporting. Record retention systems maintain documentation for appropriate timeframes based on regulatory requirements, operational needs, and risk management considerations. Retention schedules specify minimum maintenance periods for various document categories, typically ranging from 2-10 years depending on record type and applicable regulations. Storage systems balance accessibility for current operations against security and space considerations, with transition from active to archived status following defined timeframes. Destruction protocols ensure confidential information receives appropriate handling when retention periods expire. Electronic health record systems increasingly incorporate quality documentation functions through structured templates, automated data extraction for quality monitoring, clinical decision support preventing potential errors, and integrated reporting capabilities supporting improvement initiatives.

Quality Audits and External Requirements

Quality audits and external requirements provide structured evaluation of quality system effectiveness while ensuring compliance with regulatory standards. Internal audit programs systematically evaluate compliance with organizational policies, procedures, and quality standards through scheduled reviews conducted by staff independent from audited functions. Comprehensive programs include audits of physical facilities examining equipment maintenance, proper storage conditions, and security provisions; process audits evaluating adherence to established procedures for medication dispensing, compounding, and clinical services; and documentation audits reviewing completeness and accuracy of required records. Audit findings generate corrective action plans addressing identified deficiencies, with follow-up verification ensuring effective implementation. External audits conducted by regulatory agencies, accreditation organizations, or payer representatives evaluate compliance with requirements specific to each entity's jurisdiction. Preparation for external audits includes mock audit exercises identifying potential vulnerabilities; documentation organization ensuring easy retrieval during inspections; staff preparation through education regarding inspector expectations and appropriate interaction approaches; and corrective action implementation addressing previously identified deficiencies. Regulatory compliance requirements establish minimum standards for pharmacy operations through various authorities. State boards of pharmacy enforce pharmacy practice acts through inspections, complaint investigations, and disciplinary proceedings when violations occur. Federal agencies including the Drug

Enforcement Administration oversee controlled substance handling; the Food and Drug Administration regulates manufacturing and compounding activities; and the Centers for Medicare and Medicaid Services establish quality requirements for pharmacies serving Medicare/Medicaid beneficiaries. Accreditation programs provide external validation of quality through voluntary participation in evaluation against established standards. Organizations including The Joint Commission, Accreditation Commission for Health Care, URAC, and the Pharmacy Compounding Accreditation Board offer pharmacy-specific accreditation programs with distinct focus areas and standards. These programs typically involve comprehensive application documentation, on-site surveys evaluating actual practices, and ongoing reporting requirements maintaining accreditation status between full survey cycles. Accreditation often confers market advantages through quality differentiation while satisfying payer requirements for network participation.

STAFF TRAINING AND DEVELOPMENT

Staff training and development creates the foundation for consistent, high-quality pharmacy services through systematic approaches to knowledge transfer, skill building, and continuous professional growth. Effective training programs address both technical competencies and professional capabilities while adapting to diverse learning styles, evolving practice standards, and operational constraints. Strategic approaches to personnel development support both organizational objectives and individual career aspirations, enhancing performance while improving staff engagement and retention.

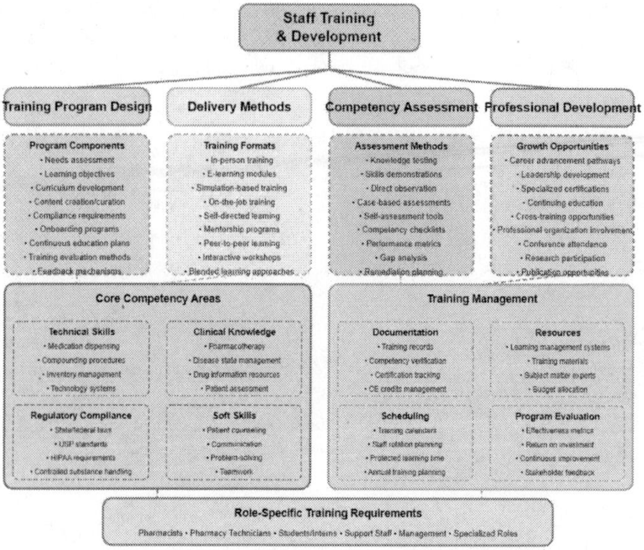

Figure 13.3: Staff Training and Development

Training Needs Assessment and Program Design

Training needs assessment identifies knowledge and skill gaps through systematic evaluation of current capabilities against required competencies. Job analysis provides the foundation by defining essential functions, required skills, and performance standards for each position within the pharmacy organization. Competency mapping extends this analysis by identifying specific knowledge areas, technical abilities, and professional behaviors necessary for successful performance, creating detailed frameworks against which individual capabilities can be assessed.

Table 13.4: Staff Training and Development

Training Component	Elements	Implementation Methods
Orientation Program	Pharmacy operations overview Safety and security procedures Regulatory requirements Company policies and culture	Structured schedule Mentor assignment Job shadowing Policy review
Technical Skills Training	Dispensing procedures Computer systems Equipment operation Inventory management	Hands-on practice Step-by-step guides Simulation exercises Competency checklists
Clinical Knowledge Development	Medication knowledge Disease state management Guidelines and protocols Evidence-based practice	Case studies Journal clubs CE programs Clinical rounds
Communication Skills	Patient counseling Team communication Conflict resolution Healthcare provider interaction	Role-playing Recorded interactions Feedback sessions Standardized patients
Leadership Development	Decision-making Team management Project leadership Strategic thinking	Mentoring programs Leadership assignments Workshop attendance Stretch projects
Regulatory Compliance	HIPAA requirements	Policy review Case-based learning

Training Component	Elements	Implementation Methods
	Controlled substance regulations State/federal pharmacy laws Accreditation standards	Online modules Compliance assessments
Patient Safety and Quality	Error prevention Adverse event reporting Quality improvement methods Risk management	Root cause analysis training Case reviews Simulation exercises Team-based improvement projects
Technology and Automation	Pharmacy management system Automation equipment Clinical decision support Emerging technologies	Hands-on training User guides Vendor-led training Super-user programs
Customer Service Excellence	Service standards Patient experience Service recovery Empathy and compassion	Role-playing Scenario-based training Customer feedback review Service excellence recognition
Professional Development Planning	Career goal setting Competency assessment Development planning Progress review	Individual development plans Regular coaching sessions Self-assessment tools Career pathing resources
Continuing Education	Required CE tracking Specialized certifications	In-house CE programs External CE support Certification

Training Component	Elements	Implementation Methods
	Advanced training Knowledge expansion	preparation Journal clubs
Cross-Training	Multiple role capabilities Backup coverage Operational flexibility Career development	Job rotation Shadowing opportunities Structured cross-training Competency verification

Gap analysis methodologies identify discrepancies between required and actual competencies through various approaches including direct observation of performance, knowledge assessments, self-evaluation tools, and performance data review. These assessments consider both individual variations and team-wide patterns requiring systematic intervention. Program design translates identified needs into structured learning experiences addressing specific competency gaps. Learning objectives establish measurable outcomes for each training component, using action verbs describing observable behaviors rather than vague terminology. Sequencing considerations determine logical progression through content, typically moving from foundational knowledge to application scenarios and culminating in integration activities combining multiple skill areas. Multimodal design incorporates diverse learning methodologies accommodating different learning preferences while reinforcing content through varied approaches. These might include didactic presentations conveying factual information; demonstrations modeling proper techniques; hands-on practice developing procedural skills; case studies applying knowledge to realistic scenarios; and simulation exercises integrating multiple competencies in controlled environments mimicking actual practice conditions. Technology integration enhances training effectiveness through various applications including learning management systems tracking completion and assessment results; video demonstrations providing consistent technique modeling; interactive e-learning modules allowing self-paced completion; and virtual reality applications creating immersive practice environments for complex procedures. Adult learning principles guide effective program design through several key concepts: establishing relevance by connecting content to immediate application; acknowledging and building upon existing knowledge and experience; incorporating practical problem-solving rather than purely theoretical content; and providing opportunities for self-direction appropriate to learner capabilities.

Evaluation of Training

Training implementation transforms designed programs into actual learning experiences through systematic delivery approaches. Orientation programs introduce new staff to organizational culture, essential policies, key personnel, physical facilities, and fundamental operating procedures. Comprehensive orientation balances immediate need-to-know information against the risk of overwhelming new employees, typically employing phased approaches addressing critical safety and operational requirements before advancing to more complex functions. Competency-based training focuses on demonstrable skills rather than simply exposure to information, requiring learners to practice and demonstrate specific abilities meeting established performance criteria. Skill verification through direct observation with structured assessment tools provides documentation of capability before independent practice. Preceptor and mentor programs leverage experienced staff in training roles through structured approaches including defined responsibilities, training-the-trainer preparation, recognition systems acknowledging contributions, and workload accommodation supporting dedicated teaching time. Effective preceptor selection considers both technical expertise and teaching ability, recognizing these represent distinct skill sets. Cross-training develops versatility through systematic exposure to functions outside primary responsibilities, enhancing operational flexibility while providing professional growth opportunities and building broader organizational understanding. Training evaluation assesses program effectiveness through multiple dimensions. Reaction measures gather participant feedback regarding training experience, typically through surveys addressing content relevance, instructor effectiveness, materials quality, and overall satisfaction. Learning assessment evaluates knowledge acquisition and skill development through testing, demonstration, or other performance measures administered before and after training. Behavior evaluation examines actual performance changes in the work environment following training completion, requiring observation of real-world application rather than controlled assessment scenarios. Results measurement connects training initiatives to organizational outcomes including error reduction, productivity improvements, regulatory compliance, patient satisfaction, or other strategic objectives. Continuous improvement of training programs utilizes evaluation data to refine content, adjust delivery methods, enhance assessment approaches, and address emerging needs through regular review cycles incorporating both formal evaluation results and informal feedback.

Continuing Professional Development

Continuing professional development extends beyond basic competency maintenance to support ongoing professional growth, practice advancement, and career progression through structured approaches to lifelong learning. Continuing education requirements establish minimum ongoing learning expectations through state board of pharmacy regulations specifying credit hours, content distributions, and reporting mechanisms necessary for license renewal. While providing fundamental knowledge updates, traditional continuing education often focuses on passive information receipt rather than active skill development or practice change. Professional certification programs provide specialized credentials demonstrating advanced knowledge and skills in specific practice areas including pharmacotherapy, ambulatory care, oncology, nuclear pharmacy, nutrition support, and various other specialties. These programs typically require combination of education, practice experience, and rigorous examination, with recertification maintaining current knowledge through continuing education or re-examination. Advanced training opportunities extend capabilities through structured programs including residencies providing intensive practical experience under preceptor guidance; fellowships focusing on research skills and specialized knowledge development; certificate programs offering focused training in specific clinical or administrative areas; and advanced degrees including Master of Science, MBA, or Doctor of Philosophy programs developing specialized expertise or leadership capabilities. Professional organization involvement provides both development opportunities and contributions to the profession through committee service, leadership roles, conference participation, and policy development activities. These experiences build professional networks, expose participants to emerging practice trends, and develop leadership capabilities extending beyond technical pharmacy knowledge. Self-directed learning approaches empower practitioners to guide their own development through structured processes. Learning portfolios document both formal and informal learning activities, reflection on practice experiences, identified development needs, and plans for addressing knowledge or skill gaps. Personal development plans establish specific learning objectives, action steps, resource requirements, timeline expectations, and evaluation methods for measuring progress. Implementation strategies include scheduling protected learning time, securing necessary resources, establishing accountability mechanisms, and creating supportive learning environments encouraging growth and experimentation.

Leadership Development and Succession Planning

Leadership development prepares pharmacy professionals for expanded responsibility through systematic approaches building capabilities beyond technical pharmacy knowledge. Leadership competency frameworks identify essential capabilities including strategic thinking translating organizational mission into actionable plans; people management skills building effective teams; communication abilities conveying information clearly while listening effectively; change management facilitating organizational transformation; financial acumen ensuring resource stewardship; and emotional intelligence navigating interpersonal dynamics effectively. Assessment methodologies identify leadership strengths and development needs through various approaches including personality inventories exploring behavioral tendencies; 360-degree feedback gathering perspectives from supervisors, peers, and direct reports; structured interviews exploring past experiences and approaches to leadership scenarios; and assessment centers evaluating performance in simulated leadership situations. Development strategies include formal leadership training through structured programs addressing specific competencies; developmental assignments providing practical experience with increasingly complex leadership challenges; mentorship relationships with experienced leaders providing guidance and feedback; coaching arrangements offering personalized development support; and self-directed learning through reading, reflection, and application of leadership principles. Succession planning ensures organizational continuity through systematic identification and development of talent for future leadership roles. Critical position identification focuses development efforts on roles with significant organizational impact, limited internal replacement options, or specialized knowledge requirements creating succession vulnerabilities. Talent assessment evaluates both current performance and future potential through structured reviews considering demonstrated capabilities, learning agility, aspiration for advancement, and alignment with organizational values. Individual development planning creates tailored growth experiences addressing specific capabilities needed for targeted future roles, with regular progress review and plan refinement. Knowledge transfer strategies prevent critical information loss during transitions through documentation of essential processes, cross-training initiatives, mentoring relationships, and phased retirement approaches allowing gradual responsibility transition with overlapping tenure periods. Integration with organizational planning aligns succession management with strategic objectives, ensuring development efforts prepare leaders for future organizational needs rather than simply replicating current leadership models.

FINANCIAL MANAGEMENT

Financial management in pharmacy practice balances patient care responsibilities against business sustainability requirements through systematic approaches to resource stewardship. Effective financial management extends beyond basic accounting functions to encompass strategic financial planning, revenue optimization, expense control, and performance analysis supporting informed decision-making. As pharmacy practice evolves toward more clinically focused and value-based models, financial management approaches must similarly adapt to capture, document, and optimize the economic value of pharmaceutical care services.

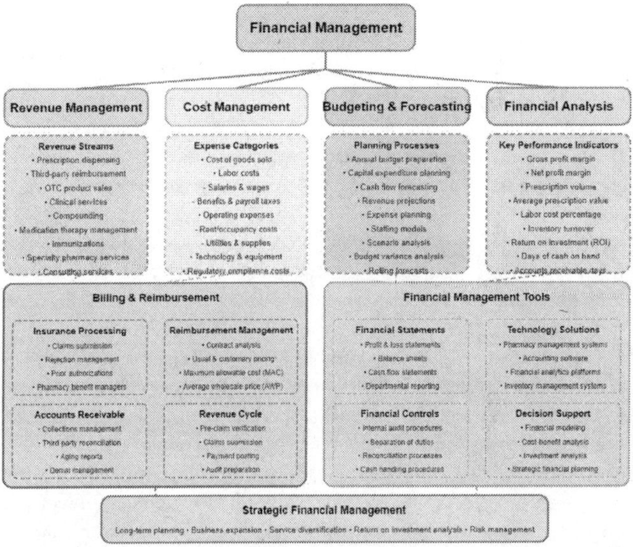

Figure 13.4: Financial Management in Pharmacy Practice

Pharmacy Financial Statements and Analysis

Financial statements provide structured representation of pharmacy economic activities, supporting both operational management and strategic planning through organized presentation of financial information. The income statement (profit and loss statement) summarizes financial performance over specific time periods, typically monthly, quarterly, and annually. Revenue sections detail income from prescription dispensing, clinical services, immunizations, durable medical equipment, and other pharmacy services. Expense categories include cost of goods sold representing actual medication acquisition costs; personnel expenses including salaries, benefits, and payroll taxes; occupancy costs covering rent, utilities, and facility maintenance; and operating expenses encompassing supplies, technology, professional liability insurance, and other administrative costs. Profitability measures include gross margin (revenue minus cost of goods sold), operating margin (revenue minus all expenses except interest and taxes), and net margin (final profit after all expenses). The balance sheet presents financial position at specific points in time through organized listing of assets, liabilities, and owner equity. Asset sections include current assets readily convertible to cash within one year (cash, accounts receivable, inventory) and fixed assets with longer-term value (equipment, fixtures, buildings). Liability sections detail current obligations due within one year (accounts payable, short-term loans, current portions of long-term debt) and long-term liabilities extending beyond one year (mortgages, equipment loans, long-term leases). Owner equity represents residual value after subtracting liabilities from assets, reflecting both invested capital and accumulated earnings. The cash flow statement tracks actual cash movement rather than accounting transactions, particularly important in pharmacy operations where timing differences between prescription dispensing, third-party reimbursement, and inventory purchasing significantly impact cash availability. Operating activities sections detail cash generated or consumed through normal business operations; investing activities cover equipment purchases or sales; and financing activities include loan proceeds, principal repayments, and owner distributions. Financial ratio analysis translates raw statement data into meaningful performance indicators supporting trend analysis and comparison against industry benchmarks. Liquidity ratios including current ratio (current assets divided by current liabilities) assess ability to meet short-term obligations. Efficiency ratios including inventory turnover (cost of goods sold divided by average inventory) evaluate operational effectiveness. Profitability ratios including return on investment measure overall financial performance relative to resources employed.

Budgeting and Financial Planning

Budgeting and financial planning translate strategic objectives into detailed financial roadmaps guiding resource allocation and operational decisions. The budgeting process typically begins with establishing assumptions regarding prescription volume, reimbursement rates, service mix, and market conditions based on historical trends, anticipated changes, and environmental scanning. Revenue projections detail expected income by category, incorporating both volume and pricing components with separate forecasting for different prescription types (new, refill, compounded), payer classes (commercial, Medicare,

Medicaid, cash), clinical services, and ancillary revenue streams. Expense budgeting addresses both fixed costs remaining relatively constant regardless of volume (base staffing, facility costs, technology infrastructure) and variable costs fluctuating with activity levels (additional staffing hours, prescription vials and labels, delivery expenses). Capital budgeting specifically addresses long-term investments in equipment, technology, facility improvements, or expansion initiatives, typically employing more sophisticated evaluation methods including payback period analysis measuring time required to recover initial investment; return on investment calculations comparing expected earnings to capital expenditure; and net present value analysis accounting for the time value of money when evaluating multi-year projects. Cash flow forecasting projects cash position throughout budget periods, identifying potential shortfall periods requiring financing arrangements or cash conservation measures while highlighting surplus periods supporting debt reduction, capital investment, or owner distributions. Effective forecasting requires attention to timing differences between service provision and payment receipt, particularly regarding third-party prescription reimbursement cycles. Variance analysis compares actual financial performance against budgeted expectations, identifying areas requiring investigation or intervention through regular review cycles. Favorable variances (better than budget) might reflect improved operational efficiency, successful new service implementation, or positive market developments, while unfavorable variances signal potential problems requiring correction. Meaningful analysis distinguishes between volume variances resulting from activity level differences and rate variances stemming from pricing or cost changes, directing attention to appropriate response strategies. Financial planning extends beyond annual budgeting to encompass multi-year strategic financial planning addressing longer-term objectives including practice expansion, ownership transition, service diversification, or technology investment. These plans typically incorporate scenario analysis examining financial implications of different potential futures, sensitivity analysis testing outcome variability based on changes to key assumptions, and contingency planning identifying specific responses to anticipated challenges or opportunities.

Third-Party Reimbursement and Revenue Cycle Management

Third-party reimbursement dominates pharmacy revenue generation, necessitating systematic approaches to payer contract management, claims processing, and revenue optimization. Payer contract management begins with thorough evaluation of proposed agreements focusing on reimbursement methodologies typically based on average wholesale price (AWP), wholesale acquisition cost (WAC), maximum allowable cost (MAC), or usual and customary pricing; dispensing fees compensating for professional services; patient copayment and coinsurance provisions; audit terms specifying documentation requirements and review procedures; and network participation requirements including hours of operation, delivery services, or specific credentialing. Contract negotiation strategies vary based on pharmacy market position, prescription volume, unique service offerings, and geographic considerations, with independent pharmacies increasingly utilizing collective negotiation through pharmacy services administrative organizations (PSAOs) leveraging aggregate volume.

Table 13.5: Financial Management in Pharmacy Practice

Financial Area	Monitoring Methods	Common Challenges
Revenue Management	Daily/weekly sales reports Payer mix analysis Reimbursement tracking Trend monitoring	Declining reimbursement rates DIR fees and clawbacks Contract complexity Payer audit risk Generic pricing fluctuations
Expense Control	Budget variance analysis Expense category tracking Benchmarking Regular financial review	Labor market pressures Rising technology costs Compliance requirements Inflation impacts Fixed cost absorption
Prescription Profitability	Script-level profitability Payer performance analysis Dispensing cost tracking Margin trend analysis	Generic effective rate challenges MAC pricing issues Preferred network pressures Specialty drug costs PBM contractual requirements

Financial Area	Monitoring Methods	Common Challenges
Cash Flow Management	Cash flow statements AR aging reports Payment cycle tracking Banking relationship	Third-party payment delays Inventory investment requirements Seasonal fluctuations Capital expenditure timing Debt service obligations
Budgeting and Forecasting	Monthly variance analysis Quarterly forecast updates Key driver monitoring Performance reviews	Market volatility Regulatory changes Competitive pressures Insurance market shifts Prescription volume uncertainty
Inventory Financial Management	Inventory valuation reports Category profitability Turn analysis by section Dead stock monitoring	Capital limitations Minimum order requirements Drug shortage management Seasonal planning Specialty drug investment
Pricing Strategies	Market basket analysis Competitor monitoring Price sensitivity testing Margin impact analysis	Price transparency demands Online/mail-order competition Consumer price sensitivity Geographic market variations Brand perception considerations
Third-Party Contract Analysis	Contract term monitoring	Limited negotiating power

Financial Area	Monitoring Methods	Common Challenges
	Performance metric tracking Reimbursement analysis DIR fee prediction	Complex contractual terms Performance metric challenges Network access requirements Retroactive adjustments
Asset Management	Asset tracking systems Depreciation scheduling Utilization monitoring Maintenance cost tracking	Technology obsolescence Capital constraints Space limitations Maintenance vs. replacement decisions Growth accommodation
Financial Risk Management	Risk assessment reviews Insurance coverage analysis Audit readiness checks Compliance cost tracking	Increasing liability concerns Cybersecurity threats Regulatory compliance costs Audit intensity growth Prescription abandonment
Productivity and Efficiency	Productivity tracking Efficiency benchmarking Process time studies Staff utilization analysis	Labor market challenges Training requirements Technology adoption barriers Staff burnout concerns Quality vs. efficiency balance
Business Development	Service financial tracking Marketing ROI analysis	Service development costs Reimbursement limitations

Financial Area	Monitoring Methods	Common Challenges
	Customer analytics Market research	Marketing effectiveness Competitive pressures Resource allocation decisions

Reimbursement monitoring identifies problematic patterns through systematic analysis comparing actual payment against expected reimbursement, with particular attention to generic medications where maximum allowable cost limits frequently fall below acquisition cost. Effective monitoring incorporates both claim-level review identifying specific problematic medications and trend analysis revealing gradual reimbursement erosion requiring contract renegotiation or inventory source adjustments. Claims adjudication optimization ensures maximum appropriate reimbursement through attention to proper coding, complete documentation, and prompt submission. Common claim rejection categories include patient eligibility issues, coordination of benefits requirements, prior authorization needs, refill-too-soon restrictions, and quantity limitations, each requiring specific resolution approaches and preventive strategies. Accounts receivable management addresses the critical interval between service provision and payment receipt through systematic tracking, aging analysis categorizing receivables by time periods since billing, and escalating intervention strategies for delayed payments. Performance metrics including days sales outstanding (average collection period), clean claim rate (percentage of claims paid without rejection), and accounts receivable aging profile provide objective measurement of revenue cycle effectiveness. Pharmacy benefit manager (PBM) relationship management addresses the intermediary organizations administering prescription benefits for health plans, self-insured employers, and government programs. Beyond basic claims processing, these relationships increasingly involve direct and indirect remuneration (DIR) fees retroactively assessed based on performance measures; preferred network participation with tiered reimbursement structures; and quality program metrics affecting both payment rates and network inclusion.

Pharmacy Business Metrics and Cost Control

Pharmacy business metrics provide quantitative measurement of financial and operational performance, supporting data-driven decision-making while identifying improvement opportunities.

Dispensing metrics track fundamental prescription department activity through measures including prescription volume trends by prescription type and payer category; average prescription value reflecting both product cost and dispensing fee components; generic dispensing rate influencing both reimbursement and acquisition cost; and prescription department labor cost per prescription reflecting staffing efficiency. Clinical service metrics quantify value-based care activities through measures including number of comprehensive medication reviews completed; immunizations administered by type; point-of-care testing volume; medication therapy management interventions; and disease-specific outcome measures demonstrating clinical impact. Productivity metrics evaluate resource utilization efficiency through measures including prescriptions dispensed per pharmacist hour; clinical services completed per clinical pharmacist hour; and revenue generated per employee. Customer metrics assess patient satisfaction and loyalty through measures including prescription abandonment rate; patient wait times; customer satisfaction scores; new patient acquisition rate; and prescription transfer patterns. Cost control strategies address expense management without compromising care quality through systematic approaches targeting major expense categories. Inventory management represents a primary focus area with strategies including optimized ordering patterns reducing excess stock; negotiated purchasing terms improving acquisition costs; enhanced monitoring identifying reimbursement challenges before significant losses accumulate; and careful management of return-to-stock medications preventing dispensing of previously filled prescriptions without appropriate credit. Personnel management balances appropriate staffing levels against labor expense through scheduling aligned with prescription timing patterns; appropriate delegation utilizing pharmacy technicians to maximum scope; workflow optimization enhancing productivity; and technology leverage automating routine functions. Operating expense control addresses the numerous smaller expense categories that cumulatively significantly impact profitability. Approaches include regular review of service contracts ensuring competitive pricing; energy efficiency initiatives reducing utility expenses; supply standardization leveraging volume purchasing; and technology solutions reducing paper, printing, and manual processing costs. Financial scenario planning prepares for contingencies through modeling potential changes in prescription volume, reimbursement rates, or expense structures, developing specific response strategies before challenges materialize.

Summary

Pharmacy management combines business principles with healthcare delivery to optimize medication services while maintaining financial sustainability. Inventory control represents a foundational management function balancing medication availability against financial constraints through strategic purchasing, storage organization, and distribution control. Effective inventory systems employ ABC classification prioritizing items by value, establish par levels triggering reordering, implement perpetual inventory tracking, and utilize just-in-time ordering to minimize carrying costs while preventing stockouts. These systems require specialized management for controlled substances through perpetual inventory maintenance, regular reconciliation processes, and secure storage systems. Quality management systems provide frameworks for continuous performance improvement through structured approaches including Plan-Do-Check-Act cycles, Lean methodology eliminating waste, and Six Sigma reducing process variation. These systems incorporate quality metrics tracking dispensing accuracy, wait times, patient satisfaction, and clinical interventions while establishing clear procedures for adverse event reporting, medication error analysis, and corrective action implementation. Staff training and development programs address both technical competencies and professional growth through structured orientation processes, competency validation methods, continuing education opportunities, and career advancement pathways. Effective training incorporates diverse learning methodologies including hands-on skill development, case-based scenarios, and technology-enhanced instruction while providing regular performance feedback. Financial management encompasses revenue cycle optimization through appropriate prescription pricing, third-party contract negotiation, and reimbursement maximization for clinical services. Expense control focuses on labor management through appropriate scheduling and productivity monitoring, while financial analysis employs metrics including prescription volume, gross margin, inventory turnover, and expense ratios to evaluate operational performance.

Multiple Choice Questions

1. Which of the following inventory management methods involves maintaining a constant inventory level with regular, fixed-quantity orders placed when stock reaches a predetermined reorder point?
   a) Just-in-time inventory
   b) Par level system
   c) Economic order quantity method
   d) First-in, first-out method
2. The formula for inventory turnover rate is:
   a) (Beginning inventory + Ending inventory) ÷ 2
   b) Cost of goods sold ÷ Average inventory
   c) Gross profit ÷ Net sales
   d) (Purchases – Ending inventory) ÷ Beginning inventory
3. Which of the following would be the most appropriate method for controlling and tracking Schedule II controlled substances in a pharmacy?
   a) Random quarterly audits
   b) Perpetual inventory system with daily verification
   c) Monthly physical inventory counts
   d) Tracking by prescription number only
4. In a quality management system, which of the following best describes the "Plan-Do-Check-Act" cycle?
   a) A one-time implementation of a quality improvement initiative
   b) A cyclical approach to continuous quality improvement
   c) A method for disciplining staff after errors occur
   d) A system for documenting regulatory compliance
5. Which of the following is a key component of a root cause analysis following a medication error?
   a) Identifying individual staff members for remedial training
   b) Implementing disciplinary actions to prevent recurrence
   c) Analyzing system factors that contributed to the error
   d) Comparing error rates to national benchmarks
6. The most effective approach to new pharmacy technician training would include:
   a) Self-directed learning through online modules only
   b) Direct instruction followed by supervised practice with feedback
   c) Observation of experienced technicians without hands-on

practice
d) Immediate independent work with periodic assessment

7. Which of the following performance metrics would be most useful in evaluating the efficiency of a pharmacy's prescription filling process?
a) Gross profit margin
b) Average prescription wait time
c) Number of prescriptions filled per day
d) Employee satisfaction scores

8. A pharmacy's gross margin is calculated as:
a) (Selling price – Cost) ÷ Selling price × 100%
b) (Selling price – Cost) ÷ Cost × 100%
c) Net profit ÷ Total revenue × 100%
d) Total revenue – Total expenses

9. Which of the following represents a variable cost in pharmacy operations?
a) Pharmacy license fees
b) Building lease payments
c) Prescription vial costs
d) Pharmacy management software subscription

10. The primary purpose of conducting a SWOT (Strengths, Weaknesses, Opportunities, Threats) analysis in pharmacy management is to:
a) Evaluate individual employee performance
b) Inform strategic planning and decision-making
c) Calculate financial ratios
d) Ensure regulatory compliance

Self-Assessment Questions

1. Explain how you would establish par levels, determine order points, implement cycle counting procedures, and evaluate inventory performance using key metrics.
2. Explain how therapeutic interchange policies, restrictive formularies, and automatic substitution protocols affect stock requirements and financial performance.
3. Explain how perpetual inventory systems, regular reconciliation processes, and diversion monitoring programs balance regulatory compliance with operational efficiency.
4. Develop a continuous quality improvement program for a pharmacy operation, explaining how you would identify quality indicators, establish measurement processes, analyze performance data, and implement targeted improvement initiatives.
5. Compare and contrast different quality management frameworks (Lean, Six Sigma, Plan-Do-Check-Act) as applied to pharmacy operations, explaining how each approach would address common quality challenges including dispensing errors and waiting times.
6. Analyze the components of a comprehensive medication error reporting and analysis system, explaining how near-miss reporting, root cause analysis, corrective action implementation, and organization-wide learning should be integrated.
7. Design an orientation and training program for new pharmacy technicians, explaining how you would structure the learning progression, assess competency attainment, provide effective feedback, and document completion of required elements.
8. Explain how continuing education requirements, credentialing opportunities, and career advancement pathways can be aligned with organizational needs and individual goals.
9. Analyze the revenue cycle in pharmacy operations, explaining how prescription pricing models, third-party contract negotiations, and reimbursement optimization strategies affect financial performance.
10. Explain key performance indicators including prescription volume, gross margin, labor cost percentage, inventory turnover, and how these metrics guide operational decision-making

Bibliography

1. Desselle SP, Zgarrick DP, Alston GL, editors. Pharmacy management: Essentials for all practice settings. 5th ed. New York: McGraw-Hill Education; 2019.
2. Wilson KA, Jetha N. Inventory management. In: Langley CA, Belcher D, editors. Applied pharmaceutical practice. London: Pharmaceutical Press; 2008. p. 39-50.
3. Mobach MP. The transformation of pharmacy concepts into building and organization. Pharm World Sci. 2005;27(4):329-338.
4. Holdford DA. Financial management in pharmacy practice. In: Chisholm-Burns MA, Vaillancourt AM, Shepherd M, editors. Pharmacy management, leadership, marketing, and finance. 2nd ed. Burlington: Jones & Bartlett Learning; 2014. p. 59-78.
5. Desselle SP, Rappaport HM. The identification of pharmaceutical care management competencies for community pharmacy practitioners. J Pharm Mark Manage. 1996;11(1):65-84.
6. McKesson Canada. Pharmacy operations - best practices. Mississauga: McKesson Canada; 2017.
7. Warholak TL, Nau DP. Quality and safety in pharmacy practice. New York: McGraw-Hill Medical; 2010.
8. Savage IT, Blenkinsopp A, Cleland JA, Mackenzie A. General practitioners' perceptions of community pharmacists' provision of 'pharmacy first' minor ailment management services. Int J Pharm Pract. 2015;23(Suppl 1):35-36.
9. Sacchetti E, Turrina C, Valsecchi P. Cerebrovascular accidents in elderly people treated with antipsychotic drugs: A systematic review. Drug Saf. 2010;33(4):273-288.
10. Tootelian DH, Gaedeke RM. Essentials of pharmacy management. 2nd ed. St. Louis: Mosby; 2005.

CHAPTER 14

CLINICAL DECISION MAKING

Author

Dr. Amit Kumar, Associate Professor, Department of Pharmacy Practice, Amity Institute of Pharmacy, Amity University, Lucknow, India

Abstract

Clinical decision making applies systematic cognitive processes to pharmaceutical care, integrating evidence evaluation with patient-specific factors to optimize therapeutic outcomes. Evidence-based practice combines research evaluation, clinical expertise, and patient preferences through structured approaches identifying answerable clinical questions, efficiently searching information sources, critically appraising literature quality, applying findings to specific patients, and evaluating outcomes, with hierarchies rating evidence from meta-analyses and randomized controlled trials to case reports and expert opinion. Clinical guidelines implementation translates consensus recommendations into practical application through identification of relevant guidelines, assessment of evidence quality and applicability, adaptation to local resources and patient populations, implementation strategies addressing barriers, and outcome monitoring evaluating adherence and clinical impact. Patient case analysis employs structured frameworks systematically evaluating subjective and objective information, including comprehensive medication reviews identifying actual and potential drug-related problems, with particular attention to indication appropriateness, effectiveness assessment, safety evaluation, and adherence factors across acute and chronic conditions. Therapeutic problem solving applies clinical reasoning models to complex medication challenges through clear problem definition, generation of multiple intervention options, systematic evaluation of alternatives against therapeutic goals, implementation of selected interventions, and ongoing monitoring with adjustment based on response, incorporating both analytical and intuitive processes while considering patient-specific contexts, preferences, and clinical variables. Decision-making principles enable pharmacists to translate theoretical knowledge into practical interventions that address individual patient needs while incorporating best available evidence and professional judgment.

Keywords: *Clinical Reasoning; Literature Evaluation; Problem Identification; Intervention Selection; Evidence-Based Practice*

Learning Objectives

After completion of the chapter, the learners should be able to:

- Formulate clinically relevant questions using PICO (Population, Intervention, Comparison, Outcome) format to guide evidence-based inquiries.
- Evaluate primary literature using critical appraisal tools to assess validity, importance, and applicability to specific patient scenarios.
- Implement clinical practice guidelines while appropriately adjusting recommendations based on patient-specific factors and comorbidities.
- Develop systematic approaches to patient case analysis using standardized frameworks that identify actual and potential drug-related problems.
- Apply clinical reasoning models to complex therapeutic problems through clear definition, option generation, intervention selection, and outcome evaluation.
- Integrate patient preferences, clinical evidence, and professional judgment when making recommendations for challenging clinical scenarios.

EVIDENCE-BASED PRACTICE

Evidence-based practice (EBP) represents the conscientious, explicit, and judicious integration of best available research evidence with clinical expertise and patient values to optimize therapeutic decision-making. This approach moves beyond tradition, intuition, or unsystematic clinical experiences to incorporate rigorous evaluation of scientific literature while recognizing the essential contributions of practitioner judgment and patient preferences. Effective implementation of evidence-based practice requires both methodological understanding for critical literature evaluation and practical strategies for integrating evidence into daily clinical workflows.

Principles of Evidence-Based Practice

Evidence-based practice rests on fundamental principles guiding both conceptual understanding and practical application. The evidence hierarchy organizes information sources according to methodological rigor and potential for bias, with systematic reviews and meta-analyses of randomized controlled trials generally occupying the highest position; individual randomized controlled trials providing strong evidence for causal relationships; observational studies including cohort and case-control designs offering insights into associations and real-world effectiveness; and case reports, expert opinion, and physiological rationale providing lowest-level evidence when stronger sources are unavailable. While this hierarchical approach provides general guidance, appropriate evidence selection must consider the specific clinical question being addressed, with different study designs offering complementary strengths for different inquiry types. The five-step EBP process offers a structured approach to clinical problem-solving: formulating clear clinical questions; searching efficiently for best evidence; critically appraising evidence quality; applying relevant findings to specific patient circumstances; and evaluating outcomes. Clinical question formulation typically employs the PICO framework identifying Patient/Problem, Intervention, Comparison, and Outcome elements, creating focused queries supporting efficient literature searching.

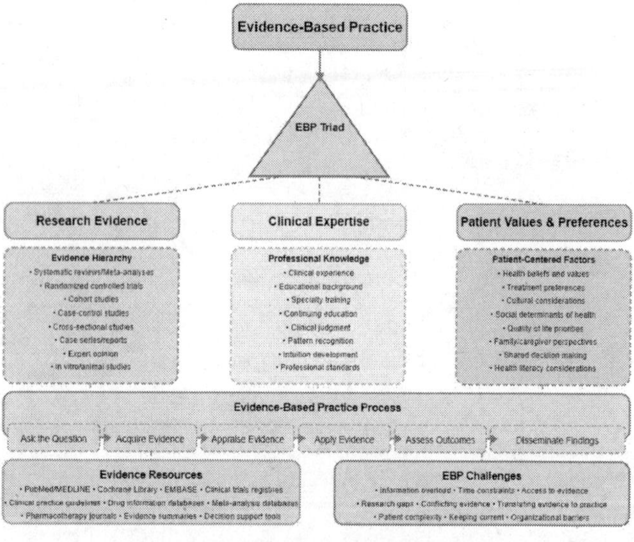

Figure 14.1: Evidence-Based Practice

Evidence searching strategies balance comprehensiveness against efficiency through selection of appropriate information resources ranging from pre-appraised sources (clinical decision support systems, evidence-based guidelines) to primary literature databases (PubMed/MEDLINE, Embase) based on question complexity, time constraints, and resource availability. Critical appraisal examines both internal validity (methodological quality) and external validity (applicability to specific patients or settings) through structured assessment of study design, execution, analysis, and reporting. Application integrates research findings with individual patient factors including comorbidities, preferences, social circumstances, and economic considerations, recognizing that even high-quality evidence requires contextual interpretation. Evaluation completes the cycle by assessing both patient outcomes and process effectiveness, creating continuous improvement opportunities in evidence application.

Table 14.1: Evidence-Based Practice Framework

Component	Description	Application Methods
Research Evidence	Systematic reviews Randomized controlled trials Cohort studies Case-control studies Case series/reports	Literature search strategies Critical appraisal tools Evidence synthesis methods Hierarchy of evidence application
Clinical Expertise	Professional knowledge Practice experience Specialized training Pattern recognition Clinical judgment	Reflective practice Experience documentation Peer consultation Skill development planning
Patient Values/Preferences	Expressed preferences Health beliefs Treatment goals Risk tolerance Quality of life priorities	Patient interviews Shared decision-making tools Preference elicitation methods Patient-reported outcomes
Clinical Circumstances	Patient-specific factors Comorbidities Medication history Social determinants Healthcare access	Comprehensive assessment Patient-specific data collection Risk stratification Contextual analysis
Critical Appraisal	Validity assessment	Structured appraisal tools

Component	Description	Application Methods
	Results interpretation Relevance evaluation Applicability determination	Quality assessment checklists Bias identification methods Statistical significance evaluation
Information Mastery	Knowledge management Efficient information access Trusted resource identification Pre-appraised evidence use	Point-of-care tools Evidence-based resources Information triage strategies Foraging vs. hunting approaches
Question Formulation	PICO framework application Focused clinical questions Searchable questions Prioritization of inquiries	PICO templates Question refinement processes Question categorization systems Priority-setting frameworks
Evidence Application	Patient-specific adaptation Contextual consideration Benefit-risk assessment Shared decision-making	Clinical pathways Decision aids Guidelines with exceptions Collaborative decision processes
Outcome Evaluation	Patient outcomes monitoring Intervention effectiveness Unintended consequences Process assessment	Outcome measurement systems Process metrics Patient feedback collection Comparative effectiveness methods
Continuous Improvement	Reflection on outcomes	Performance feedback loops

Component	Description	Application Methods
	Practice adaptation Knowledge updating System enhancement	Learning systems Continuous education Practice-based research
Evidence Implementation	Knowledge translation Practice integration System-level adoption Sustainable change	Implementation frameworks Change management strategies Educational outreach System integration approaches

Critical Appraisal of Medical Literature

Critical appraisal skills enable discrimination between robust evidence supporting practice change and flawed research potentially leading to inappropriate interventions. Randomized controlled trial (RCT) evaluation examines multiple quality dimensions including randomization adequacy protecting against selection bias; allocation concealment preventing enrollment manipulation; appropriate blinding minimizing performance and detection bias; complete outcome reporting avoiding attrition bias; predetermined analysis plans preventing selective reporting; and sufficient statistical power ensuring capability to detect clinically meaningful differences. Systematic review assessment considers comprehensive literature searching minimizing publication bias; explicit inclusion criteria ensuring appropriate study selection; rigorous quality evaluation of included studies; appropriate synthesis methods accounting for study heterogeneity; and transparent reporting of all methodological decisions. Observational study evaluation addresses design-specific considerations including representativeness of cohort studies; appropriate control selection in case-control research; adequate follow-up duration capturing relevant outcomes; comprehensive confounder identification and adjustment; and recognition of inherent limitations in establishing causality. Statistical interpretation requires understanding of both significance and clinical importance, recognizing that statistically significant findings may lack practical relevance if effect sizes remain small. Concepts including absolute risk reduction, relative risk reduction, number needed to treat, and confidence intervals provide context for determining clinical significance beyond p-value interpretation. Common methodological limitations requiring identification include inappropriate surrogate endpoints inadequately predicting clinical outcomes; insufficient study duration missing delayed benefits or adverse effects; selective population enrollment limiting generalizability; inappropriate comparators providing misleading conclusions about relative efficacy; industry funding potentially introducing bias through multiple mechanisms; and publication bias systematically overrepresenting positive findings in available literature. Practical appraisal approaches balance comprehensive evaluation against time constraints through structured assessment tools including the Cochrane Risk of Bias Tool for randomized trials; AMSTAR-2 for systematic reviews; Newcastle-Ottawa Scale for observational studies; and various critical appraisal checklists developed by evidence-based practice organizations providing guided evaluation frameworks.

Applying Evidence to Individual Patients

Translating population-based evidence to individual patient care requires thoughtful consideration of various factors influencing both appropriateness and effectiveness of interventions. Benefit-risk assessment evaluates potential therapeutic advantages against possible harms within the context of specific patient circumstances. This assessment considers absolute risk reduction rather than relative measures alone; evaluates time-to-benefit relative to patient life expectancy and treatment goals; examines number needed to treat alongside number needed to harm; and incorporates patient-specific risk factors potentially altering the intervention's benefit-risk profile. Individual patient factors significantly influencing evidence application include age-related physiological changes affecting pharmacokinetics and pharmacodynamics; organ dysfunction altering medication elimination or sensitivity; genetic variations influencing drug metabolism or receptor response; pregnancy or lactation considerations; comorbid conditions potentially introducing drug-disease interactions; and concurrent medications creating potential drug-drug interactions. Patient preferences and values constitute essential components of evidence-based decision-making, reflecting personal goals, risk tolerance, treatment burden acceptance, and quality-of-life priorities. Preference elicitation employs various approaches including direct discussion of options with associated benefits and risks; decision aids presenting information in accessible formats; and shared decision-making processes explicitly incorporating patient values alongside clinical evidence. Practical limitations affecting evidence application include financial constraints related to medication costs, monitoring requirements, or access to care; literacy and comprehension barriers affecting understanding of complex regimens; social support limitations influencing adherence capacity; and cultural factors potentially affecting treatment acceptability or implementation. Managing uncertainty represents an inherent challenge in evidence application, as available research frequently provides incomplete answers to specific clinical questions. Approaches to uncertainty include transparent communication with patients about evidence limitations; application of pathophysiological principles when direct evidence is lacking; utilization of expert consensus when appropriate; and implementation of therapeutic trials with clearly defined outcomes and stopping criteria.

Implementing Evidence-Based Practice in Clinical Settings

Implementing evidence-based practice within clinical environments requires systematic approaches addressing both individual practitioner capabilities and organizational systems supporting evidence integration. Individual barriers to implementation include knowledge limitations regarding searching and appraisal skills; time constraints within busy practice settings; difficulty accessing information resources at point of care; and challenges translating statistical concepts into practical clinical applications. Professional development strategies addressing these barriers include formal training in evidence-based practice methodology; journal club participation developing critical appraisal skills through structured discussion; and mentorship pairing less experienced practitioners with EBP-proficient colleagues. Organizational facilitators supporting evidence-based culture include leadership commitment demonstrating valuation of evidence-informed decision-making; infrastructure investments providing point-of-care information access; dedicated time allocation for literature review and evaluation; and performance expectations explicitly incorporating evidence-based practice activities. Information resource selection balances comprehensiveness against usability through strategic utilization of different resource types. Pre-appraised resources including clinical decision support systems, evidence-based textbooks, and critically appraised topics provide efficiently packaged information appropriate for many routine decisions. Primary literature databases support comprehensive searching when addressing complex or unusual clinical questions requiring deeper investigation. Mobile technology integration enhances point-of-care evidence access through smartphone applications, digital reference tools, and web-based resources optimized for clinical settings. Quality improvement integration connects evidence-based practice with performance enhancement initiatives through identification of evidence-practice gaps; development of implementation strategies addressing identified barriers; creation of audit mechanisms tracking adherence to evidence-based recommendations; and feedback systems supporting continuous improvement. Knowledge translation approaches bridge the gap between evidence generation and clinical application through development of actionable tools including clinical pathways translating evidence into structured decision algorithms; order sets incorporating evidence-based interventions for specific conditions; documentation templates prompting evidence-based care components; and clinical decision support systems delivering relevant evidence at appropriate decision points within workflow.

CLINICAL GUIDELINES IMPLEMENTATION

Clinical practice guidelines translate evidence into practical recommendations supporting consistent, high-quality care based on systematic literature evaluation and expert interpretation. Effective guideline implementation requires understanding guideline development methodology, critical evaluation of guideline quality, thoughtful adaptation to specific practice contexts, and strategic approaches to overcome implementation barriers. When appropriately applied, guidelines reduce unwarranted practice variation while allowing necessary individualization for specific patient circumstances.

Table 14.2: Implementation of Clinical Guidelines

Implementation Component	Implementation Methods	Common Barriers
Guideline Selection	Structured evaluation tools Stakeholder input Gap analysis Adaptation frameworks	Conflicting guidelines Limited applicability Resource misalignment Evidence quality concerns Outdated recommendations
Stakeholder Engagement	Advisory committees Focus groups Opinion leader identification Shared decision-making	Competing priorities Time constraints Resistance to change Power dynamics Conflicting perspectives

Implementation Component	Implementation Methods	Common Barriers
Local Adaptation	Adaptation frameworks Modified Delphi process Local consensus processes Resource mapping	Maintaining evidence fidelity Limited local expertise Resource constraints System limitations Adaptation consistency
Implementation Strategy	Educational outreach Clinical decision support Audit and feedback Practice facilitation	Resource limitations Competing initiatives Staff turnover Change fatigue Implementation expertise gaps
Educational Interventions	Interactive workshops Case-based learning Academic detailing Just-in-time resources	Time constraints Varied learning styles Knowledge-practice gap Educational effectiveness Sustainability of learning
Clinical Decision Support	EHR integration Order sets/templates Mobile applications Point-of-care tools	Alert fatigue Technical limitations Workflow disruption Maintenance requirements Implementation costs
Audit and Feedback	Automated data extraction Performance dashboards Benchmarking Facilitated feedback sessions	Data availability Measure attribution Feedback effectiveness Resource requirements Defensive reactions
Environmental Restructuring	Workflow redesign Visual cues/reminders	Physical constraints Cost limitations Workflow

Implementation Component	Implementation Methods	Common Barriers
	Resource provision Default option changes	complexity System rigidity Competing demands
Patient-Focused Strategies	Patient education programs Decision aids Self-monitoring tools Motivational approaches	Health literacy barriers Material accessibility Time limitations Patient engagement challenges Cultural considerations
Performance Monitoring	Quality dashboards Regular reporting Variance analysis Continuous feedback loops	Data collection burden Measure validity concerns Resource limitations Feedback ineffectiveness Improvement sustainability
Sustainability Planning	Integration into policies Resource commitment Continuous education Monitoring systems	Leadership changes Competing priorities Resource reallocation Initiative fatigue System changes
Deimplementation Strategies	Choosing Wisely integration Academic detailing Decision support modification Alternative pathways	Practice inertia Patient expectations Revenue implications Defensive medicine Risk aversion

Guideline Development and Evaluation

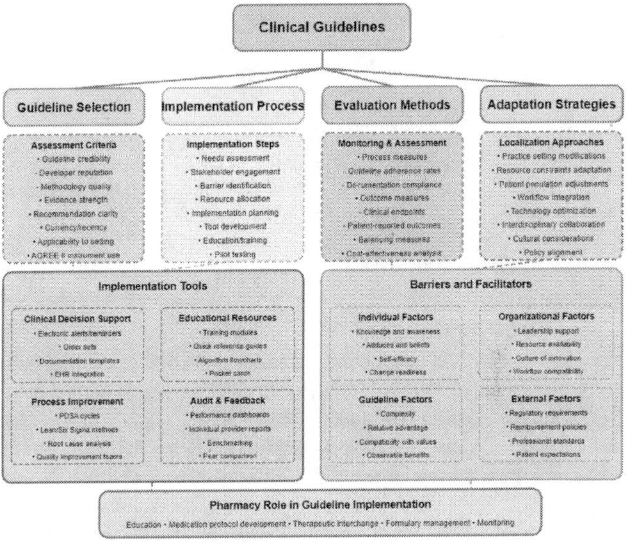

Figure 14.2: Clinical Guidelines Implementation

The knowledge about guideline development processes and quality evaluation methods provides foundation for appropriate implementation decisions. Guideline development methodologies have evolved significantly, with rigorous approaches including systematic evidence review establishing the evidence base; explicit linkage between recommendations and supporting evidence; multidisciplinary development teams incorporating diverse perspectives; transparent consensus processes resolving areas of disagreement; and clear specification of recommendation strength reflecting both evidence quality and benefit-risk assessment. Recommendation grading systems communicate both evidence quality and recommendation strength, though specific systems vary across guideline developing organizations. The GRADE approach (Grading of Recommendations Assessment, Development and Evaluation) represents an increasingly adopted framework categorizing recommendations as strong or conditional/weak based on evidence quality, benefit-risk balance, resource considerations, and patient preferences. Quality evaluation employs structured assessment tools examining methodological rigor. The AGREE II instrument (Appraisal of Guidelines for Research and Evaluation) evaluates six domains: scope and purpose clarity; stakeholder involvement; development rigor; presentation clarity;

applicability considerations; and editorial independence from funding sources. This structured assessment guides implementation decisions by identifying guidelines meeting quality standards warranting clinical application. Guideline limitations requiring recognition include evidence gaps necessitating expert opinion for certain recommendations; potential conflicts of interest influencing recommendation formation despite disclosure requirements; rapid evidence evolution potentially outdating recommendations between revision cycles; and inherent tensions between population-focused recommendations and individual patient needs requiring clinical judgment in application. Guideline sources demonstrate variable quality and focus requiring selective utilization. Professional society guidelines typically address specific disease states or therapeutic areas within specialty domains, often incorporating practical clinical perspectives but potentially limited by resource constraints affecting methodological rigor. Government agency guidelines frequently employ comprehensive development processes with substantial methodological support but may involve lengthy development timelines affecting currency. International guidelines offer valuable perspectives but require evaluation for applicability across different healthcare systems and patient populations. Commercial guideline producers may provide user-friendly formats and frequent updates but require careful evaluation for potential commercial influences on recommendations.

Adapting Guidelines to Specific Practice Settings

Adaptation translates guidelines developed for general application into practical protocols addressing specific practice environment characteristics, patient populations, and resource constraints. Local adaptation processes typically begin with guideline selection identifying high-quality guidelines addressing relevant clinical questions, followed by systematic adaptation rather than complete redevelopment conserving limited resources. Stakeholder engagement ensures incorporation of perspectives from all affected parties including pharmacists, physicians, nurses, administrators, and when appropriate, patient representatives. This multidisciplinary approach identifies potential implementation barriers while building consensus supporting successful adoption. Adaptation frameworks provide structured approaches guiding modification processes. The ADAPTE framework offers systematic methodology including scope definition, guideline assessment, decision processes for accepting or modifying recommendations, and external review of adapted guidelines ensuring quality maintenance throughout modification. Contextual factors influencing adaptation include patient population characteristics potentially affecting intervention appropriateness or effectiveness; formulary constraints limiting medication recommendations; resource availability affecting diagnostic testing or monitoring capabilities; staff expertise and scope of practice determining implementation feasibility; and existing workflows requiring alignment with guideline recommendations. Practical adaptation strategies include recommendation prioritization focusing implementation on high-impact, strongly supported interventions rather than attempting comprehensive adoption; recommendation modification addressing necessary contextual adjustments while preserving core evidence-based principles; algorithm development translating narrative recommendations into visual decision pathways supporting clinical application; documentation standardization integrating guideline elements into routine clinical documentation; and performance measure identification establishing metrics evaluating successful implementation. Maintaining guideline currency represents an ongoing challenge requiring systematic approaches to evidence monitoring and update triggering. Surveillance mechanisms include literature monitoring identifying practice-changing research; automated alerts from guideline developing organizations signaling updates; and feedback systems capturing implementation challenges potentially indicating needed modifications. Predetermined review cycles establish maximum intervals between comprehensive reassessments while allowing accelerated updates when significant evidence changes occur.

Implementation Strategies and Challenges

Implementation strategies address the complex challenge of translating guideline recommendations into sustained practice change through multifaceted approaches targeting identified barriers. Educational approaches build knowledge and understanding through various modalities including didactic sessions explaining guideline recommendations and supporting evidence; interactive workshops developing practical application skills; academic detailing providing individualized education addressing specific practitioner questions; and case-based learning demonstrating guideline application in realistic scenarios. While necessary for building understanding, education alone typically produces modest and temporary practice changes without additional implementation components. Structural interventions modify practice environments supporting guideline adherence through system changes including computerized decision support embedding recommendations within electronic health records; standardized order sets incorporating guideline-based interventions; clinical pathways structuring care processes around evidence-based recommendations; and documentation templates prompting guideline-concordant assessment and treatment. These approaches reduce reliance on memory and conscious decision-making by integrating recommendations into workflow. Behavioral interventions address practitioner motivation and decision patterns through strategies including audit and feedback comparing individual performance against guideline recommendations; opinion leader influence leveraging respected colleagues supporting guideline adoption; champion identification developing internal advocates promoting implementation; and public commitment creating social expectations supporting adherence. Implementation barriers occur at multiple levels requiring targeted strategies. Guideline-level barriers include excessive length and complexity limiting usability; conflicting recommendations between guidelines creating uncertainty; and inadequate tools supporting practical application. Practitioner-level barriers include knowledge deficits regarding recommendations; disagreement with specific guideline elements; concerns about applicability to specific patient populations; and skepticism regarding development processes. Organizational barriers include time constraints limiting guideline review and application; inadequate resources supporting implementation; workflow misalignment with recommendations; and competing priorities reducing implementation focus. Patient-level barriers include preferences conflicting with guideline recommendations; adherence challenges with recommended interventions; and financial constraints limiting access to suggested therapies. Implementation science frameworks provide structured approaches to barrier identification and strategy development. The Consolidated Framework for Implementation Research (CFIR) organizes influential factors across domains including intervention characteristics, outer setting, inner setting, individual characteristics, and implementation process. The Theoretical Domains Framework identifies behavioral determinants of guideline adherence, supporting targeted intervention development addressing specific barriers.

Evaluating Guideline Implementation and Outcomes

Evaluation provides essential feedback regarding implementation effectiveness, guideline impact, and unintended consequences through systematic assessment approaches. Evaluation planning ideally occurs concurrent with implementation design, establishing clear objectives, appropriate metrics, measurement methodologies, and analysis approaches before implementation begins. Process evaluation assesses implementation fidelity examining the degree to which planned activities occurred as intended; penetration measuring adoption breadth across targeted settings and practitioners; adaptation tracking modifications made during implementation; and sustainability evaluating continued adherence beyond initial implementation period. These measures provide insight into implementation effectiveness independent of clinical outcomes. Outcome evaluation examines guideline impact on clinical results, typically employing measures directly addressed by guideline recommendations such as achievement of therapeutic targets, symptom improvement, disease progression, or complication rates. Comprehensive evaluation includes both intermediate process measures (medication utilization patterns, monitoring frequency, intervention timeliness) and patient-oriented outcomes (mortality, morbidity, functional status, quality of life) providing complementary perspectives on guideline value. Measurement approaches balance feasibility against comprehensiveness through strategic data collection. Chart review provides detailed information but requires significant resources; administrative data offers broader coverage with limited clinical detail; electronic health record extraction combines reasonable clinical detail with efficient collection when properly designed; and patient-reported outcomes capture experience dimensions inaccessible through other methods. Unintended consequences assessment identifies potential negative impacts including treatment burden from guideline-recommended interventions; care fragmentation when multiple condition-specific guidelines apply to patients with multimorbidity; resource diversion from non-guideline care areas; and potential overtreatment when guidelines are applied without appropriate individualization. Monitoring for these effects ensures guideline implementation enhances rather than compromises overall care quality. Quality improvement integration connects guideline implementation with broader performance enhancement initiatives through Plan-Do-Study-Act cycles testing implementation strategies; statistical process control methods tracking performance trends; and continuous feedback mechanisms supporting ongoing refinement. This integration transforms guideline implementation from isolated events into continuous improvement processes responding to implementation experience, emerging evidence, and evolving practice contexts.

PATIENT CASE ANALYSIS

Patient case analysis represents the systematic process of evaluating individual patient situations to develop optimal pharmaceutical care plans addressing identified medication-related needs. This complex cognitive process integrates clinical information gathering, problem identification, therapeutic evaluation, and care plan development within patient-centered frameworks. Effective case analysis requires both analytical thinking applying clinical knowledge to specific situations and critical thinking questioning assumptions and exploring alternative perspectives throughout the decision-making process.

Comprehensive Patient Assessment

Comprehensive patient assessment establishes the foundation for effective case analysis through systematic information gathering addressing all factors potentially influencing medication therapy outcomes. Patient interview techniques elicit essential information while building therapeutic relationships through approaches including open-ended questioning encouraging detailed responses; active listening demonstrating engagement with patient concerns; empathic communication acknowledging emotional aspects of health experiences; and non-judgmental discussion of potentially sensitive topics including adherence challenges, substance use, or complementary therapy utilization. Structured information gathering typically follows organized frameworks while remaining flexible enough to explore unexpected findings. The patient profile encompasses demographic factors potentially influencing therapy selection including age, gender, pregnancy/lactation status, race/ethnicity when pharmacogenomic implications exist, occupation when relevant to medication timing or adherence, and living situation affecting medication management capabilities. Chief complaint and history of present illness explore the patient's primary concerns and symptom progression, providing context for current therapy evaluation. Medical history review identifies comorbid conditions influencing medication selection, dosing, or monitoring requirements while establishing therapeutic priorities among multiple health concerns. Medication history includes comprehensive review of prescription medications, over-the-counter products, dietary supplements, and complementary therapies, with specific attention to medication allergies, previous adverse effects, efficacy of current and past treatments, and adherence patterns with contributing factors. Social history examines lifestyle factors including tobacco, alcohol, and recreational drug use; dietary patterns; physical activity; occupation-related exposures; and social support systems potentially influencing both health status and medication management capabilities. Family history identifies genetic predispositions potentially affecting medication response or disease progression. Physical examination findings relevant to medication therapy include vital signs, weight for dose calculations, organ function indicators, and specific findings related to therapeutic problems under evaluation. Laboratory and diagnostic test interpretation provides objective measures of disease control, organ function affecting medication clearance, therapeutic drug levels when applicable, and monitoring parameters related to medication safety and efficacy. Information organization employs structured frameworks supporting comprehensive assessment while maintaining efficiency, with problem-oriented approaches organizing findings around specific health conditions and medication-oriented approaches examining each therapy's appropriateness, effectiveness, safety, and adherence characteristics.

Table 14.3: Patient Case Analysis

Analysis Component	Assessment Methods	Clinical Application
Patient Demographics	Medical record review Patient interview Family/caregiver input Social determinants assessment	Age-appropriate treatments Social support needs Cultural adaptations Access solutions
Chief Complaint	Patient interview Symptom assessment tools Functional assessments Quality of life measures	Problem prioritization Urgency determination Patient-centered focus Treatment goal alignment
History of Present Illness	Chronological history taking Symptom diaries Previous records review Treatment response assessment	Disease progression understanding Treatment response patterns Modifiable triggers Self-management opportunities
Past Medical History	Medical record review Patient interview Previous provider communication Family history assessment	Comorbidity management Contraindication identification Risk factor assessment Genetic risk considerations
Medication History	Medication reconciliation Prescription records Adherence	Drug interaction checking Adherence barrier identification Side effect

Analysis Component	Assessment Methods	Clinical Application
	assessment Side effect evaluation	management Therapeutic duplication avoidance
Allergies/Adverse Reactions	Allergy assessment Reaction characterization Timing/causality evaluation Cross-sensitivity assessment	Avoidance planning Alternative selection Risk-benefit assessment Desensitization consideration
Review of Systems	Structured interview Symptom checklists Body system review Pattern recognition	Complete clinical picture Differential diagnosis expansion Symptom pattern recognition Comprehensive assessment
Physical Examination	Focused examination Measurement tools Comparison to norms Trend analysis	Diagnosis confirmation Disease severity assessment Treatment monitoring Complication detection
Laboratory/Diagnostic Data	Laboratory data review Imaging interpretation Diagnostic report analysis Trend analysis	Diagnosis confirmation Treatment monitoring Complication detection Response assessment
Problem Assessment	Clinical judgment application Differential diagnosis Evidence	Treatment planning focus Resource allocation Intervention

Analysis Component	Assessment Methods	Clinical Application
	integration Risk stratification	prioritization Risk-appropriate care
Therapeutic Assessment	Guideline comparison Literature evaluation Risk-benefit analysis Individualization assessment	Therapy optimization Guideline implementation Individualized approaches Monitoring plan development
Patient-Specific Factors	Patient interview Goal setting discussion Barrier identification Health belief assessment	Patient-centered planning Adherence strategy development Goal alignment Individualized approaches
Treatment Plan	Evidence-based planning Shared decision-making Risk-benefit consideration Monitoring design	Evidence-based treatment Patient-specific adaptations Appropriate monitoring Systematic follow-up

Identification of Drug Therapy Problems

Drug therapy problems represent the core focus of pharmaceutical care, defined as undesirable events or risks involving medication therapy that actually or potentially interfere with desired health outcomes. Systematic identification employs structured categorization frameworks while requiring clinical judgment in application to specific patient situations. Comprehensive classification systems typically include unnecessary drug therapy (medication without valid indication); need for additional drug therapy (untreated indication or preventive therapy requirement); ineffective drug (inappropriate selection for condition or patient factors); dosage too low (suboptimal dose, frequency, duration, or administration timing); adverse drug reaction (undesirable effect from appropriate or inappropriate medication); dosage too high (excessive dose causing toxicity or unnecessary cost); and nonadherence (patient not taking medication as intended due to various factors).

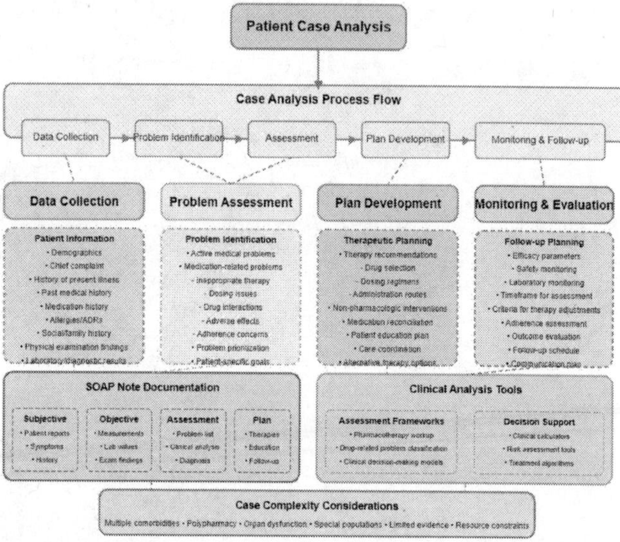

Figure 14.3: Patient Case Analysis

Problem identification methodologies include systematic medication review comparing current therapy against evidence-based standards for specific conditions; trigger tool application identifying high-risk medications, laboratory values, or clinical findings warranting detailed evaluation; and comprehensive medication therapy management processes examining each medication for appropriateness, effectiveness, safety, and adherence considerations. Problem prioritization addresses the reality that many patients present with multiple actual or potential drug therapy problems requiring sequenced intervention. Prioritization factors include problem severity considering potential clinical consequences; urgency based on time sensitivity for intervention; patient-specific risk factors potentially exacerbating problem impact; patient preferences regarding which problems most significantly affect quality of life; intervention feasibility within available resources; and likelihood of successful resolution through pharmaceutical care interventions. Causality assessment distinguishes between correlation and causation when evaluating potential adverse drug effects through structured approaches including temporal relationship evaluation, dechallenge/rechallenge information when available, alternative explanations assessment, and known reaction patterns with specific agents. Documentation of identified problems employs clear, specific language describing the problem, contributing factors, supporting evidence, and clinical significance. Effective documentation facilitates intervention planning, communication with other healthcare providers, justification of pharmacy services, and outcomes tracking over time.

Therapeutic Plan Development

Therapeutic plan development translates problem identification into concrete action steps addressing medication-related needs through patient-specific interventions. Goal setting establishes clear, measurable objectives for each identified problem, ideally incorporating both clinical parameters (laboratory values, symptom control, functional status) and patient-centered outcomes reflecting individual priorities and preferences. Well-constructed goals specify the targeted outcome, measurement method, timeframe for achievement, and threshold for success in specific, measurable terms. Intervention selection considers multiple options for addressing identified problems, including initiating new medications for untreated indications; discontinuing unnecessary or harmful therapies; modifying doses, frequencies, or formulations of existing medications; recommending monitoring parameters for efficacy and safety evaluation; providing patient education enhancing understanding and adherence; implementing adherence support systems; and coordinating care across multiple providers. Selection among these options involves evaluating evidence supporting each intervention, patient-specific factors influencing likely effectiveness, resource requirements, and patient preferences regarding treatment approaches. Patient engagement in plan development supports both ethical principles of autonomy and practical benefits of enhanced adherence through shared decision-making. This process involves providing information about therapeutic options in understandable language; eliciting patient preferences regarding potential benefits, risks, and treatment burdens; addressing questions and concerns influencing treatment decisions; and reaching mutual agreement on implementation steps. Monitoring plan development establishes specific parameters evaluating intervention effectiveness and safety, including objective measures (laboratory values, physical findings, symptom scales); subjective assessments (patient-reported symptoms, functioning, quality of life); timeframes for follow-up evaluation; criteria for determining success or failure; and contingency plans for inadequate response or adverse effects. Documentation communicates the care plan to patients, caregivers, and other healthcare providers through structured formats specifying problems addressed, interventions implemented, goals established, monitoring parameters, follow-up timing, and responsibility assignments for various plan components.

Case Presentation

Case presentation and documentation translate patient assessment, problem identification, and care planning into effective communication supporting clinical decision-making and continuity of care. Oral case presentations concisely communicate essential information supporting therapeutic decision-making through organized structures balancing comprehensiveness against time constraints. Common formats include subjective-objective-assessment-plan (SOAP) organizing information into patient-reported symptoms, objective findings, clinical assessment, and intervention plans; problem-oriented presentations focusing on specific medication-related issues with supporting data and recommendations; and case-based presentations examining complex patient situations through detailed analysis of multiple factors influencing therapeutic decisions. Presentation adaptation considers audience characteristics (clinical specialty, professional background, familiarity with patient), presentation purpose (information sharing, consultation request, intervention justification), and setting constraints (formal rounds, informal consultation, interprofessional team meeting). Effective presentations prioritize relevant information supporting clinical decisions while avoiding extraneous details; employ precise clinical terminology appropriate to the audience; present logical reasoning connecting assessment findings to therapeutic recommendations; anticipate questions regarding therapeutic alternatives; and provide specific, actionable recommendations rather than general observations. Written documentation serves multiple purposes including communication among healthcare team members; legal documentation of professional services; justification for interventions and reimbursement; and longitudinal tracking of patient progress. Documentation formats vary across practice settings but typically include standardized elements: patient demographics and clinical characteristics; subjective information from patient interview; objective findings from examination, laboratory results, and other data sources; assessment analyzing medication-related problems with supporting rationale; and plan detailing specific interventions with responsibilities and follow-up parameters. Electronic health record documentation integrates pharmacy case analysis into shared clinical records through various mechanisms including dedicated pharmacy notes; contribution to interdisciplinary progress notes; structured medication management documentation; care plan development within shared platforms; and documentation within specific clinical pathways or protocols. Quality documentation demonstrates multiple characteristics: factual accuracy distinguishing between direct observation and inference; clinical relevance focusing on information supporting therapeutic decisions; logical organization following consistent structure; appropriate detail balancing comprehensiveness against usability; objectivity separating observation from interpretation; professional terminology appropriate to healthcare communication; and timeliness supporting clinical decision-making when needed.

THERAPEUTIC PROBLEM SOLVING

Therapeutic problem solving applies systematic approaches to complex medication-related challenges, integrating clinical knowledge, critical thinking, and problem-solving methodology to develop optimal pharmaceutical care interventions. This process extends beyond simple application of guidelines or protocols to address situations requiring nuanced judgment, balancing multiple factors, and navigating uncertainty. Effective therapeutic problem-solving employs both analytical approaches decomposing complex situations into manageable components and creative thinking generating innovative solutions when standard approaches prove inadequate.

Clinical Reasoning in Pharmacy Practice

Clinical reasoning encompasses the cognitive processes pharmacists employ when evaluating patient-specific medication therapy situations and developing appropriate interventions. Diagnostic reasoning identifies underlying causes of medication-related problems through hypothetico-deductive approaches generating potential explanations for observed findings and systematically evaluating supporting and contradicting evidence. This process typically begins with problem recognition noting deviations from expected patterns; proceeds through hypothesis generation considering potential explanations; continues with targeted information gathering testing specific hypotheses; and concludes with hypothesis evaluation weighing evidence for competing explanations. Pattern recognition complements analytical reasoning by identifying characteristic presentations based on previous experience, allowing rapid problem identification in familiar situations while requiring verification to avoid premature conclusion. Decision analysis structure complex therapeutic decisions through systematic approaches including defining the decision context; identifying available options; determining potential outcomes for each option with associated probabilities; assigning values to different outcomes based on patient preferences and clinical significance; calculating expected utility for each option; and selecting the approach maximizing desired outcomes while minimizing unacceptable risks. These formal approaches prove particularly valuable for high-stakes decisions with significant uncertainty. Information processing approaches examine how pharmacists organize and utilize clinical knowledge, with concepts including illness scripts (structured mental representations of disease presentations and treatments); semantic networks connecting related clinical concepts; and clinical algorithms providing decision pathways for specific therapeutic situations. Expert-novice differences in clinical reasoning reflect development progression from reliance on explicit rules and limited pattern libraries among novices toward sophisticated pattern recognition, efficient information gathering, and tolerance of uncertainty characteristic of expert practitioners. Development of reasoning skills occurs through deliberate practice with varied cases; explicit articulation of reasoning processes; feedback addressing both conclusions and underlying thought processes; reflection on challenging cases; and progressive independence with appropriate supervision. Metacognition—thinking about one's own thinking—plays crucial role in clinical reasoning quality through awareness of cognitive biases, recognition of knowledge limitations, and deliberate strategy selection appropriate to specific problem types.

Table 14.4: Therapeutic Problem-Solving Approaches

Problem-Solving Phase	Activities	Common Pitfalls
Problem Identification	Recognize clinical issues Identify medication-related problems Determine problem significance Establish problem context	Focusing on symptoms not causes Missing underlying issues Overlooking patient perspective Premature problem definition Confirmation bias
Data Gathering	Collect relevant information Identify missing data Assess data reliability Organize information systematically	Incomplete data collection Overreliance on single sources Disorganized information Excessive data without focus Missing critical information
Problem Analysis	Determine potential causes Identify contributing	Superficial analysis Single-cause assumption

Problem-Solving Phase	Activities	Common Pitfalls
	factors Establish relationships between factors Evaluate problem impact	Overlooking system factors Premature conclusion Failure to prioritize factors
Solution Generation	Develop potential solutions Consider multiple approaches Identify evidence-based options Generate creative alternatives	Limited option generation Premature commitment to solutions Overlooking novel approaches Failure to consider evidence Resource constraint ignorance
Solution Evaluation	Assess solution feasibility Evaluate benefit/risk ratio Consider patient-specific factors Compare solution alternatives	Inadequate risk assessment Failure to consider patient factors Overlooking implementation barriers Insufficient comparison of options Optimism bias
Solution Selection	Choose optimal solution Consider patient preferences Incorporate feasibility factors Ensure evidence support	Failure to involve patient Resource constraint ignorance Evidence-practice gap Overconfidence in solution Implementation barrier oversight
Implementation Planning	Develop specific action steps Assign responsibilities	Inadequate specificity Unrealistic timelines Insufficient resource allocation

Problem-Solving Phase	Activities	Common Pitfalls
	Establish timeline Identify potential barriers	Overlooking potential barriers Inadequate responsibility
Monitoring Design	Establish outcome measures Define monitoring parameters Set evaluation timepoints Create follow-up plan	Inadequate outcome measures Vague monitoring parameters Inappropriate timepoints Insufficient follow-up planning
Contingency Planning	Anticipate potential issues Develop alternative approaches Establish thresholds for action Create response strategies	Failure to anticipate problems Inadequate alternative planning Unclear action thresholds Insufficient response strategies Overconfidence in primary plan
Communication	Document recommendations Communicate with team members Educate patient/caregivers Ensure understanding	Incomplete documentation Communication gaps Inadequate patient education Failure to verify understanding Jargon/complexity
Evaluation & Adjustment	Assess implementation success Evaluate outcomes Identify improvement opportunities Adjust approach as needed	Inadequate outcome assessment Implementation evaluation failure Resistance to adjustment Delayed identification of issues Insufficient improvement processes

Structured Problem-Solving Techniques

Structured problem-solving techniques provide methodical frameworks addressing complex therapeutic challenges through systematic processes reducing the risk of overlooking important factors or prematurely narrowing solution consideration. The pharmaceutical care process represents a fundamental problem-solving framework including assessment gathering comprehensive patient information; problem identification recognizing actual and potential drug therapy problems; care planning developing interventions addressing identified problems; implementation executing planned interventions; and follow-up evaluating intervention outcomes and adjusting plans as needed. This patient-centered approach ensures comprehensive consideration of medication-related needs while maintaining focus on patient-specific outcomes rather than abstract pharmacotherapy principles. Clinical decision-making models provide structured approaches to therapeutic decisions, including evidence-based decision models integrating research evidence, clinical expertise, and patient values; risk-benefit analysis frameworks explicitly weighing potential therapeutic benefits against possible harms; and collaborative decision models incorporating multiple stakeholder perspectives including patients, caregivers, and interdisciplinary team members. The ASHP Pharmacists' Patient Care Process offers a standardized approach including collect (gathering subjective and objective information); assess (analyzing information to identify problems and determine priorities); plan (developing patient-centered care plans addressing problems); implement (performing interventions in collaboration with other providers); and follow-up (monitoring and evaluating progress toward goals). Root cause analysis techniques identify underlying factors contributing to medication-related problems rather than addressing superficial manifestations. The "five whys" technique involves repeatedly asking why a problem occurs, moving progressively deeper toward fundamental causes. Fishbone diagrams (Ishikawa diagrams) systematically explore potential contributing factors across categories including patient factors, medication characteristics, provider issues, system processes, and environmental conditions. These approaches support development of interventions addressing fundamental causes rather than symptoms, enhancing likelihood of sustainable improvement. Algorithms and decision trees provide visual representations of decision pathways for specific therapeutic situations, explicitly mapping the logical progression from assessment findings through intervention selection. These tools support consistent decision-making while accommodating patient-specific factors through appropriate branching points incorporating relevant clinical variables.

Managing Complex Therapeutic Situations

Complex therapeutic situations require specialized approaches addressing multiple interacting factors, competing priorities, and significant uncertainty. Polypharmacy management addresses the challenges of multiple medication regimens through systematic approaches including comprehensive medication review identifying all current therapies; medication reconciliation resolving discrepancies between information sources; assessment of each medication's ongoing indication, effectiveness, safety, and adherence characteristics; deprescribing evaluation identifying medications appropriate for discontinuation; and regimen simplification enhancing adherence through reduced complexity. These approaches balance disease-specific treatment guidelines against overall medication burden, recognizing that guideline-concordant care for multiple conditions often creates unsustainable regimen complexity. Multimorbidity considerations address interactions between coexisting conditions affecting therapeutic decisions. Approaches include prioritizing conditions based on severity, symptom burden, and treatment effectiveness; identifying condition-condition interactions where one disease affects the course or management of another; recognizing condition-treatment interactions where therapy for one condition affects another; and evaluating treatment-treatment interactions beyond simple drug-drug interactions to include competing treatment goals or cumulative side effect burdens. Therapeutic decision-making under uncertainty addresses situations with incomplete information, evolving evidence, or unpredictable outcomes. Strategies include explicit acknowledgment of uncertainty with transparent communication to patients and colleagues; threshold approaches identifying the level of certainty required before implementing specific interventions based on benefit-risk profiles; provisional decision-making with clear monitoring and reassessment plans; and development of contingency plans for alternative scenarios. Conflicting guideline recommendations frequently emerge in complex cases, particularly involving multimorbidity or special populations excluded from guideline development evidence base. Resolution approaches include evaluating guideline quality and currency to prioritize more robust recommendations; assessing applicability of different guidelines to specific patient characteristics; identifying underlying principles and evidence supporting conflicting recommendations; conducting explicit benefit-risk assessment for each approach; and when appropriate, seeking expert consultation for particularly challenging conflicts.

Table 14.5: Clinical Decision-Making Models and Applications

Decision-Making Model	Pharmacy Applications	Strengths and Limitations
Analytical (Hypothetico-Deductive)	Complex medication reviews Atypical presentation analysis Drug-related problem investigation Diagnostic dilemmas	Strengths: Systematic, thorough, explicit reasoning Limitations: Time-consuming, cognitive load, may miss pattern recognition opportunities
Pattern Recognition	Common medication issues Recognized adverse effects Typical drug interactions Standardized therapy selection	Strengths: Efficient, effective for common situations, experience utilization Limitations: Bias vulnerability, premature closure, limited for novel situations
Intuitive	Red flag identification Patient deterioration recognition Urgent intervention needs Potential medication errors	Strengths: Speed, pattern integration, expert-level functioning Limitations: Difficult to explain, bias vulnerability, experience-dependent
Dual Process	Complex but familiar problems High-stakes decisions Time-pressured situations Clinical teaching	Strengths: Flexible, context-appropriate, efficient yet thorough Limitations: Cognitive switching challenges, calibration difficulties, expertise demands
Bayesian	Diagnostic test interpretation Therapeutic	Strengths: Quantitative, evidence-based, uncertainty management

Decision-Making Model	Pharmacy Applications	Strengths and Limitations
	decision thresholds Risk assessment Screening program evaluation	Limitations: Probability data requirements, complexity, time demands, numerical literacy needs
Clinical Decision Rules	Risk stratification tools Treatment algorithms Dosing protocols Therapeutic interchange	Strengths: Standardization, evidence-based, reduced variation, efficiency Limitations: Inflexibility, limited to specific situations, validation concerns, may oversimplify
Shared Decision-Making	Medication selection Risk-benefit discussions Treatment discontinuation Adherence challenges	Strengths: Patient-centered, autonomy respect, adherence promotion, satisfaction Limitations: Time requirements, patient capacity variations, information complexity, preference elicitation challenges
SOAP Framework	Medication therapy management Pharmaceutical care planning Documentation systems Clinical pharmacy services	Strengths: Organized, comprehensive, standardized, communication facilitation Limitations: Rigid structure, problem-oriented focus, implementation variations, length
Evidence-Based Medicine	Therapy selection Protocol development Formulary decisions Clinical guideline implementation	Strengths: Evidence grounding, systematic approach, critical thinking promotion, transparency Limitations: Evidence gaps, application challenges,

Decision-Making Model	Pharmacy Applications	Strengths and Limitations
		time demands, expertise requirements
Narrative-Based Approach	Medication experience understanding Adherence exploration Culturally sensitive care Chronic disease management	Strengths: Patient-centered, context-rich, meaning exploration, relationship building Limitations: Time-intensive, standardization challenges, scientific integration difficulties, subjective elements
Casuistry (Case-Based)	Rare adverse effect management Complex medication regimens Special population considerations Non-standard dosing situations	Strengths: Practical wisdom application, complexity management, experience utilization Limitations: Case availability, relevance determination, principles extraction, generalizability
Heuristics and Biases	Diagnosis verification Therapy selection scrutiny Decision quality improvement Clinical reasoning education	Strengths: Error reduction, decision improvement, cognitive insight, self-awareness Limitations: Bias persistence, overcompensation risk, implementation challenges, cognitive effort

Continuous Learning and Improvement in Problem Solving

Continuous learning and improvement in problem-solving capabilities occurs through deliberate approaches developing both knowledge base and reasoning processes. Reflective practice involves systematic examination of clinical experiences to extract learning and improve future performance. Structured reflection frameworks include the "What? So what? Now what?" sequence examining what happened, analyzing implications, and identifying future applications; critical incident analysis examining particularly challenging or instructive cases through detailed review; and learning portfolios documenting significant cases, insights gained, and application plans. These approaches transform experience into learning through deliberate processing rather than simple accumulation of cases. Feedback seeking actively solicits input from colleagues, preceptors, and patients regarding therapeutic decision quality, communication effectiveness, and intervention outcomes. Effective feedback utilization requires openness to potentially uncomfortable information, skillful processing separating personal worth from specific performance aspects, and deliberate application to future situations. Case-based learning employs structured examination of patient cases to develop problem-solving capabilities through various formats including case presentations with peer discussion; paper cases with guided analysis questions; simulation experiences providing realistic decision-making opportunities without patient risk; and retrospective case review examining actual patient outcomes relative to therapeutic decisions. Knowledge management strategies organize and update clinical information supporting problem solving through approaches including personal knowledge systems organizing information for efficient retrieval; deliberate knowledge gap identification through self-assessment; targeted learning addressing identified gaps; and integration of new information into existing knowledge structures through concept mapping, teaching others, or application to sample cases. Peer consultation and collaborative problem-solving leverage collective expertise through case discussions, formal consultations, or team-based approaches to complex cases. Beyond immediate problem resolution, these collaborative approaches expose participants to alternative thinking patterns, novel solution approaches, and diverse knowledge bases, enhancing individual problem-solving capabilities through cognitive apprenticeship. Error analysis examines suboptimal decisions for learning opportunities through approaches including prospective risk identification before implementing interventions; immediate review when interventions fail to achieve expected outcomes; and systematic analysis of significant adverse events identifying contributing factors and prevention strategies for future situations.

Summary

Clinical decision-making transforms pharmaceutical knowledge into optimal patient care through systematic evaluation processes and reasoned therapeutic judgments. Evidence-based practice forms the foundation of clinical decision making by integrating best available research evidence, clinical expertise, and patient preferences. This approach begins with formulating answerable clinical questions using PICO framework (Population-Intervention-Comparison-Outcome), followed by efficiently searching appropriate information sources ranging from primary literature to systematic reviews and meta-analyses. Critical appraisal skills enable assessment of study validity, clinical importance, and applicability to specific patient situations through understanding of research methodology, statistical significance versus clinical relevance, and generalizability limitations. Clinical guideline implementation translates evidence into practice through standardized recommendations developed by expert panels following rigorous methodology. Effective implementation requires understanding guideline development processes, critically evaluating recommendation strength, appropriately adapting guidelines to local contexts, and identifying patient-specific factors warranting deviation from standard approaches. Patient case analysis applies systematic frameworks to individual situations, typically following problem-oriented approaches identifying active medical conditions, medication-related problems, and monitoring parameters. Comprehensive analysis incorporates medical history evaluation, current medication assessment including prescription and non-prescription therapies, relevant physical findings, laboratory parameter interpretation, and social/behavioral factor consideration. Therapeutic problem-solving employs structured decision-making processes including clear problem definition, identification of therapeutic goals, generation of potential interventions, evaluation of options against patient-specific factors, implementation of selected therapy, and outcome monitoring. This process balances evidence-based recommendations with patient-specific considerations including comorbidities, pharmacogenetic factors, previous medication experiences, adherence capabilities, and personal preferences.

Multiple Choice Questions

1. Which of the following best describes the final step in the evidence-based practice process?
   a) Formulating a clinical question
   b) Searching for the best evidence
   c) Critically appraising the evidence
   d) Evaluating the outcomes of the decision
2. When evaluating a randomized controlled trial, which of the following would most strongly suggest the presence of selection bias?
   a) Lack of blinding
   b) Significant differences in baseline characteristics between groups
   c) Use of subjective outcome measures
   d) High dropout rate
3. Which of the following represents the highest level of evidence in the traditional evidence hierarchy?
   a) Expert opinion
   b) Case series
   c) Randomized controlled trial
   d) Systematic review and meta-analysis
4. When evaluating a study's results, the number needed to treat (NNT) represents:
   a) The number of patients who need to receive the intervention for one patient to benefit
   b) The total sample size needed for statistical significance
   c) The minimum number of patients required to detect side effects
   d) The number of patients excluded from analysis
5. Which of the following best describes how clinical practice guidelines should be applied in patient care?
   a) Guidelines should be followed exactly as written for all patients
   b) Guidelines should be applied considering patient-specific factors and preferences
   c) Guidelines are only relevant for research purposes, not clinical practice
   d) Guidelines should only be used when other treatment options have failed
6. A major barrier to implementing clinical practice guidelines in pharmacy practice is:

a) Insufficient guideline publication in pharmacy journals
b) Pharmacists' lack of diagnostic abilities
c) Lack of awareness and familiarity with guideline recommendations
d) Guidelines are rarely relevant to medication therapy

7. Which of the following is the most appropriate approach when clinical guidelines provide conflicting recommendations?
a) Always follow the most recently published guideline
b) Evaluate the quality of evidence supporting each recommendation
c) Follow the guideline from the most prestigious organization
d) Average the recommendations from different guidelines

8. In patient case analysis, which of the following data would be most relevant when evaluating a potential drug-induced liver injury?
a) Red blood cell count
b) Serum creatinine
c) Alanine aminotransferase (ALT)
d) Blood glucose

9. When applying a clinical decision support alert recommending dose adjustment for renal impairment, the pharmacist should:
a) Override the alert if the physician has already approved the dose
b) Evaluate the patient's actual renal function and the specific medication properties
c) Always implement the recommended dose adjustment
d) Ignore the alert if the patient has been on the medication previously

10. Which of the following factors is most important when determining the clinical significance of a potential drug interaction?
a) The publication date of the interaction information
b) The patient-specific risk factors and the consequence of the interaction
c) Whether the interaction appears in multiple drug interaction references
d) If both medications are in the same therapeutic class

Self-Assessment Questions

1. Provide examples of well-structured questions addressing therapy, diagnosis, prognosis, and harm, and explaining how question formulation guides effective literature searching.
2. Explain how study designs ranging from case reports to systematic reviews and meta-analyses differ in methodological rigor and appropriate applications to clinical questions.
3. Design a systematic approach to critical appraisal of randomized controlled trials, explaining how to evaluate internal validity through assessment of randomization, blinding, allocation concealment, intention-to-treat analysis, and appropriate statistical methods.
4. Explaining how to identify and address potential sources of bias including study design, endpoint selection, comparison groups, and reporting of results.
5. Analyze the process of clinical practice guideline development, explaining how evidence is gathered, evaluated, and translated into recommendations with appropriate consideration of strength of evidence and benefit-risk assessment.
6. Evaluate strategies for implementing clinical guidelines in diverse practice settings, explaining how barriers including resource limitations, competing priorities, clinician resistance, and patient factors can be addressed through effective implementation science principles.
7. Design a systematic approach to patient case analysis, explaining how subjective and objective information should be organized, interpreted, and prioritized to identify medication-related problems requiring intervention.
8. Explain how electronic alerts, order sets, and decision algorithms can enhance therapeutic decision making while addressing potential limitations including alert fatigue.
9. Explaining how to resolve conflicting guideline recommendations, manage potential drug interactions, and incorporate patient preferences into care plans.
10. Explain how genetic testing results should be interpreted, how therapeutic recommendations should be modified, and how to balance genetic information with other clinical factors.

Bibliography

1. Sackett DL, Rosenberg WM, Gray JA, Haynes RB, Richardson WS. Evidence based medicine: What it is and what it isn't. BMJ. 1996;312(7023):71-72.
2. Guyatt G, Rennie D, Meade MO, Cook DJ. Users' guides to the medical literature: A manual for evidence-based clinical practice. 3rd ed. New York: McGraw-Hill Education; 2015.
3. Straus SE, Glasziou P, Richardson WS, Haynes RB. Evidence-based medicine: How to practice and teach EBM. 5th ed. Edinburgh: Elsevier; 2019.
4. Institute of Medicine (US) Committee on Standards for Developing Trustworthy Clinical Practice Guidelines; Graham R, Mancher M, Miller Wolman D, Greenfield S, Steinberg E, editors. Clinical practice guidelines we can trust. Washington, DC: National Academies Press; 2011.
5. Grol R, Grimshaw J. From best evidence to best practice: Effective implementation of change in patients' care. Lancet. 2003;362(9391):1225-1230.
6. Cabana MD, Rand CS, Powe NR, Wu AW, Wilson MH, Abboud PA, et al. Why don't physicians follow clinical practice guidelines? A framework for improvement. JAMA. 1999;282(15):1458-1465.
7. DiCenso A, Bayley L, Haynes RB. Accessing pre-appraised evidence: Fine-tuning the 5S model into a 6S model. Evid Based Nurs. 2009;12(4):99-101.
8. Bader JD, Shugars DA, Bonito AJ. Systematic reviews of selected dental caries diagnostic and management methods. J Dent Educ. 2001;65(10):960-968.
9. Ebell MH, Siwek J, Weiss BD, Woolf SH, Susman J, Ewigman B, et al. Strength of recommendation taxonomy (SORT): A patient-centered approach to grading evidence in the medical literature. Am Fam Physician. 2004;69(3):548-556.
10. Malone PM, Kier KL, Stanovich JE, Malone MJ. Drug information: A guide for pharmacists. 6th ed. New York: McGraw-Hill Education; 2018.

ANSWERS TO THE MCQS

Chapter 1: 1. b 2. a 3. c 4. b 5. c 6. b 7. c 8. c 9. b 10. c

Chapter 2: 1. a 2. a 3. b 4. c 5. b 6. d 7. b 8. a 9. b 10. c

Chapter 3: 1. c 2. b 3. c 4. c 5. c 6. b 7. c 8. b 9. c 10. b

Chapter 4: 1. b 2. c 3. c 4. d 5. b 6. d 7. b 8. c 9. c 10. b

Chapter 5: 1. b 2. b 3. c 4. c 5. b 6. b 7. c 8. b 9. d 10. d

Chapter 6: 1. b 2. d 3. b 4. b 5. c 6. b 7. a 8. b 9. c 10. b

Chapter 7: 1. b 2. c 3. b 4. b 5. b 6. b 7. b 8. b 9. c 10. b

Chapter 8: 1. b 2. b 3. c 4. b 5. b 6. c 7. b 8. c 9. c 10. b

Chapter 9: 1. d 2. b 3. a 4. c 5. c 6. a 7. c 8. b 9. d 10. c

Chapter 10: 1. a 2. c 3. c 4. c 5. c 6. b 7. d 8. c 9. b 10. b

Chapter 11: 1. c 2. a 3. b 4. c 5. b 6. b 7. c 8. c 9. c 10. c

Chapter 12: 1. b 2. b 3. c 4. c 5. c 6. c 7. b 8. b 9. c 10. a

Chapter 13: 1. b 2. b 3. b 4. b 5. c 6. b 7. b 8. a 9. c 10. b

Chapter 14: 1. d 2. b 3. d 4. a 5. b 6. c 7. b 8. c 9. b 10. b

ABOUT THE EDITORS

Dr. AMIT KUMAR

Dr. Amit Kumar is an Associate Professor at the Amity Institute of Pharmacy, Amity University, Lucknow. He received his Ph.D. in Pharmacy Practice from BPUT, Odisha, M.Pharm from Royal College of Pharmacy and Health Sciences, Berhampur, and B.Pharm from CNK Reddy College of Pharmacy, Bengaluru. He has over 40 research publications in prestigious journals, he has mentored 76 PharmD, 26 B.Pharm, and 10 M.Pharm scholars. He is a life member of the Association of Pharmaceutical Teachers of India (APTI) and the Indian Pharmaceutical Association (IPA).

Dr. RAVI PRAKASH DEGALA

Dr. Ravi Prakash Degala is working as an Associate Professor and Head of Department in Pharmacy Practice at Pydah College of Pharmacy, Patavala, Kakinada with over 8 years of academic and clinical experience. He holds a Doctor of Pharmacy (Pharm.D) from Rajiv Gandhi University of Health Sciences and has contributed significantly to pharmaceutical research through multiple publications in reputed journals. His expertise spans pharmacovigilance, clinical research, and drug safety, with a particular focus on patient counseling and clinical pharmacy services. He has guided numerous research projects and received recognition for his contributions to pharmacy education and research.

Mr. PRAKASH NATHANIEL KUMAR SARELLA

Mr. Prakash Nathaniel Kumar Sarella is working as an Associate Professor and Controller of Examinations at Aditya College of Pharmacy, Aditya University with over 9 years of experience in teaching and research. His expertise includes nanomedicine, liposomes, polymer therapeutics, antibody-drug conjugates, specialized pharmaceutical packaging solutions, microneedle technologies, and other innovative drug delivery solutions. He published over 42 research papers and life member of APTI and IPGA.

Mrs. VINNY THERISSA MANGAM

Mrs. Vinny Therissa Mangam is an Assistant Professor working at Aditya College of Pharmacy, Aditya University with over 5 years of experience in teaching, analytical method development and validation. She published 8 research papers and lifetime member of APT and IPGA. Her expertise lies in optimizing techniques, comparing methods, and transferring procedures to enable enhanced standards in pharmaceutical analysis.

Dr. AJMAL TARIQ HUSSAIN

Dr. Ajmal Tariq Hussain is working as an Assistant Professor at the Amity Institute of Pharmacy, Lucknow. After completing his Doctor of Pharmacy from Integral University, he gained clinical experience as a clinical pharmacologist at Medanta Super Speciality Hospital and completed his internship at the prestigious Fortis Escorts Heart Institute in New Delhi. His contributions to pharmacy practice are reflected in his numerous publications in leading journals and his awarded patents. He is a dedicated educator who mentors Pharm.D and B.Pharm students in their research endeavors while maintaining an active presence in national and international pharmaceutical conferences.

INDEX

Made in the USA
Monee, IL
07 November 2026

68086783R00242